OPEN WATER LIFESAVING

THE UNITED STATES LIFESAVING ASSOCIATION MANUAL

SECOND EDITION
B. CHRIS BREWSTER, EDITOR

PEARSON
Custom
Publishing

Cover Photo: *Water Stair,* by Angela Sciaraffa.

Taken from:

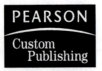

PEARSON CUSTOM PUBLISHING
75 Arlington Street, Suite 300, Boston, MA 02116
A Pearson Education Company

We gratefully dedicate this text
to the men and women who have
risked their lives in the water
to save the lives of others,
and to those who lost their lives in the effort.

Contents

Preface

This manual is intended to be used as a guide in the instruction and training of open water lifesavers, a reference for professional lifeguards, and a yardstick against which lifesaving agencies can measure their performance. It is the product of the combined knowledge of the members of the United States Lifesaving Association (USLA), the only national association of open water lifeguards at both surf and inland beaches. While there have been many texts written for instruction of pool lifeguards, some of which also reference inland beaches, we know of no other text which has focused on the role of lifesaving at ocean and inland beaches in a comprehensive manner.

In many countries of the world, lifesaving evolved under the umbrella of national organizations, which set standards from the beginning. That was not the case in the United States, where many lifesaving organizations emerged independent of each other. Eventually however, there were calls for the establishment of clear, objective training programs for professional lifesavers.

One of the most significant events in the development of lifeguard training programs occurred in 1980, when leaders of water safety organizations across the country gathered at Texas A&M University in Galveston for a *Conference to Develop Guidelines for Establishing Open-Water Recreational Beach Standards*. This conference was conducted in an effort to address the extraordinary challenge of creating nationwide standards for the diversity of conditions found at beaches throughout the United States.

Armed with the findings of the conference, and with hundreds of aggregate years of open water lifeguard management experience, members of the USLA National Certification Committee began meetings to develop a national lifeguard training program. Problems with a project of this scope surfaced immediately. How could one training program meet the needs of every lifeguard agency in the United States? Could one program be applicable at both a large, urban, year-round beach operation in Southern California and at a small, seasonal beach operation in the Northeast? How should local variances in water conditions, climate, aquatic life, beach attendance, and other aspects of beach management be handled?

USLA moved ahead in 1981 with the publication of our first manual, *Lifesaving and Marine Safety*, and the USLA National Certification Committee began to assemble a list of standards to accompany it. The most immediate product of their labors was the 1983 publication of a booklet entitled *Guidelines for Open Water Lifeguard Training*. The contents of this booklet immediately served as a model for beach lifeguard agencies throughout the United States, but there remained a desire on the part of USLA and open water lifeguard agencies for more—a program to certify beach lifeguards and the standards of beach lifeguard agencies.

In 1992 a newly composed National Certification Committee amended and added to the 1983 guidelines to create *Guidelines for Open Water Lifeguard Training and Standards,* along with the national USLA Lifeguard Agency Certification Program. This program creates a set of clearly defined guidelines and minimum recommended standards for beach lifeguard agencies and allows agencies in compliance to become nationally certified. These agencies are then empowered to certify the lifeguards they train as having successfully completed a USLA certified training course.

During the many years of work by the National Certification Committee, another committee was formed to revise the original textbook. The task of rewriting the text was assumed by Tim Hall of New England, who did a yeoman's job in beginning a compilation of the aggregate experience of lifeguards from throughout the United States into a single, authoritative text. Mr. Hall completed a draft update in 1991, but several obstacles to publication remained and the effort was delayed until development of the Lifeguard Agency Certification Program in 1992 created an impetus to finally bring about publication of an updated USLA manual.

When the National Certification Committee updated the guidelines in 1992, the committee chair was B. Chris Brewster, Lifeguard Chief for the City of San Diego. He was asked to chair the USLA National Textbook Committee, with a goal of updating the text a final time and bringing about publication. A newly composed National Textbook Committee, made up of representatives from across the United States, convened in Chicago in February of 1994. Subsequently, thousands of hours of research and editing coalesced in the second USLA textbook, *The United States Lifesaving Association Manual of Open Water Lifesaving,* published in 1995. When it became evident that progress in lifesaving demanded a new edition, another meeting of the National Textbook Committee was convened, this time in Austin, Texas. The book you now hold is a result of the tireless work of the members of that committee.

The extraordinary efforts required to compile this manual were not the work of paid USLA staff members, for there were none. Rather, it was a labor of love and dedication to the lifesaving profession. The lifeguards involved gave of their free time unselfishly and with a common purpose—Lifeguards for Life.

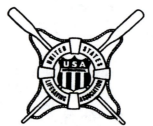

About the United States Lifesaving Association

We are America's nonprofit, professional association of beach lifeguards and open water rescuers. USLA works to reduce the incidence of death and injury in the aquatic environment through public education, national standards, training programs, promotion of high levels of lifeguard readiness, and related means. Membership is critical to support USLA's mission and is open to anyone.

To qualify for *Regular Membership* an individual must be a current member of an ocean, bay, river, or other open water lifesaving or rescue service. Our regular membership includes seasonal lifeguards, full time lifeguards, lifeguard supervisors, and lifeguard chiefs from virtually every major ocean lifeguard service in the U.S., along with those of the Great Lakes and many inland open water areas.

Associate Membership is available to those who do not qualify for regular membership.

Junior Lifeguard Membership is available to youths who are active participants in a junior lifeguard program affiliated with a local USLA Chapter.

Corporate Membership, *Honorary Membership*, and the position of *Chief Patron* may be designated by the Board of Directors.

For further information, visit our website at: *www.usla.org*

Editor's Note

- This text represents the collective knowledge of recognized leaders associated with the most highly regarded lifesaving agencies in the United States. It is intended to be a comprehensive text essential to the effective training and retraining of those involved in open water lifesaving. Each open water lifesaving agency in America faces unique challenges posed by the local environment and the particular assignments of its personnel. Therefore, this text will only be fully effective when used in conjunction with a training program in compliance with the USLA Lifeguard Agency Certification Program or the USLA Aquatic Rescue Response Team program, and supplemented by appropriate specialized training addressing local conditions.

- This text does not and cannot stand alone as a lifesaving training manual. It has been deliberately written to be used in conjunction with an agency's manual, which must contain the specific policies and procedures pertaining to the information provided in this text.

- THE MATERIAL CONTAINED IN THIS TEXT CONSTITUTES THE CONSIDERED AND EXPERT OPINION OF THE AUTHORS AND USLA. THE AUTHORS AND USLA MAKE NO EXPRESS OR IMPLIED WARRANTY OR GUARANTEE AS TO THE MATERIAL, OPINIONS, OR METHODS CONTAINED IN THIS TEXT.

- The procedures, techniques, and equipment used in open water lifesaving are constantly changing and improving. It has only been through experimentation over the years by innovative lifesavers that improved techniques have been developed. This process must continue if we are to effectively meet the challenge of the future.

Acknowledgments

USLA National Textbook Committee

B. Chris Brewster (Chair)—Lifeguard Chief (ret.), San Diego Lifeguard Service
Julian K. "Duke" Brown, M.Ed.—Beach Safety Director, Horry County, South Carolina
Jerry Gavin—Lifeguard Captain, Chicago Park District Lifeguard Service
Nick Lerma—Lieutenant, San Diego Lifeguard Service
Dan McCormick (Photo Editor)—Aquatics Manager, East Bay Regional Park District, California
James H. McCrady V—Lieutenant, Ft. Lauderdale Beach Patrol
David M. Shotwell, Sr.—Beachfront Supervisor (ret.), Ocean Grove, New Jersey
Kim W. Tyson—Aquatic Coordinator, University of Texas at Austin
Peter Wernicki, M.D.—Medical Advisor, United States Lifesaving Association

Ad-Hoc National Textbook Committee Members

Eric Bauer—Lifeguard Captain, Newport Beach Fire Department, California
Carl Martinez—USLA National Curriculum Accreditation Program
Dr. Alfred W. (Bud) McKinley, Ph.D.—Operations Chief, Ocean City Beach Patrol, New Jersey
Robert Ogoreuc—Training Officer, Ocean City Beach Patrol, New Jersey

Additional Contributors and Reviewers

Michael J. Bascom—Deputy Director, Office of Emergency Management, Neptune Township, NJ
Fred Carter—Beachfront Coordinator, City of Rochester Hills, Michigan
Divers Alert Network
Peter Fenner, M.D.—National Medical Officer, Surf Life Saving Australia
Rick Gould—USLA National Lifesaving Statistics Coordinator.
Jim Howe—Operations Chief, Ocean Safety Division, Honolulu, Hawaii
Kenna Kay—Artiste Extraordinaire
Tom Matheson—Warning Coordination Meteorologist, National Weather Service
Jerome Modell, M.D.—Emeritus Professor of Anesthesiology, University of Florida

John "Chip" More—Legal Advisor, United States Lifesaving Association
Mark J. Ringenary—Water Quality Specialist, Gateway National Recreation Area
Bruce Schmidt—Statistician, U.S. Coast Guard Office of Boating Safety
David Szpilman, M.D.—Drowning Resuscitation Center, Rio de Janeiro (Brazil) Fire Department
John T. Tanacredi, Ph.D.—Chief of Natural Resources, Gateway National Recreation Area
Eric Wayman—Lifeguard II, Newport Beach Fire Department

Chapter 1
Lifesaving History

In this chapter, you will learn how lifesaving began with the rescue of people shipwrecked along coastal shores. It progressed to involve the rescue of swimmers and other recreational water users. The first open water lifeguards were strong swimmers who used their aquatic skills, with little formal training or equipment, to rescue others. Over a period of decades, as you will see, they formed local, national, and international organizations, exchanged knowledge, invented and improved lifesaving equipment, and created standards that have transformed lifesaving into a highly professional public safety service. The United States Lifesaving Association and its associated lifeguard agencies follow the traditions of the first lifesavers to this very day.

CHAPTER EXCERPT

One of the most gallant and skillful crews in the [U.S. Life-Saving] service was lost at Point aux Barques, Lake Huron, in October, 1880, and the heart-rending details of the calamity are known to the world through its sole survivor. These loyal men went out in the surf-boat in prompt response to a signal of distress displayed upon a vessel three miles away. The boat was capsized and righted several times, but finally remained capsized, the men clinging to it; but the cold was such that one after another perished, until six were gone ... These heroic men had during the same year saved nearly a hundred lives. (Merryman & Jones, 1882)

The First American Lifesavers

The first lifesavers in America rarely worked during summer. Most of their work came during fall, winter, and spring and much of it was accomplished in the dead of night. There were cold and lonely vigils, sometimes in snowstorms as they met each other on foot patrols along desolate beaches. Consider the following passage from an annual report of the U.S. Life-Saving Service describing one of the scores of dramatic rescues that year. This one took place April 3, 1884 in Wellfleet, Massachusetts on the outer shore of Cape Cod. It involved the schooner Viking, "on her way from George's Bank with a fare of fish, for Boston."

> "At a few minutes after 2 in the morning, the weather being rainy and dark, with a strong northeast wind blowing and a rough sea, Surfman F.H. Daniels, of the Cahoon's Hollow [Life-Saving] Station ... saw a bright light ahead which he at first supposed to be the station on fire, but which after a moment's reflection he concluded from its bearing must be the distress signal of a stranded vessel. He at once started on a run and in a short time arrived abreast of a schooner aground in the breakers about 50 yards from the beach ... two miles north of the station [and any assistance from other surfmen].
>
> His first thought was to keep on and alarm his comrades, but upon considering the time it would take to get to the station he determined on a bold effort to save the vessel's crew single-handed. The bright light that had attracted his attention was still burning when he arrived, and proved to be some clothing saturated with kerosene oil, which the crew had ignited as a signal for aid.
>
> The whole scene was brilliantly illuminated by it, and the sailors, seeing Daniels arrive, watched their opportunity and threw him the end of a lead line. This he managed to secure by rushing down into the surf, and in a few minutes the end of a larger line was bent to it and drawn ashore. One of the men then secured the bight of the rope around his body, and, with a shout to Daniels to haul away, plunged into the boiling surf.
>
> The gallant surfman was equal to the task, and, with the water waist deep around him, he pulled on the rope and succeeded in landing the man all right, the latter exclaiming, as he staggered to his feet upon reaching the beach, "For God's sake, who are you?" The reply of Daniels was brief and to the point: "I am a life-saving man, and you must lend me a hand to save the rest."
>
> At a signal from Daniels the line was quickly hauled back, and in a short time the entire crew, twelve in all, were safely landed ... It was about 3 o'clock when the last man was drawn ashore and then Daniels, after turning the water out of his hip boots, started with the wrecked crew for the station ...." (U.S. Life-Saving Service, 1884)

After this rescue, the schooner's owner wrote, "The circumstances under which this crew was saved were those of the most extreme peril, not only to themselves but also to the gallant man who, single-handed, attempted and providentially achieved their rescue. His name is not known to us, but we think his deed one worthy to be widely known and well rewarded." (U.S. Life-Saving Service, 1884)

The Early Days

During the late 1700s, much of the American coastline was totally uninhabited. Life was hard and recreational swimming was of little interest. Yet loss of life due to drowning was a serious problem. Shipwrecks were the reason.

With today's modern navigational aids and high-powered vessels, shipwrecks are relatively uncommon, but prior to these advancements, sailing ships were navigated by compass, sextant, and educated guess. They were always at the mercy of nature. Storms and inclement weather, particularly in winter, brought tragedy time and time again as ships foundered along the American coastline. In the mid-1800s on Massachusetts' Cape Cod alone, shipwrecks occurred at an estimated frequency of once every two or three weeks. (Quinn, 1973) Few people could swim and the sometimes frigid waters were unmerciful to even the most hardy swimmer. Passengers were often left to drown as their ships broke up a short distance from shore.

The earliest organized lifesaving efforts in the world began with China's Chinkiang Association for the Saving of Life, established in 1708. It eventually came to involve staffed lifesaving stations with specially designed and marked rescue vessels. (Shanks, York, & Shanks, 1998) In the Netherlands, the Maatschappij tot Redding van Drenkelingen (Society to Rescue People from Drowning) was established in Amsterdam in 1767, primarily to address problems of drowning in the numerous, open canals in Amsterdam. Across the English Channel, British lifesaving efforts began in 1774. (Shanks et al., 1998)

In the United States, the first organized efforts at lifesaving began with the founding of the Massachusetts Humane Society in 1786. The Humane Society built houses of refuge along the Massachusetts coast for shipwreck survivors, and in 1807 the Society set up the nation's first lifeboat station on Cape Cod. By the mid-1800s, the Massachusetts Humane Society operated 18 stations with lifeboats and line-throwing equipment. (Johnson, 1988)

In 1790, the U.S. Government created the Revenue Cutter Service as an arm of the Treasury Department with a goal of protection of revenue by enforcing payment of customs and tonnage duties on ships importing goods to America. The founding of the Revenue Cutter Service is today viewed as the birthday of the United States Coast Guard. (Johnson, 1988) Initially, the service was not expected to engage in rescue activities, but beginning in 1832, its vessels were assigned to cruise the coast during winter months to assist ships in distress. It was sometime later though, that they came to join forces with shore-based lifesavers.

In 1839 Dr. William A. Newell witnessed a shipwreck near Long Beach, New Jersey and watched as 13 people drowned trying to swim 300 yards to safety. He remembered this tragedy and later, as a New Jersey Congressman, helped persuade the U.S. government to become involved in lifesaving. In 1848, Congress passed the Newell Act and appropriated $10,000 to be spent to build and equip eight small lifeboat stations along the New Jersey coast between Sandy Hook and Little Egg Harbor. The Massachusetts Humane Society provided assistance in the endeavor. (Johnson, 1988) The next year, $20,000 was appropriated and provided to the Life-Saving Benevolent Association of New York for the purpose of building lifesaving stations on Long Island.

At first, lifesaving stations were simple unstaffed houses of refuge containing basic lifesaving equipment. Keys to the stations were left with local townspeople who, by following a list of printed instructions, were expected to rig and use the equipment to save those stranded aboard foundering ships. While this system resulted in some success and occasionally heroic rescues, without a posted watch from shore many shipwrecks went undetected along uninhabited stretches of the coast. The occupants often perished before any lifesaving efforts could be mounted. In addition, volunteer lifesavers from local towns were sometimes unable to effectively employ the lifesaving equipment due to lack of skill and training. Occasionally, lifeboat stations were vandalized and lifesaving equipment stolen. Many became run down and of little use.

By 1854 the magnitude of the problem could no longer be ignored. Congress appropriated additional funds to hire a superintendent for the Long Island and New Jersey coasts and a keeper for each station. (Johnson, 1988) The keepers were initially paid an annual salary of $200. (Quinn, 1973) Patrols were organized and station keepers were expected to walk the coastline at night, regardless of weather, to detect shipwrecks. Despite these advances however, there were no funds for maintenance, no paid lifesaving staff who could be depended upon to assist the keeper in emergencies, and no regulations to follow. Without a paid lifesaving staff, regular drills could not be effectively organized to prepare the volunteers for rescues.

During the Civil War the system deteriorated, but once the war was over, Congress again turned its attention to lifesaving. In 1869 the Revenue Marine Division was established to combine administration of lifesaving stations, the Revenue Cutter Service, steamboat inspection, and marine hospitals. (Johnson, 1987) Sumner Increase Kimball was appointed to administrate the Revenue Marine Division in 1871 and eventually came to be the single most important influence in early lifesaving.

Congress appropriated additional funds to staff lifesaving stations on a seasonal basis, but as Kimball toured the stations shortly after his appointment, he was disappointed to find many in deplorable condition. Some keepers were not even living at the stations to which they were assigned. Kimball embarked upon a crusade to improve the quality of the service. He enacted regulations, inspected the stations on a regular basis, and discharged those who failed to measure up.

Creation of the U.S. Life-Saving Service

Despite advances, funding continued to be a serious problem. The appropriation for 1877-78 was so low that the lifesaving stations could not open until December. Unfortunately, in late November of that year the steamer Huron grounded along the North Carolina coast and in the absence of lifesavers, 98 people drowned. In the wake of this disaster, in 1878 Congress appropriated funds to create a separate organization, the U.S. Life-Saving Service, with Sumner Kimball to be its first and, it turned out, only leader.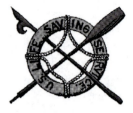

During Kimball's tenure, crews were employed to staff each station and the stations' size and comfort facilities were expanded. Most stations were staffed with six surfmen and an Officer in Charge (the station keeper). Professionalism grew too, as strict regulations were set for competence, performance, routine beach patrols, and physical conditioning. The system eventually grew to comprise 189 lifesaving stations—139 on the Atlantic coast from Maine to Florida, 37 on the Great Lakes, seven on the Pacific coast, and one in Ohio. (Johnson, 1988)

Like other emergency responders, lifesavers worked long and often tedious shifts, with daily drills and monotonous foot patrols throughout the night. But once the cry, "Ship Ashore!" was sounded, the boredom was often replaced by heroism in harrowing and exhausting struggles with the sea to save lives. When this happened, the primary tools of the early lifesavers were the breeches buoy and lifeboats.

Lifesaving Apparatus

The lifeboats which are now most commonly associated with early lifesavers were those used along the Atlantic coast. These wooden boats weighed 700 to 1,000 pounds and were about twenty-five to thirty feet long. Some had air chambers at either end to help prevent swamping, but they were not self-righting or self-bailing. They were generally rowed by a crew of six surfmen, with the station keeper at a sweep oar at the stern that served as a rudder.

Atlantic lifeboats were stored inside the lifesaving stations. When duty called, they were rowed by lifesavers wearing primitive lifejackets and water repelling oilskins. Since lifesaving stations were miles apart, Atlantic coast lifeboats had to be moved along the beach in wagons drawn through the soft sand. This effort alone could sap the strength of lifesavers, so some stations acquired horses to draw the wagons. (Ryder, 1990)

Lifeboats used on the Great Lakes and most of the Pacific coast were self-righting and self-bailing with air chambers to prevent capsizing. They weighed about four thousand pounds and were generally launched from safe harbors. In some cases, tugs would pull them to the mouth of a harbor, where the lifesavers aboard would take over using eight oars for propulsion. According an 1880 article in *Scribner's Monthly*, "It is a common occurrence for the life-boats to go under sail and oars ten or twelve miles from their stations to the assistance of vessels in distress." (Merryman, 1981)

Most Atlantic coast rescues involved ships aground on bars near the beach, having been driven there by storm surf or through disorientation of the

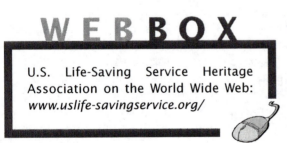

WEBBOX

U.S. Life-Saving Service Heritage Association on the World Wide Web: *www.uslife-savingservice.org/*

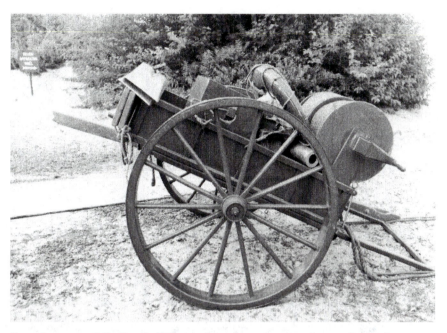

Beach cart with the full breeches buoy apparatus aboard. Lifesavers would pull this cart through the sand to the point of the rescue.

Credit: Brian Feeney, National Park Service

skipper. Since the Atlantic coast lifeboats were vulnerable to capsizing, when seas were high and the wrecked vessel near shore lifesavers turned instead to the breeches buoy apparatus.

The breeches buoy itself was actually a large life ring. Canvas was slung loosely across the center with two holes for the legs of a victim, forming a sort of trousers. The victim could hang securely in the breeches buoy with legs through the holes and the life ring under the armpits. The device used to deploy the breeches buoy was more complex.

The lifesavers transported the breeches buoy apparatus on a beach cart. The apparatus consisted primarily of a wooden crotch, extensive amounts of heavy line on large reels, strong linen thread in a faking box, and apparatus to deliver this thread through the air to the vessel in distress. The linen thread served as a lead line, which was light enough to be thrown or shot through the air to the shipwrecked vessel and to which the heavier line could then be fastened and pulled aboard by the shipwreck victims. The wooden faking box had upturned, gently pointed pegs inside, around which the lead line was neatly laid, ready to easily play out.

The first step was to get the lead line to the foundering vessel. If the ship was close enough, a *heaving stick* was used. With light lead line attached to this weighted stick, it could reportedly be thrown up to 50 yards. (Dalton, 1967) When the ship was out of reach of a heaving stick, the Lyle gun was employed.

The Lyle gun was a small 163 pound canon, developed by Captain David A. Lyle of the U.S.

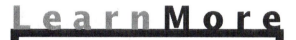

You can learn more about the Lyle gun in *The Lifesaving Guns of David Lyle* by J.P. Barnett (1974).

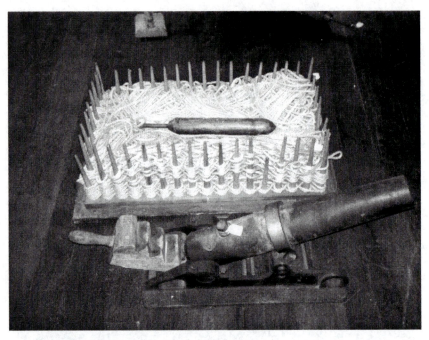

A Lyle gun, faking box, and projectile.

Credit: B. Chris Brewster

Army in 1877. The lifesavers would fire a metal projectile from the Lyle gun toward the rigging of the foundering ship. Attached to the projectile was one end of the lead line from the faking box. With the lead line attached, the projectile could reach up to 400 yards. (Ryder, 1990) If the shot was a good one, the lead line would become entangled in the rigging or simply drape over the foundering ship. If not, the line was retrieved and another attempt made. Sometimes, repeated attempts were required.

One hazard of the Lyle gun was its violent recoil. In the interest of keeping the gun light and portable, Lyle eliminated much of the weight normally used to minimize a canon's recoil. Tests on flat ground suggest that in some cases recoil of the gun may have been as much as 16 feet. (Barnett, 1974) On the beach, the Lyle gun was positioned so that its recoil was absorbed by the sand itself.

Once a connection was made to the ship with the lead line, the heavier line would be attached to the lead line by the lifesavers ashore and persons aboard the ship would pull it aboard. Rudimentary directions on a wooden pallet attached to the line instructed the shipwrecked victims to make the heavy line fast to a high point in the rigging. Meanwhile, the lifesavers erected the wooden crotch on the beach to provide a high point for the shore end of the line and anchored it in the sand. Eventually, both ends of the line were made fast and it was drawn taught.

The breeches buoy was hung from the line on a pulley and drawn back and forth by use of a separate line. When it worked properly, victims board the ship could be pulled ashore one at a time sitting in the breeches buoy without touching the water.

Lifecars were also used in some cases. Like the breeches buoy, these devices were hung from the line and pulled back and forth. They were made of copper or iron and enclosed with bolts. Three to four adults could be squeezed inside.

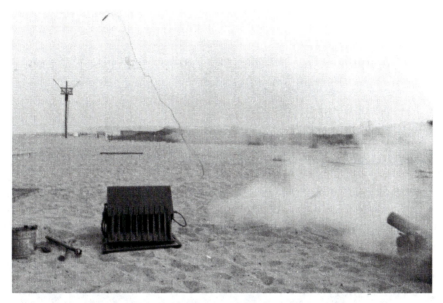

The Lyle gun is fired during a drill toward a practice target intended to simulate ships rigging. Note heavy projectile with line attached and faking box in the foreground with upturned pegs.

Credit: Brian Feeney, National Park Service

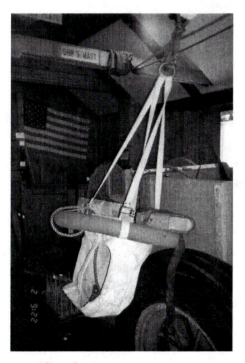

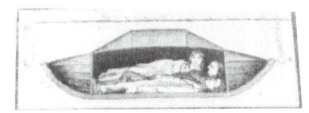

Breeches buoy

Credit: B. Chris Brewster

Lifecar

Credit: Dave Foxwell

U.S. Life-Saving Service Procedures

Lifesavers patrolled the beaches on foot throughout the night, awakened in turn for their watch. They would walk to a halfway point to the next station, exchange a brass "check" with a lifesaver from the neighboring station, and return to wake up the next lifesaver whose turn it was to patrol. The check proved that the patrol had been completed. If a ship was sighted near shore, the lifesavers would burn a red coston signal (a flare) as a warning to turn away.

Although the work was sometimes tedious, the rescues were often harrowing and sometimes lethal. Regulations stated, "You have to go out." (Quinn, 1973) Discretion in the face of adversity was not an option. J. H. Merryman, writing in *Scribner's Monthly* quoted a lifesaver as saying, "When I see a man clinging to a wreck, I see nothing else in the world, and I never think of family and friends until I have saved him." (Merryman, 1981)

Heroism of the lifesavers became legendary, particularly considering the fear of open water that many people of the day harbored. *Harpers Monthly* reported the following of one incident, "One of the most gallant and skillful crews in the service was lost at Point aux Barques, Lake Huron, in October, 1880, and the heart-rending details of the calamity are known to the world through its sole survivor. These loyal men went out in the surf-boat in prompt response to a signal of distress displayed upon a vessel three miles away. The boat was capsized and righted several times, but finally remained capsized, the men clinging to it; but the cold was such that one after another perished, until six were gone. The keeper drifted upon the beach, insensible, and was found steadying himself by the trunk of a tree ... These heroic men had during the same year saved nearly a hundred lives." (Merryman et al, 1882)

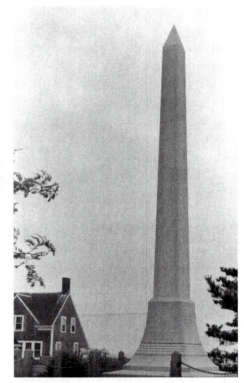

Memorial to the Monomoy lifesavers, Chatham, Massachusetts.

Credit: Kenna Kay

Another famous incident was known as the Monomoy disaster. On March 17, 1902 a lifeboat crewed by eight lifesavers had picked up five victims from the Wadena, a distressed vessel off Monomoy Point on Cape Cod, Massachusetts. As the lifesavers were making their way back to shore, the victims panicked and the lifeboat was overcome in high seas. All but one of the lifesavers perished, as did all of the victims.

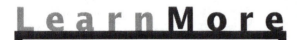

You can learn more in *The U.S. Life-Saving Service* by Ralph Shanks, Wick York, and Lisa Woo Shanks (1998).

According to the report of the U.S. Life-Saving Service for 1902, "The loss of the 7 lifesaving men who so nobly perished created everywhere a sense of profound sorrow. There was no more skillful or fearless crew on the whole coast, and ... there was a general conviction that the men were practically a sacrifice ... to their own high sense of duty, which would not permit them to turn their backs upon a signal of distress. "We must go," said the keeper,

At 2:30 a.m. [in December 1879] the patrol of Station No. 14, Second District, Massachusetts, discovered a vessel at anchor about a mile and a half east-northeast of the station, burning a torch as a signal of distress. He answered the signal and returned to the station for help. The lifesaving crew on reaching the shore found it impossible to launch the boat through the breakers. The keeper then sent to Station No. 13 for assistance, and in the meantime went north abreast of the distressed vessel and showed signals to her and caused fires to be built to show her the deepest water in case her chains should part. The wind was blowing a strong gale with blinding snow squalls, and a heavy sea was running.

When the crew of No. 13 arrived it was evident that the vessel was dragging toward shore. The lifesaving men now brought the mortar cart with the Lyle gun and equipment abreast of the vessel, which was now near the breakers. The first shot took the line across the headstays, but the crew were so exhausted and benumbed that they were unable to get to it. The second shot laid the line over the fore-yard and was happily made fast.

The breeches buoy was then taken aboard, and in thirty minutes the entire crew, eight men, were landed in safety, though five of them were in such a helpless condition that they had to be assisted to the station, where they were furnished with hot drinks, dry clothing, and comfortable beds.

— From the 1880 Annual Report of the U.S. Life-Saving Service

"there is a distress flag in the rigging." Over $45,000 was raised to help the widows and orphans of the drowned men and a monument was placed ashore in memory of the victims. It can be found today at the Coast Guard Station in Chatham, Massachusetts. (Quinn, 1973)

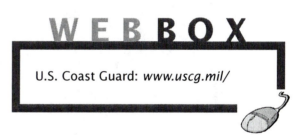

U.S. Coast Guard: *www.uscg.mil/*

The Life-Saving Service even performed inland rescues in some circumstances. For example, during serious flooding in the Midwest during early 1913, lifesavers were dispatched with their boats to perform rescues. In an after-action report published by the House of Representatives, Sumner Kimball reported that the Life-Saving Service rescued 3,509 persons from flooding in Ohio, Kentucky, Indiana, and Illinois. (Kimball, 1918)

In its short lifetime, the U.S. Life-Saving Service amassed a truly extraordinary record—28,121 vessels aided and 178,741 people saved. In 1915, the Life-Saving Service was merged with the Revenue Cutter Service, this time to form the United States Coast Guard. Sumner Kimball retired after 43 years of service, but the lifesavers continued on in their duties as part of the Coast Guard for many years thereafter. As navigational aids improved and powered vessels became the norm, shipwrecks occurred with diminishing frequency. The need for skilled persons to go out through the surf in lifeboats slowly dwindled. The last known use of the breeches buoy was in 1962. (Ryder, 1990) As will become evident to the reader though, the United States Lifesaving Association and its associated lifeguard agencies follow the traditions of the U.S. Life-Saving Service to this very day.

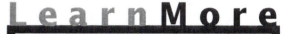

You can learn more in *Guardians of the Sea, History of the United States Coast Guard* by Robert E. Johnson (1987).

To the General Superintendent

United States Life-Saving Service

Dear Sir: The undersigned hereby wish to make known that the keeper and crew of Peaked Hill Bar Life-Saving Station (Cape Cod) have rendered such assistance and exposed themselves to such risk of their own lives during the wreck of the schooner W.H. Mailer, of Calais, Maine, that we cannot go on our way without a word in their praise.

We struck on the inner bar ... in a blinding snow-storm and dense fog. Land was scarcely visible at the time, but the patrolman, having good eyes, discovered us and signaled to us, and we answered him. We then saw him start on a run along the beach. In a short time our masts went over the side and then we began to drift over the bar.

We could then see the crew with their apparatus, coming along the beach ... The sea made quick work, and in a short time broke us all up, except a small part of the stern, to which, with the captain's wife, we were all hanging. The crew were then three hundred yards distant.

The keeper, seeing there was no time to lose, ran ahead with lines, and, with great daring and terrible risk, succeeded in getting on part of the wreck and passing a line to us. We then made the line fast around the woman, and the keeper, with great pluck, took her off, and both were hauled ashore by the brave men on the beach, through a tremendous sea, the men being at times almost washed off their feet. They then passed the line to us again, and after a lot of courageous work got us all ashore alive, not a minute too soon, as she all broke up just as the last man got ashore ...

No human beings could do more for us than the keeper and his men, and they are deserving of great praise.

— A letter reprinted in the 1884 Annual Report of the U.S. Life-Saving Service

Roots of Modern Lifeguarding

During the 1800s, life in America began to change as the country grew. Americans became more prosperous and less dependent on constant work for survival. Recreation time was on the rise and Americans discovered that recreational swimming, once widely thought to be a sure cause of death, was an enjoyable pastime. Beach resorts sprang up along the coastline and on lakes. Governments began to acquire beachfront property and guarantee public access specifically for the purpose of recreation. Open water swimming was all the rage, but it was not without risk.

Newspapers buzzed with reports of drownings, particularly when several lives were lost in storm surf or rip currents. In Atlantic City, New Jersey there were 13 drownings in 1865. (Methot, 1988) In many areas, lifeboats were positioned onshore for use by citizen rescuers. *Lifelines*—ropes to which swimmers could cling—were sometimes fastened between shore and upright poles driven into the ocean bottom. As was found in earlier efforts to save shipwreck victims though, provision of equipment alone was inadequate to prevent drowning without the presence of trained lifesavers to employ it.

Some volunteers stepped forward in Atlantic City to rescue persons in distress, but their motives were questionable. According to Talese (1996), this group was, "… composed of a few petty brigands who received no municipal salary and therefore supported themselves in summer by unsubtly soliciting donations from the proprietors and patrons of bathhouses and the largess of anyone they rescued from drowning. When their funds ran low, they would fake rescues."

The First Lifeguards

In response to the drownings, beach resorts and local governments began to hire especially good swimmers to "guard" the beach. In Atlantic City, municipal police were initially assigned to lifesaving duties, but police resources soon became strained by this responsibility. So in 1892, a corps of lifeguards was employed. (Methot, 1988) The term "beach patrol" is said to have been coined in Atlantic City. (Atlantic City Beach Patrol, 2002)

Down the Jersey Shore, in Cape May, drowning prevention efforts began with rescue rings hung on bathhouses and the provision of dories on the beach that could be used for rescue. By 1865, hotels began hiring persons to staff the dories. Later, a municipal lifeguard operation was begun that continues to the present day. (Cape May Beach Patrol, 2001)

On the West Coast, a similar trend was followed, with seaside bathhouses hiring lifeguards to ensure safety of their patrons. It was not until 1908 though, that the first municipal lifeguard, Hinnie Zimmerman, was hired by the city of Long Beach, California. (D'Arnall, Shea, Rohrer, & Mark, 1981)

One approach to lifesaving was public education and the provision of swimming lessons. The Young Men's Christian Association (YMCA) began building pools at their facilities in 1885, with 17 reported built that year. Mass swim lessons were initiated at the Detroit YMCA in 1907 by George Corsan, who helped promote swimming lessons by providing bronze buttons as rewards for swimming proficiency to any boy who could swim 50 feet. By 1909, his learn-to-swim programs had developed into the first nationwide effort to teach every boy in the U.S. and Canada to swim. (YMCA of the USA, 2001)

In 1911, lifesaving work and research was established at the YMCA's national college in Springfield, Massachusetts. There, in 1913, the first American work on lifesaving was written (and later published as a lifesaving textbook in 1916) by George Goss, as his college thesis. In 1919, the YMCA published the *YMCA Swimming and Lifesaving Manual*.

In 1914, Commodore Wilbert E. Longfellow formed the Life-Saving Service of the American Red Cross, a corps of volunteers recruited and trained to provide rescues at beaches not regularly patrolled by lifeguards. Not satisfied that this adequately addressed the drowning problem, Commodore Longfellow recruited the strongest swimmers from the corps to teach swimming to beach visitors. He began a program to "waterproof America" by teaching people to swim and by training lay people in the skills necessary to rescue a drowning person. His slogan, "Everyone a swimmer, every swimmer a lifesaver," became the motto of early Red Cross programs that taught swimming, water safety, and lifesaving to many children and adults.

At the same time these efforts took hold, professional open water lifeguard services gradually spread along the shores of the United States. As in the case of the first lifesavers, great tragedies sometimes precipitated the creation of America's public lifeguard services. For example, a municipal lifeguard service was not initiated in San Diego, California until 1918, when 13 people drowned on a single day in flash rip currents. (The San Diego Union, 1918) By the end of the 1930s, publicly employed lifeguards had become a common site at many beaches across the United States.

There was little consistency among these services, largely due to the lack of a national organization charged with setting standards for the new profession. This was unusual compared to other countries, such as those of the British Commonwealth, where societies were chartered and mandated to set standards for lifesaving operations.

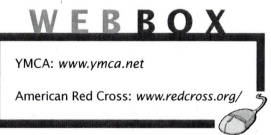

WEBBOX

YMCA: *www.ymca.net*

American Red Cross: *www.redcross.org/*

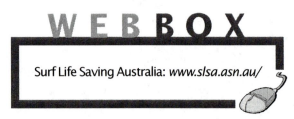

Surf Life Saving Australia: www.slsa.asn.au/

In some countries, lifesaving societies actually supervised and ran lifeguard operations, regardless of who owned or had responsibility for the open water recreation site. In Australia, for example, the first volunteer lifesaving "club" was founded at Bondi in 1906, followed by the development of other local clubs and, eventually, Surf Life Saving Australia. (Longhurst, 2000) Today, some Australian lifesavers are paid, but most are still volunteers associated with SLSA.

A club or society based lifesaving system did not proliferate in the U.S. The YMCA and Red Cross initially declined to become involved in professional lifeguarding, contending that their programs were intended to promote safe swimming and provide training in personal rescue techniques for lay people, not professional lifeguards. There were however, exceptions. One of these, the American Red Cross Volunteer Lifesaving Corps was founded in 1912 and still exists today, in Jacksonville, Florida.

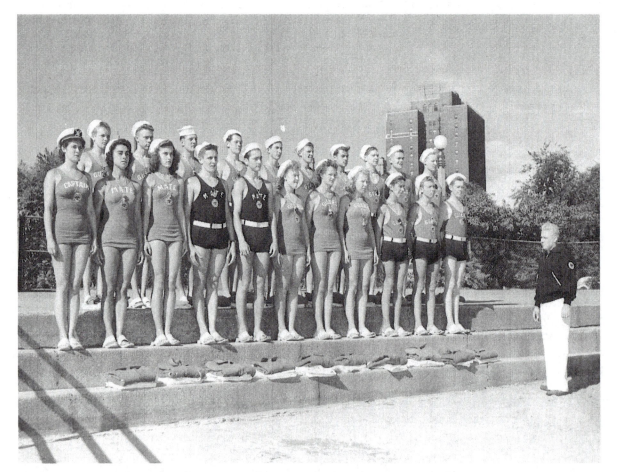

It was during World War II that the Chicago Park District first employed female lifeguards to work the beaches.

Credit: Chicago Park District

Professional open water lifeguards employed techniques that had evolved from the U.S. Life-Saving Service, along with the growing body of knowledge being developed by the lifesaving programs of the American Red Cross and the YMCA. The rescue equipment, what there was of it, was adapted from other disciplines, such as the devices that had been used by the U.S. Life-Saving Service to rescue sailors from the sea. Surfboats, similar to those used by the U.S. Life-Saving Service, were adapted for use by lifeguards to row to swimmers in trouble. They remain in use in a few areas of the U.S. The predominant method of rescue though, was by swimming to the victim.

With open water recreation established as a major national pastime, acquisition of park systems and provision of recreational opportunities came to be seen as an important role of government. Recreation programs and departments were created on a national and local level. During the Great Depression, numerous federal public works projects involved construction of recreation facilities. After the Depression, many of these facilities were turned over to local and state recreation agencies and lifeguards were added to operation staffs.

During World War II, the male dominated profession of lifeguarding was impacted by recruitment of men into the armed forces. In some areas of the country, where beach lifeguards were seen as essential public safety providers, draft waivers were issued to keep trained and experienced lifeguards on the beaches. As was the case in other professions, women sometimes filled the vacancies that were created when male lifeguards enlisted in the armed forces.

Unlike police and fire services with centuries of history, professional lifeguards were relatively new providers of public safety and their place in governmental structures varied greatly. In areas where lifeguards were on duty year round, some lifeguard services became divisions of other public safety services or were organized into departments unto themselves. These organizational structures gave the lifeguards a stature equivalent to that of police officers or firefighters.

In other areas, open water lifeguard services were administered as part of recreation programs or park systems and lifeguards were sometimes titled as "recreation assistants" or "program aides." This perception of lifeguards persisted in many areas of the United States well into the 1960s until two events changed the course of professional lifeguarding: the creation of a national association of open water lifeguards and the increased attention of Americans to accident prevention and treatment.

Birth of the United States Lifesaving Association

Decades after professional lifeguard agencies had been established at beaches throughout America, Australia was chosen to host the 1956 summer Olympics. The volunteer lifesavers of Australia decided to use the occasion to hold the Australian Olympic International Surf Championships at Torquay, outside the city of Melbourne. California lifeguards and a contingent from the Territory of Hawaii agreed to participate. The California lifeguards organized themselves under the banner of the Surf Life Saving Association of America (SLSA), although they were solely from the Los Angeles County, Santa Monica, and Los Angeles City lifeguard agencies.

The event drew a crowd of 115,000 spectators, with "Duke" Kanhanamoku as the honorary Chairman. In addition to the Americans and Australians, teams from South Africa, Great Britain, Ceylon, and New Zealand participated.

The U.S. lifeguards brought rescue tubes and rescue buoys along, exposing the Australians to these devices for the first time. U.S. team members also introduced Malibu Bolsa Surfboards to Australia. When they departed, the boards were left behind, which revolutionized surfing in Australia. (Burnside, 2001)

Just as the Americans introduced new lifesaving equipment to the Australians, the Australians introduced the concept of a national organization of lifesavers. Surf Life Saving Australia impressed them and they considered the value of a similar national organization in the U.S. After they returned, the Surf Life Saving Association of America was maintained as a viable organization, with the strong support of Los Angeles County Lifeguard Chief Bud Stevenson. He appointed one of his lifeguards, Bob Burnside, as president of the organization.

In 1963, efforts were commenced to expand the scope of SLSA. Burnside called for representatives from as many Southern California lifeguard agencies as possible to attend a concept meeting at City of Santa Monica Lifeguard Headquarters. In attendance were Vince Moorhouse (Huntington Beach), Max Bowman (Huntington Beach), Don Rohrer (LA City), Dick Heineman (LA City), Tim Dorsey (Seal Beach), Jim Richards (California State Central), and Rudy Kroon (Santa Monica). (Burnside, 2001)

The group agreed that they should expand SLSA to a truly national organization, based on the structure of the Australian association. They established a temporary Executive Board to develop a constitution, bylaws, and method of representation.

In 1964, Howard Lee of LA County designed the SLSA logo, still in use today with minor modifications. His design was influenced by a similar design that Tad Devine of the 1956 Australia team had created for the team uniform. Both are similar to the logo of the U.S. Life-Saving Service. (Burnside, 2001)

Many milestones can be traced to these early years. In 1965, the organization changed its name to the National Surf Lifesaving Association. That year, ABC's Wide World of Sports invited members to participate in an East Coast/West Coast/Australian lifesaving championship at Montauck on Long Island, New York. Dramatic video of a surfboat surfing careening down a wave became part of the standard lead-in to Wide World of Sports. Also in 1965, the newsletter *Ocean Lifeguard* was first published and proposed written examinations for beach lifeguards were forwarded to civil service departments, to encourage standardization.

In 1967, NSLSA sent a competition team to Ft. Lauderdale, Florida, for the first East vs. West Coast championships. The following year, Lt. Jim Holland of the Miami Beach Patrol was appointed to act as East Coast Liaison.

In 1969 Dade County, Florida requested that NSLSA representatives journey to Miami and make recommendations for improvements in their lifeguard program. The outcome included suggestions that resulted in installation of a communication system, new vehicles and equipment, new qualification requirements, and increased funding. It was the first demonstration of the potential power of NSLSA to improve lifesaving standards nationwide.

In 1971, NSLSA became a founding member of World Lifesaving, which also included the national surf lifesaving federations of Australia, Great Britain, New Zealand, and South Africa. The following year, NSLSA hosted a meeting of World Lifesaving in Huntington Beach, California—the first international lifesaving meeting in the U.S. That same year NSLSA was granted tax exempt status as a charitable/educational organization. A few years later, in 1976, Vince Moorhouse of Huntington Beach was appointed World Lifesaving's president, and in 1978 NSLSA hosted a World Lifesaving Educational Congress in Newport Beach, California.

There was much discussion during these times, about expanding the reach of the organization to embrace all open water lifeguards, whether at surf or non-surf beaches. NSLSA President Sheridan Byerly chaired a Board of Directors meeting in Santa Cruz, California in May of 1979 thick with heated and passionate discussion about the course of the organization's future. Ultimately, the NSLSA Board of Directors voted to change the name of the organization to the United States Lifesaving Association (USLA) and adopt various bylaw changes that set the stage for a broader and more embracing organization. It was agreed that USLA members could now include any member of an ocean, bay, lake, river, or open water lifesaving or rescue service, including chiefs, directors, and their equivalent.

American lifeguard agencies and professional lifeguards now had a national organization they could use to exchange information on professional techniques, lifesaving equipment, lifeguard agency organization, and other items of concern. Two primary goals have been maintained by U.S.L.A since its inception: 1) to establish and maintain high standards of professional open water lifesaving; and 2) to educate the public in water safety and the role of lifeguards.

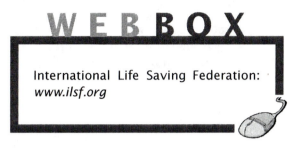

WEBBOX

International Life Saving Federation: *www.ilsf.org*

On the international scene, USLA was one of the founding members of World Life Saving and, when it merged to become the International Life Saving Federation, USLA became the United States' full member to this worldwide lifesaving body. Thus, USLA helps shape the face of lifesaving internationally, as well as in the U.S.

Emergency Medical Aid Advances

In 1966, the National Academy of Sciences published a document entitled, *Accidental Death and Disability: The Neglected Disease of Modern Society.* This document outlined a poor state of training and service standards for emergency medical care providers in the United States, where many ambulance attendants had little or no training beyond basic first aid. It helped to spur passage of the nation's Highway Safety Act of 1966, which charged the U.S. Department of Transportation with the development and establishment of an Emergency Medical Service Standard. This led to the establishment of standards in emergency medical care now taken for granted in the United States. The document also recommended, "Active exploration of the feasibility of designating a single nationwide telephone number to summon an ambulance." Many now take 9-1-1 for granted, but the 9-1-1 system only gradually came into being over a period of many years after this recommendation. (National Academy of Sciences, 1966)

Recognizing the problems in the nation's emergency medical services also motivated citizen groups and government organizations to carefully evaluate training and service standards for other emergency services, including police, fire, and open water lifeguard services. It became evident that some lifeguard agencies worked with little or no formal training. Others required their lifeguards to undergo only rudimentary training aimed at "drown proofing" the general public, rather than preparing professional rescuers. Many had wrongly considered pool lifesaving training adequate for open water lifeguards, even those assigned to the most treacherous surf beaches. National standards were needed and U.S.L.A. was to provide them.

Lifesaving Devices

One of the greatest difficulties for swimming lifesavers was the struggle sometimes required to overpower a panicked victim before the rescue could be completed. The line and reel (landline), was an early solution. A lifeguard would swim out to the victim while attached to the line, clutch the victim, and would be rapidly pulled back to shore by others.

This method had the advantage of quick retrieval, but there were some disadvantages too. The line produced drag, which could slow approach to the victim; it required two or more persons to operate; it was inadequate in cases of multiple rescues simultaneously occurring at different locations; and, it could become tangled. Nevertheless, it was widely used for decades and is still in use in a few areas.

As an alternative, Atlantic City lifeguards developed what may be the first rescue floatation device (RFD) by fastening an eight-foot line and shoulder harness to a life ring. The lifeguard would swim out with the life ring, throw it to the victim, and tow the victim to a dory or to shore. This avoided contact with the victim, but like the line and reel, the life ring created significant drag in the water. (Burnside, 1973)

The Rescue Buoy

Captain Henry Sheffield, an American with a variety of aquatic accomplishments to his credit, was touring Durban, South Africa in 1897 when he designed another type of RFD, the first "rescue can" (also called the "rescue cylinder") for a lifesaving club there. It was made of sheet metal and pointed on both ends, with the same over-the-shoulder harness and line used by lifeguards towing life rings. The advantage was that it moved much more smoothly through the water, producing little drag. A disadvantage was that the heavy metal and pointed ends sometimes caused injuries, both to rescuers and those being rescued. The design was later modified in the United States, where the heavy sheet metal was eventually replaced with copper, then aluminum—rounded on both ends. (Burnside, 1973)

Aluminum rescue buoys, even with their rounded ends, still caused injuries. It wasn't until the mid-1960s though, that the next major advancement in design of these devices occurred. As Los Angeles County lifeguard Lieutenant Bob Burnside was typing up the second injury report in a week for a lifeguard injured after being struck by an aluminum rescue can, he noticed a plastic statuette sitting on his desk. He wondered if the metal rescue can could instead be constructed of plastic and thereby made safer for both lifeguard and victim. He sent a lifeguard to the University of California at Los Angeles (UCLA) Industrial Arts Department to inquire as to the feasibility of such a design.

Professor Ron Rezek, familiar with a manufacturing process called rotational molding, coordinated with Lt. Burnside to develop the design. In 1968, a wood prototype was submitted to the Board of Directors of the National Surf Life Saving Association (the forerunner of U.S.L.A.) and received with great enthusiasm. Professor Rezek subsequently won a design award and entered into production with Lt. Burnside for the first plastic rescue buoy. These RFDs are now a basic tool of open water lifeguards and still known to many as *Burnside buoys*, but more commonly referred to as *rescue buoys*. (Burnside, 1973) (Rezek, 1999) (Burnside, 2001)

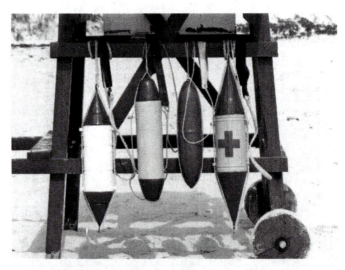

Some original rescue buoys. They were often known as "can" buoys because of their metal construction.

Credit: Mike Hensler

The Rescue Board

In 1907, George Freeth of Hawaii arrived in Redondo Beach, California and was engaged to help promote a seaside resort. Billed as, "the man who walks on water," Freeth was one of the first persons to surf on the American West Coast and helped greatly to popularize surfing. He is considered by some to be the first open water lifeguard in California, but that is difficult to establish with certainty. (The first municipal lifeguard was Hinnie Zimmerman in Long Beach.) Although it appears that he was not specifically employed as a lifeguard, he was unquestionably an extraordinary ocean swimmer and surfer. He reportedly made many rescue rescues of people in distress, sometimes using his surfboard. In one case, in December 1908, Freeth reportedly rescued as many as seven fishers whose boats capsized in a sudden, violent storm off Venice beach. When the legendary Hawaiian "Duke" Paoa Kanhanamoku visited California in 1913 and introduced his redwood surfboard to Long Beach, California lifeguards, the surfboard was adopted as a rescue tool. Later, the term "rescue board" would be coined. (D'Arnall et al., 1981)

The Rescue Tube

In 1935, based on a design by Reggie Burton and Captain George Watkins, former Santa Monica lifeguard Pete Peterson produced an inflatable, bright yellow rescue tube with a snap hook molded onto one end and a 14 inch strap on the other. A line and harness were then attached. This highly visible RFD was used by many lifeguard services into the early 1960s. (Burnside, 1973)

In response to the buoyancy problems related to punctures and climactic conditions, Peterson redesigned the tube, constructing it of flexible foam rubber with an orange skin to keep water out of the interior. While this was an improvement, the skin was still subject to piercing and the open cell foam would then act like a sponge, becoming waterlogged. By the late 1960s however, closed cell foam rubber was invented and the tube was manufactured with this material so that punctures to the skin no longer resulted in water absorption. This device is still known to some as the *Peterson tube*, but is more commonly known as the *rescue tube*.

Developing National Open Water Lifeguard Standards

It became clear that the pool and open water environments are incomparable for purposes of training or standards. As a result, open water lifeguards began to seek specialized training for their unique environment. None being available, more progressive lifeguard agencies developed their own standards, networking with each other for consistency and validation of their practices. Nevertheless, the open water lifeguard profession suffered greatly for lack of state or national standards.

In 1980, a conference held at the University of Texas A & M brought together all of the major American organizations concerned with promoting public safety in and around the aquatic environment. The intent of the conference was to discuss ways to develop standards for open water lifeguards. The result was a Sea Grant funded publication entitled, *Guidelines for Establishing Open-Water Recreational Beach Standards* (McCloy & Dodson, 1981).

In 1981, the first USLA lifesaving text, *Lifesaving and Marine Safety*, was published. (D'Arnall, Shea, Rohrer, & Mark). In 1983, based on the work accomplished in Galveston, USLA published a booklet entitled *Guidelines for Open Water Lifeguard Training*, which set the first nationwide recommended standards for open water lifeguards at both inland and surf beaches.

Ten years later, USLA revised the original guidelines and published *Guidelines for Open Water Lifeguard Training and Standards*, which now formed the basis for the first national certification program for both inland and surf open water lifeguard training programs. (Brewster, 1993) Rather than certifying the lifeguards themselves, USLA created the *Lifeguard Agency Certification Program*. This program provides an independent review of open water lifeguard programs and encourages lifeguard agencies across the country to meet the standards recommended by USLA. By the end of the decade,

WEBBOX

You can download a copy of *Guidelines for Establishing Open-Water Recreational Beach Standards* from the Lifeguard Library section of: *www.usla.org*.

You can download a current version of *Guidelines For Open Water Lifeguard Agency Certification* from the Certification section of *www.usla.org*

You can download a current version of *Training and Standards of Aquatic Rescue Response Teams* from the Certification section of *www.usla.org*

the guidelines had been revised again and retitled, *Guidelines For Open Water Lifeguard Agency Certification.* (Brewster, 2000) By the year 2000, over 100 U.S. lifeguard agencies, large and small, had been certified.

The first edition of the text you now read, *The United States Lifesaving Association Manual of Open Water Lifesaving,* was published in 1995 to provide a core reference for the training of America's open water rescuers. It was followed by development of a second certification program for open water rescuers who are not lifeguards, which is known as the *Aquatic Rescue Response Team* (ARRT) certification program. It is described in the USLA publication *Training and Standards of Aquatic Rescue Response Teams.* (Brewster, 1996)

These publications, along with the ongoing work of USLA training committees, have greatly added to the body of knowledge used by open water lifeguard agencies and enhanced development of an image of the lifeguard as a professional emergency provider. The 1997 development of the USLA website—*www.usla.org*—has further helped disseminate information to lifeguards and provided a forum for exchange of lifesaving ideas. Today, USLA is known nationally and internationally as an authoritative body in the field of open water lifeguarding and marine safety. USLA guidelines are required by law in some areas for training newly hired lifeguards.

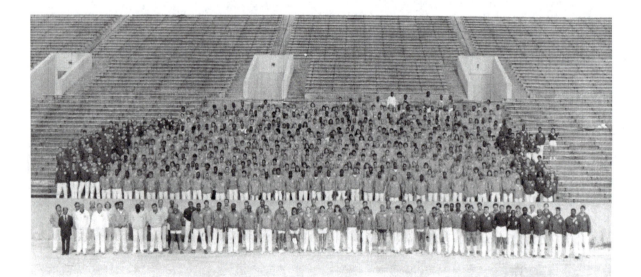

Chicago Park Service lifeguard staff.
Credit: Bob Burtog

Modern Lifeguarding

The profession of lifeguarding will always be unique among emergency services due largely to its highly seasonal nature. While in Florida, California, and Hawaii hundreds of open water lifeguards work year round on a career basis, open water lifeguards in most other states work seasonally. Nevertheless, whether year round or seasonal, professional lifeguard services have perhaps the most direct and profound impact on public safety per employee of any emergency service providers.

Open water lifeguards consistently and continually make the difference between the life and death of otherwise healthy people through timely preventive acts. While other emergency services are largely reactive, responding once an emergency has occurred, alert lifeguards can often prevent the emergencies from developing in the first place or pluck unsuspecting people from harm's way.

In the warmer states, lifeguards have particularly broad responsibilities. Some American lifeguards are armed police officers serving a dual role of rescuer and law enforcer. Others are called upon to perform duties such as marine firefighting, coastal cliff rescue, paramedic services, flood rescue, and scuba search and recovery.

Several American lifeguard agencies keep their personnel on duty 24 hours a day to provide response to nighttime aquatic emergencies. In some areas, when a citizen calls 9-1-1 to report an aquatic emergency, the reporting party is connected directly to a lifeguard dispatcher. In other areas, even those lacking regular off-summer lifeguard protection, aquatic emergency response systems are in place to dispatch qualified open water lifeguards whenever the need arises.

Lifesaving equipment continues to evolve as lifeguards experiment and innovate. The inshore rescue boat (IRB), pioneered in Australia and New Zealand has been employed in many areas, as have personal watercraft (PWC), replacing the traditional dory. Hard hull rescue boats up to 32' in length, some with firefighting equipment, are also used. The Baywatch vessels of the Los Angeles County lifeguards, after which the popular television show was named, represent perhaps the best prepared fleet of open water rescue vessels maintained by a local government in the United States.

Increasing expectations of the general public for emergency medical care have resulted in dramatic improvements in the quality of emergency medical training. USLA minimum recommended standards require that all lifeguards have emergency medical aid training well beyond the basic levels available to the general public. More advanced open water lifeguard agencies now require their personnel to be certified at the level of Emergency Medical Technician or the equivalent of Department of Transportation First Responder. Medical equipment, such as spineboards, cervical collars, and oxygen, have become a must for open water lifeguard agencies. Cardiac defibrillators, once a highly specialized device, are becoming common tools

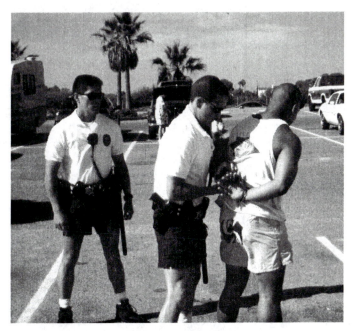

California State Lifeguards make an arrest.
Credit: Ken Kramer

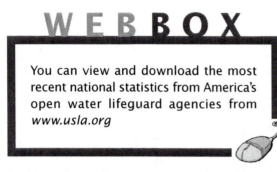

You can view and download the most recent national statistics from America's open water lifeguard agencies from *www.usla.org*

of lifeguards. It is no longer acceptable to wait precious minutes for an ambulance to deliver essential pieces of equipment such as these.

Facilities too, have improved. Properly designed lifeguard facilities minimize stress and fatigue by providing refuge from the elements. Most larger lifeguard stations include areas with private, sterile treatment areas for persons requiring medical attention. Some include garages, offices, workout rooms, kitchen areas, and other facilities commonly found in the stations of other emergency service providers.

Thus, the period from the 1960s to the present has brought a great change to the role of the professional lifeguard. Lifeguarding has emerged as a true emergency service with the same charge as that of other emergency services—the protection of lives and property. In a typical year in this country, well over 80,000 lives are saved by open water lifeguards and many millions of dollars in property protected.

Historical Lessons

Despite these advances, not all of today's open water lifeguard agencies can boast of modern equipment and facilities. Many seasonal agencies still operate following years of tradition based on equipment developed for lifesaving more than 100 years ago. Other lifeguard services employ the most basic equipment and training. At some parks and beaches, solitary lifeguards work long hours without assistance; while at others administrators struggle over how, or even if, lifeguards should be employed.

The lessons of the past are hard learned and oft forgotten. On Memorial Day 1994, five people drowned at American Beach in northern Florida. No lifeguards were present because they had been eliminated in a cost saving measure. Shortly after the drownings and ensuing nationwide attention, lifeguard protection was restored.

More recently, at San Francisco's Ocean Beach where the National Park Service (NPS) had declined to provide lifeguards, three persons drowned on the first day of summer in 1998. The United States Lifesaving Association, the International Life Saving Federation, and others, conducted a campaign to bring about the staffing of lifeguards at this beach.

Although several more persons drowned that summer in the face of a continued reluctance to provide safety protection, by the following summer NPS had relented. Open water rescue personnel, in a program later certified by the United States Lifesaving Association, were staffed. No drownings were reported that year. Unfortunately, in these cases, as in many others in American history, lifeguard staff was provided only after avoidable tragedy dramatically punctuated the need for prevention.

There was a time that common public perception of lifeguards was that of sun worshippers with little more to offer than directions and sun tan lotion. It has changed through the efforts of open water lifeguards who understand that recognition of their essential public safety role is directly tied to their own level of professionalism. Lifeguards who willingly accept the old stereotypes directly contribute to their perpetuation, seriously harming not only their own image, but that of their fellow lifeguards. On the other hand, lifeguards who demonstrate respect for their occupation through preparedness, maturity, and dedication help ensure that lifeguards will be recognized, trained, equipped, and compensated at appropriate levels.

The first lifesavers who walked the beaches of America in search of shipwrecked victims were not fully respected or funded until they adopted regulations, drilled regularly, and demonstrated an abil-

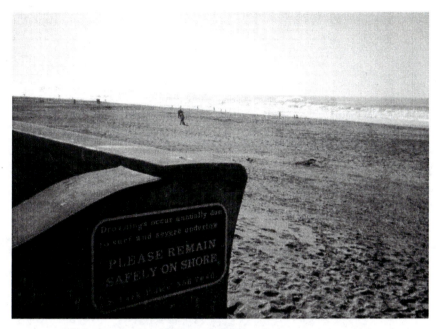

At one time, at treacherous Ocean Beach in San Francisco, no lifeguards were provided. Instead, the National Park Service chose to simply accept the fact that "drownings occur annually." This was changed as a result of work by USLA and others.

Credit: B. Chris Brewster

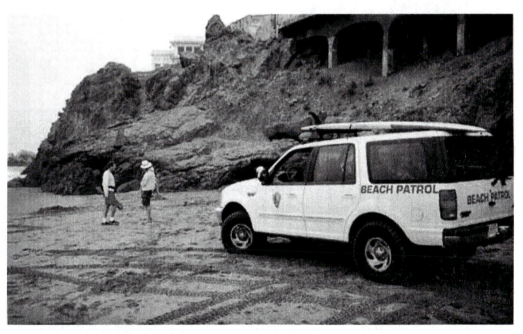

An Ocean Beach lifeguard makes a public contact.

Credit: Bob Airey-Van Diem

ity to handle the most complex rescues with the ease of professionals. It was through their own actions that their profession became recognized as essential to the safety and well-being of the public. The same is true today. Every open water lifeguard is directly responsible for the professional image of all open water lifeguards.

Chapter Summary

In this chapter, we have learned that organized lifesaving efforts began in America in the 1700s to rescue shipwrecked sailors. As the shipwrecks diminished in number, interest in swimming grew, and open water lifeguards were first hired in the U.S. in the late 1800s to rescue swimmers.

Many innovations have taken place since that time, including the invention of the rescue tube, rescue buoy, and the rescue board. Lifeguards have evolved their skills to include advanced medical aid and a variety of other emergency services. The United States Lifesaving Association was created after American lifeguards visited Australia and saw the benefits of a national lifesaving association. Later, USLA developed national standards for open water lifeguard training. Today, USLA is a world leader in lifesaving and, as a result of the efforts of lifeguards throughout the United States, lifeguarding has evolved to become a true emergency service.

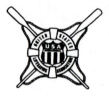

Discussion Points

- Why were lifesavers first needed in the U.S.?
- Why didn't the first U.S. lifesavers work during summer months?
- The Massachusetts Humane Society was founded for what purpose?
- What prompted Congress to pass the Newell Act?
- Who was Sumner Increase Kimball?
- What were the rescue implements of the U.S. Life-Saving Service and how were they used?
- What were lifelines?
- How did World War II impact lifesaving?
- What event prompted creation of the Surf Lifesaving Association of America?
- What prompted the decision to adopt the name United States Lifesaving Association?
- What were some advantages and disadvantages of the first rescue "can"?
- How did plastic revolutionize rescue buoy design?
- How do lifeguards compare with other emergency service providers?
- Why is it important for lifeguards to maintain a professional image?

References

Atlantic City Beach Patrol (2002). Retrieved December 12, 2002 from the World Wide Web: *www.acbp.org/acfame.html*

Barnett, J. (1974). *The lifesaving guns of David Lyle.* Plymouth, Indiana: Town and Country Press.

Brewster, B.C. (Ed.). (1993). *Guidelines for open water lifeguard training and standards.* Huntington Beach, California: United States Lifesaving Association.

Brewster, B.C. (Ed.). (1996). *Training and standards of aquatic rescue response teams.* Huntington Beach, California: United States Lifesaving Association.

Brewster, B.C. (Ed.). (2000). *Guidelines for open water lifeguard agency certification.* Huntington Beach, California: United States Lifesaving Association.

Burnside, R. (1973). History of the American rescue can. *Ocean Lifeguard*

Burnside, R. (2001). The early history of the United States Lifesaving Association. Palm Desert, California: Burnside.

Cape May Beach Patrol (2001). Retrieved January 4, 2001 from the World Wide Web: *www.capemay beachpatrol.org/*

Councilmen Visit Scene of Ocean Beach Disaster. (May 7, 1918) *The San Diego Union*, p. 1.

D'Arnall, D., Shea, B., Rohrer, D., & Mark, R. (1981). *Lifesaving and marine safety.* Piscataway, New Jersey: New Century Publishers.

Dalton, J. (1967). *The life savers of Cape Cod.* Chatham, Massachusetts: Chatham Press.

Johnson, R. (1988). *Guardians of the sea: history of the United States Coast Guard.* Annapolis, Maryland: United States Naval Institute.

Kimball, S. (1913); *Rescuing flood victims in the middle western states.* Report to 63rd Congress, First Session, Document No. 94. Washington, D.C.: Library of Congress.

Longhurst, R. (2000); *The lifesaver—images of summer.* Caringbah, NSW, Australia: Playright Publishing.

McCloy, J. &. Dodson, J. (Eds.). (1981). *Guidelines for establishing open-water recreational beach standards.* Galveston, Texas: Texas A&M University.

Merryman, J. & Jones, W. (Ed.). (1981). *The United States Life-Saving Service—1880.* Silverthorne, Colorado: Vistabooks.

Methot, J. (1988). *Up and down the Jersey Shore.* Navesink, New Jersey: Whip Publishers.

National Academy of Sciences (1966). *Accidental Death and Disability: The Neglected Disease of Modern Society.* Washington, D.C.: National Academy of Sciences Printing and Publishing Office.

Quinn, W. (1973). *Shipwrecks around Cape Cod.* Orleans, Massachusetts: Lower Cape Publishing.

Rezek, R. (1999). Personal correspondence.

Ryder, R. (1990). *Old Harbor Station.* Norwich, Connecticut: Ram Island Press.

Shanks, R., York, W., & Shanks, L. (Ed.). (1998). *The U.S. Life-Saving Service.* Petaluma, California: Costano Books.

Talese, G. (1996, September 8). One more spin of the wheel for Atlantic City. *The New York Times.*

U.S. Life-Saving Service (1880). Annual report to Congress. Washington, D.C.: Library of Congress.

U.S. Life-Saving Service (1884). Annual report to Congress. Washington, D.C.: Library of Congress.

YMCA of the U.S.A (2001). Retrieved January 4, 2001 from the World Wide Web: *www.ymca.net/*

Chapter 2
Use and Protection of America's Beaches

In this chapter, you will learn that open water beaches are one of the great natural resources of our nation. People have always been drawn to the water, but beaches have experienced an explosion in popularity over the past several decades. In fact, they are the most popular tourist destination in the United States by a wide margin. Some impacts of humans upon the beach environment include pollution and development. Lifeguards play an important role in mitigating negative impacts, protecting both the environment and the people who use it for recreation.

CHAPTER EXCERPT

It is sometimes forgotten that our beaches are a fragile resource that must be carefully protected. In addition to protecting visitors from beach and water hazards, a major role of lifeguards is to protect the beach itself.

Beach Popularity

Beaches are the leading tourist destination in the United States. In fact, their popularity far exceeds other tourist attractions. For example, one study found that Miami Beach alone reported more annual visits than any single national park—twice as many as the combined annual visitation of Yellowstone, Grand Canyon, and Yosemite National Parks. (Houston, 1995) Beach tourism contributes $170 billion annually to the U.S. economy (Houston, 1995) and 85% of tourist-related revenues are generated by the coastal states (Cicin-Sain & Knecht, 1999).

The beach has become a magnet for all socioeconomic groups. They flock to the shore for myriad reasons. Some come merely to relax, contemplate, perhaps read a book. Many come to recreate. Most will benefit by the oversight and assistance of a professional lifeguard.

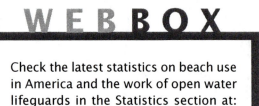

WEB BOX

Check the latest statistics on beach use in America and the work of open water lifeguards in the Statistics section at: *www.usla.org*

Part of the seemingly ever-increasing popularity of the beach stems from the tremendous interest in aquatic recreation. Each year more than 80 million Americans participate in open water swimming and some 77 million participate in boating. (Cicin-Sain & Knecht, 1999) There are many other poplar aquatic recreational activities though. Participation in activities such as surfing, skin and scuba diving, windsurfing, and kite boarding, are just a few examples. Beaches are also popular venues for non-aquatic activities like sunbathing, volleyball, walking, running, skating, biking, hiking, backpacking, climbing, and a host of others. Some municipalities even permit vehicle traffic on their beaches. All of these have created added demands on the limited recreational space available and on the lifeguards who manage these areas.

The popularity of the beach lends itself to the occasional conflict between users, which lifeguards are often called upon to mediate. For example, lifeguards must be prepared to help resolve the dispute that may arise when a nearby primary school camps out for a picnic in front of a surfing spot favored by locals, or a volleyball group sets up next to a group of older citizens practicing tai chi, or a visiting college group unaware of the local prohibition of alcohol on the beach arrives with several large coolers of beer. All these problems can be solved, but require the social, diplomatic and managerial skills of the professional lifeguard.

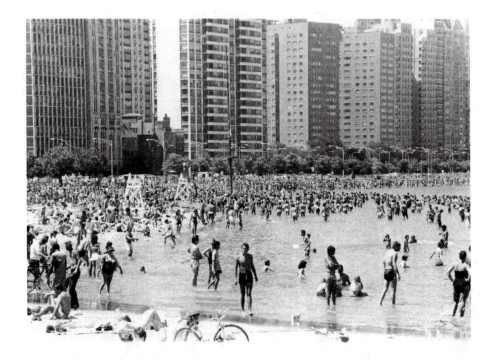

Oak Street Beach, Chicago.
Credit: Joe Pecoraro

Every beach activity, even walking along the shore, involves some risk. Beach visitors place their trust in lifeguards and, as the closest emergency responders, lifeguards must be prepared to manage and respond to any which occur within their jurisdiction.

Protecting the Beach Environment

The beach is more than a natural, sandy amusement park. It is a complex ecosystem that can be irreparably damaged through misuse. Litter, development, sand loss, and water pollution are just a few examples of potential threats to the beach environment. Each of these can also threaten the safety of visitors. It is sometimes forgotten that our beaches are a fragile resource that must be carefully protected. In addition to protecting visitors from beach and water hazards, a major role of lifeguards is to protect the beach itself.

Litter

Visitors to the beach sometimes seem to think they are visiting an amusement park, and that someone will always pick up after them. Some leave food, paper products, cans, bottles, and all other forms of litter. Not only does the appearance of these items sully the beach, it also threatens the safety of people and animals. People can be injured by stepping on sharp items of discarded waste. Animals may be injured by ingesting or becoming entangled in waste. The problem is compounded when people actually use the sand to cover and dispose of litter such as glass containers, which may break and provide a hidden hazard to other visitors. Many communities ban glass containers or even food for these reasons. In any case, lifeguards can play an important role in discouraging conduct of this nature.

Flotsam

Flotsam is debris floating in the water. Such objects can be in the form of harmless seaweed or can be large, dangerous objects containing sharp edges or surfaces. Flotsam may take the form of hazardous materials or substances, which can cause a health threat to beach visitors. It is most evident after a storm or storm surf. At surf beaches, flotsam is particularly dangerous since it can be washed in at high velocity by surf action, injuring swimmers in its path. At both surf and flat water areas, flotsam that washes ashore without incident can continue to be dangerous, especially if it becomes buried and therefore hidden to beach visitors. Landed flotsam can cut, stab, and stick visitors walking along the beach.

Lifeguards should scan their water areas for flotsam and immediately investigate any unexpected floating objects. At surf beaches, it may be necessary to clear a water area until a large object floats in, so that it does not strike anyone. Regular patrols of beach areas by lifeguards are important to check for all hazards, including flotsam.

Sand

Sandy beaches are unique environments, seemingly perfect for recreation. Sand sometimes seems to be ever-present, but when shorelines are reinforced to protect adjacent structures, the result is sometimes a significant loss of sandy beach frontage. Most sandy beaches are created and regenerated by erosion of coastline, by sand that flows to the sea from inland rivers, and by movement of sand along the shoreline. When this natural process is impeded by development, beaches suffer. At some beaches,

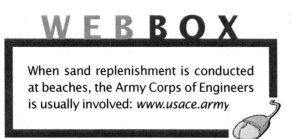

When sand replenishment is conducted at beaches, the Army Corps of Engineers is usually involved: *www.usace.army*

jetties and groins have been constructed in an effort to save the beach. One extreme solution, increasingly employed, involves importing sand or pumping it onshore from an offshore location. These efforts have a high price tag. Although nature seems to eventually undo sand replenishment efforts, the cost is often considered well spent because of the tremendous enjoyment the beach provides.

Sand can be dangerous. Blowing sand, thrown sand, and uneven sand can all cause injuries. One of the most serious problems involving sand occurs when visitors dig holes or tunnels in the sand. Sand is an inherently unstable substance, as is evident from the constantly shifting sands at most beaches. While digging in the sand may be a common pastime, beachgoers have been buried alive and died when these pits or tunnels have collapsed over them. Lifeguards can reduce the potential for injury by discouraging the digging of deep holes and tunnels. Some areas have ordinances which forbid it. A related problem involves lifeguard emergency vehicles. Children often enjoy covering each other with sand up to their necks. Unfortunately, this can camouflage the covered child from a lifeguard driving a beach emergency vehicle. Great caution is essential in all beach driving.

Disposal of hot charcoal or fire ashes is a particularly dangerous situation at some beaches. Visitors may prepare picnics using small charcoal grills, disposing of the used but still hot coals in the sand and burying them. Buried coals can retain their heat for many hours, later causing second and third degree burns to the feet of unsuspecting visitors. This is a particular problem for infants who may wander away

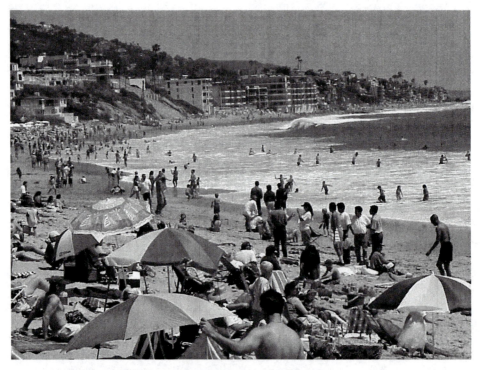

Coastal development in Laguna Beach, California.
Credit: Laguna Beach Lifeguards

from their mothers and walk on discarded coals, but who may not understand how to get away from the burning sensation. Serious injuries causing lifelong deformity to children occur this way every year. A solution employed by some agencies is to maintain containers for disposing of hot coals.

Development Pressure

A home with a view of the water, any open body of water, is often the most sought after in a community. So just as the beach draws short-term visitors, it also attracts development, like homes, restaurants, and streets. Waterfront property can sometimes obstruct public access to the beach. Development pressure, added to the increasing popularity of beaches and water activities, can threaten the fragile beach environment.

To prevent over-development, concerned citizens have pressed for government action. In some cases, the result has been public acquisition of oceanfront property. Another method of protection is through coastal zoning laws enacted to protect not only the beach resource, but all aspects of life by the nation's oceans, lakes and waterways. This has included protection of the right of persons to access their beaches. In California, for example, voters enacted the Coastal Conservation Initiative in 1972 to plan for and regulate land and water uses in the coastal zone in the interests of the public. This resulted in creation of the California Coastal Act and the California Coastal Commission, which wields significant power over coastal development. Its very existence serves to demonstrate public interest in protecting the coastline.

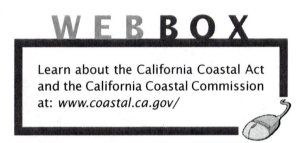

WEBBOX

Learn about the California Coastal Act and the California Coastal Commission at: *www.coastal.ca.gov/*

Water Quality

Many events can influence water quality. A malfunctioning sewage treatment system may cause an inadvertent release of untreated waste. Industrial effluents may be allowed into the water, either accidentally or on purpose. Even natural events can result in changes in water quality. Rain and other forms of precipitation can cause pollutants on land to be washed into the water, introducing "shock loads" of pollutants, often through storm drains that channel runoff into an open water area. Other contributing factors may include tidal mixing, vertical mixing in the water column (by currents, wind, sun, and waves), bioturbation of bottom sediments, biological oxygen demand, photosynthesis by phytoplankton, and water temperature.

Water pollution threatens both the environment and the health of recreational water users. Literature indicates that swimmers stand a much greater risk of contracting disease from polluted water than non-swimmers, when swimmers are defined as those who undergo total immersion. The health of any water user though, may be threatened. Consider the board sailor, who occasionally falls off the board, or the person who eats fish from a contaminated body of water. Infectious diseases, such as cholera and typhoid fever, whose agents are excreted in feces, are spread by water and food contaminated with fecal wastes or sewage.

Numerous parameters can be used to evaluate the quality of a waterbody. The most commonly used indicators in determining risk to human health are bacteria levels. Bacteria called coliforms and enterococcus (marine waters) are specific microorganisms whose elevated densities can cause human health hazards for water users. They should be frequently monitored at aquatic recreation areas.

WEBBOX

Both the National Resources Defense Council *www.nrdc.org/* and the Environmental Protection Agency *www.epa.gov/* publish annual reports on water quality monitoring results.

Government agencies concerned about protecting public and environmental health have implemented laws and procedures to reduce the level of pollutants entering the water. When a body of water declines below levels considered safe, health authorities typically direct that the area be closed to water contact.

Testing of recreational water quality historically varied greatly from state to state and even from county to county. Some community leaders, in areas where regular monitoring resulted in occasional closures of recreational water areas, were frustrated to see other communities that did little or no testing suggest that their waters were cleaner. Of course, without testing, there was no way to compare, and it is likely that swimmers were sometimes unknowingly exposed to pathogens (disease causing agents). Not surprisingly, according to the Environmental Protection Agency (2002), "You are less likely to be exposed to polluted water at beaches that are monitored regularly and posted for health hazards."

Federal legislation aimed at ensuring a more consistent level of testing and public notification was signed into law in 2000. Known as the Beaches Environmental Assessment and Coastal Health (B.E.A.C.H.) Act, it amended the federal Clean Water Act. The BEACH Act was coauthored by Member of Congress Brian Bilbray, a former open water lifeguard. It requires the Environmental Protection Agency to oversee a program whereby a minimum national water quality testing standard must be met or exceeded by the coastal states, and to ensure public notification of the results. Thus, it can be expected that a more standardized system of testing, reporting, and notifying the public about water quality will occur nationwide. In addition to helping water users make decisions about whether the water is clean enough for their activities, this process is likely to put pressure on governments and pollution sources to minimize contamination of aquatic recreation areas.

Lifeguard agencies should have established procedures in effect for recognizing and reporting possible contamination events. They should also have procedures for notifying the public and protecting them from exposure. Normally, once the local department of health determines that water is unsafe for human contact, the beach will be officially closed by public notice, including verbal warnings, signs, media advisories, etc.

Some incidents may cause a lifeguard agency to close a beach to public contact even before the local health authority makes a determination of severity. For example, oil, grease, or sewage in the water or

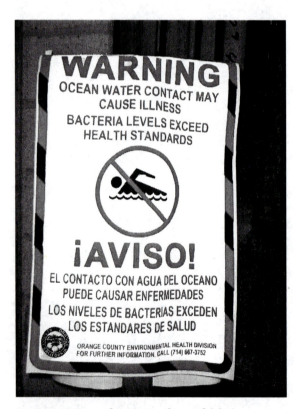

A temporary sign warning of high bacteria levels.

Credit: Ken Kramer

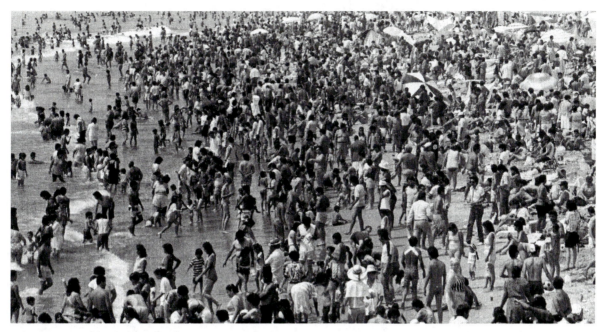

A busy day at the beach in Los Angeles County.

Credit: Los Angeles Times

on the beach may cause a preemptive closure. In more serious cases, even aquatic areas not designated for recreation may be closed.

When a beach is closed due to contamination, everyone suffers. Those who enjoy water recreation are prevented from recreating. The economy of the local community may be negatively impacted because of a reduction in visitors. Lifeguard staff may be reduced. There are therefore many reasons for lifeguards and the communities they serve to be very concerned about maintaining the best possible levels of water quality.

Chapter Summary

In this chapter we have learned that beach popularity is on the rise as well as activities centered on the beach and the surrounding areas. We have learned that our beaches are a fragile resource which needs protection. In coming years, as a result of the BEACH bill, we can expect heightened awareness of water contamination events and pressure to reduce their frequency and severity. Lifeguards can be protectors and advocates for the beach environment by encouraging people to recognize the beach as an irreplaceable natural resource of inestimable value. In doing so, lifeguards help protect the future enjoyment of generations of beach visitors and even their own jobs.

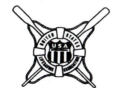

Discussion Points

- What are some conflicts among users you have observed at the beach?
- What activities do you know of that put pressure on the beach environment?
- How might lifeguards discourage littering?
- Why should flotsam be removed?
- What dangers are posed by digging in the sand?
- Why are hot coals a problem at the beach?
- What agencies, in beach areas you know of, are responsible for testing water quality and responding to contamination events?
- What are some regulations you know of that help protect the beach?
- What sand loss have beaches in areas you visit experienced over the years?
- What actions have been taken to prevent sand loss or replace sand lost?
- How are lifeguards impacted by water quality problems?

References

Cicin-Sain, B., & Knecht, R. W. (1999). *The Future of U.S. Ocean Policy: Choices for the New Century.* Washington, D.C.: Island Press.

Houston, J. R. (1995). The economic value of beaches. *The CERCular, CERC-95-4.* Vicksburg, Mississippi: Coastal Engineering Research Center.

U.S. Environmental Protection Agency (2002). Frequently asked questions (beaches). Retrieved December 20, 2002 from the World Wide Web: www.epa.gov/waterscience/beaches/faq.html#public

Chapter 3
The Role of the Professional Lifeguard

In this chapter you will learn that the professional lifeguard has many responsibilities. Primarily, they involve lifesaving and other forms of public safety, but they include providing many other public services to beach users, like finding lost persons. The professional lifeguard serves as a manger of both public safety and general activities. Professional lifeguards should always perform their duties ethically. By performing their duties professionally and ethically, lifeguards can expect to enjoy extraordinary rewards.

CHAPTER EXCERPT

The stress of a lifeguard's responsibilities can sometimes be immense. The challenges however, make lifeguarding one of the most diverse and rewarding jobs available. How many people can go home after work with the satisfaction of knowing that they have performed the most important act of all in our society—the saving of human life?

Responsibilities and Expectations

The United States Lifesaving Association is an organization largely composed of professional lifeguards. Why then is USLA not known as the United States *Lifeguard* Association? The answer is that all lifeguards are dedicated to a key goal—lifesaving. Our organization is named for that goal. In truth, anyone can be a lifesaver. Heroic acts are not the sole province of lifeguards or other emergency responders. Many of the most impressive and selfless acts of heroism are performed by persons with little or no training in lifesaving. Unfortunately, these acts all too often result in tragedy.

Unlike untrained citizens who may bravely or impulsively respond to an unexpected emergency, lifeguards are specially prepared to anticipate, prevent, and respond to emergencies in and around the

WEBBOX

Awards for heroism, many of which are for aquatic rescue efforts, are given every year by the Carnegie Hero Fund Commission: *www.carnegiehero.org*

USLA offers the Medal of Valor to lifeguards and its Heroic Act Award to non-lifeguards whose actions meet extraordinary criteria. For a list of recipients, visit the Heroic Acts area of the USLA website at: *www.usla.org*

You can review the latest statistics on lifeguard rescues, beach attendance, and related information in the Statistics section of the USLA website at: *www.usla.org*

aquatic environment. Most lifeguards who spend any significant time in the profession will perform many, many lifesaving acts with little recognition or expectation thereof. This is as it should be, since a lifeguard who is properly trained and prepared will prevent loss of life as a daily routine. It is, after all, the basic job of a lifeguard to help ensure that those who visit the nation's beaches, waterways, adjacent parks, and campgrounds return home alive. Not all accidents can be prevented, but well trained professional open water lifeguards rescue tens of thousands of people from drowning in America each year and perform many times that number of preventive actions to intercede before emergencies develop.

Accomplishing these core tasks of prevention and rescue has a significant impact, not only on the individual who is saved from injury or death, but also on the families of those rescued, and even on the nation's economy. It has been estimated that for every 10,000 beach visitors there is a national monetary savings of between $705,000 and $16,000,000 as a result of professional lifeguards doing their job.

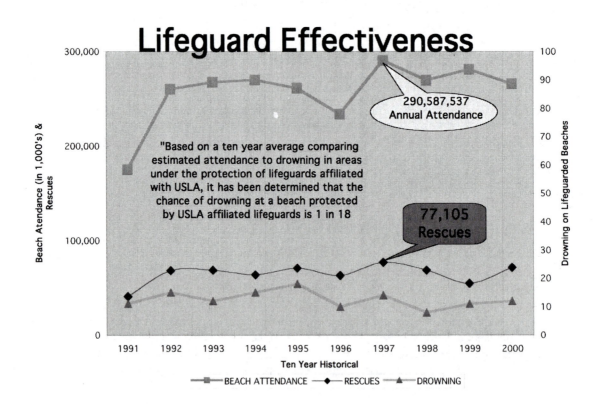

Lifeguard Effectiveness

290,587,537 Annual Attendance

"Based on a ten year average comparing estimated attendance to drowning in areas under the protection of lifeguards affiliated with USLA, it has been determined that the chance of drowning at a beach protected by USLA affiliated lifeguards is 1 in 18

77,105 Rescues

Ten Year Historical

BEACH ATTENDANCE   RESCUES   DROWNING

(Mael, Seck, & Russell, 1998) This figure includes not only the direct economic cost of accidental death or injury but also measures the value of lost quality of life associated with death or injuries. In other words, it assesses what society would be willing to pay to prevent such a loss. These numbers rise to astounding levels when multiplied by the many millions of people who visit beaches each year and very clearly demonstrate the value of open water lifeguards as emergency service professionals.

In 2001, the Centers for Disease Control and Prevention's National Center for Injury Prevention issued a report entitled, *Lifeguard Effectiveness: A Report of the Working Group.* This extensive report covered many topics and included numerous findings. Among them: "Most drownings are preventable through a wide variety of strategies, one of which is to provide lifeguards in public areas where people are known to swim and to encourage people to swim in those protected areas ... There is no doubt that trained, professional lifeguards have had a positive effect on drowning prevention in the United States." (Branche & Stewart 2001)

In the United States, open water lifeguards have worked hard to be recognized as equals to other emergency services professionals—police officers, firefighters, and emergency medical personnel. This has been accomplished through a steady process of improving the quality of the services provided and a constant dedication to public safety. As a result, Americans have come to expect lifeguards on their beaches, just as they have come to expect professional police, fire, and emergency medical services in their communities.

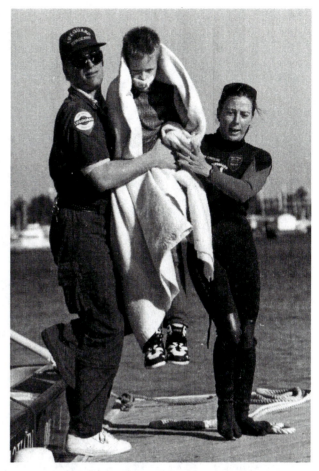

San Diego lifeguards assist one of five victims of a boat fire. Lifeguards extinguished the fire, but the boat was a total loss.

Credit: San Diego Union-Tribune—John Gibbins

Lifeguarding is viewed by many as the most physically demanding job among the various emergency services. This is because unlike other emergency services, which are able to rely heavily on mechanized support, lifeguarding in its purest form comes down to a simple struggle against the forces of nature by one human being endeavoring to save the life of another. Even with new developments in motorized rescue equipment, many rescue situations depend on the sheer strength, physical endurance, running ability, and swimming skills of the lifeguard.

The primary job of a professional open water lifeguard in the United States is public safety. While the core drowning prevention role is well defined, job descriptions can vary dramatically from one locale to the next. This is particularly true as local employers seeking to stretch thin budgets ask their lifeguards to perform increasingly diverse public safety functions. At one agency a lifeguard may find that the job is a blend of several aquatic related public safety responsibilities. At another, the job may be defined more narrowly, emphasizing the more traditional aspects of lifeguarding.

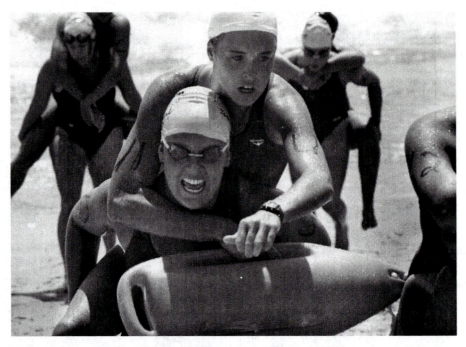

Competitors in the annual All Women Lifeguard Tournament carry victims from the water.

Credit: National Park Service

Persons hired as lifeguards are typically intimately familiar with all facets of the aquatic environment and adjacent land areas. This familiarity leaves lifeguards uniquely prepared to handle a variety of functions that serve to protect public safety in these areas, such as emergency medical services, scuba search and recovery, cliff rescue, boat rescue, marine firefighting, swiftwater rescue, and flood rescue. Many open water lifeguards are given law enforcement powers and responsibilities to help maintain public safety within their jurisdiction.

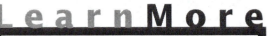

You can learn more about the financial impact of lifesaving by reading, *A Work Behavior-Oriented Job Analysis for Lifeguards,* which is posted in the Lifeguard Library section of the USLA website at: *www.usla.org*

You can download and read a copy of *Lifeguard Effectiveness: A Report of the Working Group* by visiting the Lifeguard Library section of the USLA website at *www.usla.org*

Lifeguards have additional functions. Among these are the responsibilities to provide public information and education, complete required documentation, locate missing persons, and throughout to maintain a professional demeanor. Lifeguards should never be assigned or assume duties beyond those directly related to their public safety role. Such assignments only serve to diminish attention to safety and can result in serious, life-threatening consequences.

The professional lifeguard is reliable, mature, consistent, and maintains an expert knowledge of the aquatic environment. A professional appearance and readiness to respond is critical to professional open water lifeguarding. Lifeguards must train diligently in order to maintain their skills and readiness.

The first professional beach lifesavers rescued victims stranded aboard foundering boats, not recreational swimmers. The wide-ranging responsibilities of America's open water lifeguards show that they have the ability to adapt to providing the aquatic oriented emergency services needed by the American public, whatever they may be.

The Lifeguard as Manager

Experienced lifeguards know that the job includes more than just watching the water and responding to emergencies. Lifeguards act as managers for the areas they oversee. This means managing safety and managing the interactions of people, both with the environment and with each other. High levels of coordination with other emergency service providers are needed to help protect people from themselves and their fellow beach users.

One day the lifeguard may be expected to arbitrate in a dispute among beach patrons as tempers rise to the boiling point over a seemingly minor conflict. Another day, the lifeguard must allay the terror of a mother whose child has been lost in a sea of beachgoers. When a beach patron collapses, the victim of a heart attack, everyone turns to the lifeguard to perform lifesaving CPR or to employ an Automatic External Defibrillator (AED). Each day of work, the pressure is on, the public is watching, and lifeguards hold the lives and welfare of the people they watch over in their hands. Constant vigilance is imperative; a momentary distraction may mean that a person in lifeguard care could die or be seriously injured.

Managing Safety

Water is not a natural environment for humans. With proper skills, people can recreate safely in water, but they are ill equipped for surviving in all water conditions. Many beach visitors have never learned that fact. Others simply forget. Many emergencies occur because people visiting an area presume that conditions will be similar to those near their home or the same as the last time they visited the beach.

Lifeguards should never assume that beach visitors are familiar with a beach's particular hazards or energy conditions, such as waves, currents, or dams. With today's mobile society, lifeguards must always anticipate lack of experience and poor judgment on the part of the beach visitor.

Lifeguards must also be cognizant of their regional demographics. People often behave differently in groups and some may push themselves beyond their capability just to impress one another. For example, young teenage boys are prone to risk taking behavior, which can lead to emergency situations for lifeguards.

Lifeguards are sometimes drawn away from the water to handle problems or emergencies involving medical aids, law

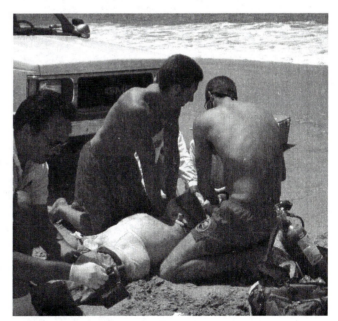

Credit: Ken Kramer

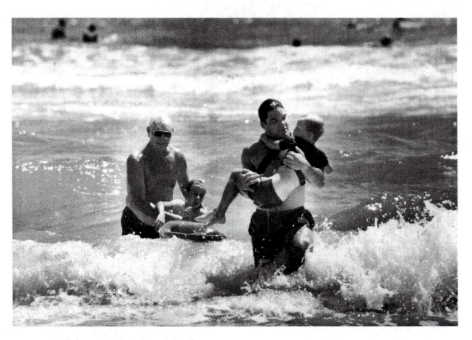

Rescue from an inshore hole.
Credit: Mike Hensler

enforcement contacts, and so on. Good managers will be sure adequate backup is available to maintain watch over the water and that lifeguards are trained to conclude any contact which diverts attention from the water as soon as possible. Attention directed away from the water, even for short periods of time, can create a situation where simple problems become serious ones, including a possible drowning.

Managing Conflict

Wherever people gather, there are occasionally conflicts. As beach use intensifies, so does the potential and prevalence of conflict. Problems of human interaction at the beach may be as simple as verbal disputes, or more serious, like vandalism, drug and alcohol abuse, theft, or assault. Today, a major aspect of beach management is people management. This means protecting people from themselves and each other, in addition to protecting them from the hazards of the aquatic environment.

Beach activities frequently conflict with one another. Therefore, lifeguarding can involve mediating among differing uses. Lifeguards will often find themselves in the position of social referee in a game where the rules are not always clear. In a recreational setting, people do not always feel obligated to adhere to established norms. Use of alcohol exaggerates these problems.

Effective beach management includes preventing conflicts by separating incompatible activities whenever possible. For example, participants in a game of horseshoes being set up near an area where small children are playing might be asked to move, or the Frisbee player who inadvertently, but consistently allows his disc to strike others might similarly be relocated. This obviates the need to intervene later, when tempers may flare.

When disputes do arise, lifeguards, as the most prominent and available source of authority, are often expected to mediate. The best approach, in these cases, is a calm demeanor, complete objectivity, and a goal of finding a way for both parties to feel that they have been heard.

Sometimes it is a good idea to separate the parties, out of earshot of each other, so that the conflict does not intensify as each tells their side of the story. First, tell each party you will hear them out, but that you want to talk to them privately. Listen patiently to both parties. Don't give an opinion until you have heard from each. If there is a large group involved, avoid conversing in front of all of them. Ask first who the group leader or representative is and take that person aside. Otherwise, a very real sense of group resistance may arise with many members of the group yelling out their opinions and exciting each other further. The ideal resolution is one which allows both parties to continue their activity, perhaps in some modified manner. Can you find a resolution like this?

Sometimes, one party or the other will need to be told that they must discontinue what they are doing, perhaps because it violates a beach rule or regulation. Disputes involve ego and any resolution that requires someone to change their behavior may cause them to "lose face." Minimizing this outcome will help greatly. Talk to the person or the group representative quietly, to avoid drawing a crowd or undue attention. Most beach disputes can be resolved by a patient and calm lifeguard without the need for summoning police, but in some cases, there may be no choice.

USLA Code of Ethics

The United States Lifesaving Association maintains a code of ethical principles, which we believe all lifeguards should follow. These are the core principles which every professional open water lifeguard should seek to maintain.

USLA Code of Ethics

In recognition of the fundamental responsibilities of a professional open water lifeguard, the trust and confidence placed in the lifeguard, the unwavering devotion to duty required of the lifeguard, and the dignity commensurate with the lifeguard's position, the United States Lifesaving Association recognizes ethical principles.

Lifeguards will:

- Maintain an unwavering dedication to the safety of those they are assigned to protect.
- Recognize and accept that heightened personal dangers are an unavoidable aspect of the job.
- Maintain high standards of fitness, recognizing that their strength, stamina, and physical skill may mean the difference between life and death.
- Make every reasonable effort to prevent accidents before they occur.
- Avoid any undue distraction which may deter them from their primary responsibility.
- Proudly carry out the duties they are assigned, providing the highest possible levels of courtesy, respect and assistance to those whom they watch over.
- Take proactive steps to educate the public about the hazards of the aquatic environment and ways to safely enjoy aquatic recreation.
- Promote their profession through personal actions which serve to demonstrate that lifeguards everywhere are deserving of the trust placed in them by the public they serve.
- Diligently follow established policies and procedures set forth by their employing agency to promote the best possible public service.

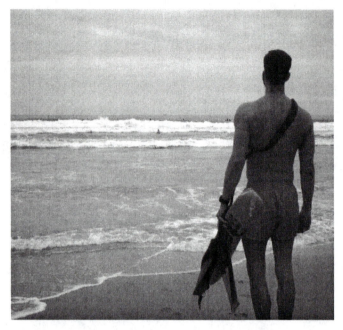

Credit: Ken Kramer

Lifeguard Rewards

A lifeguard's stress and challenges can sometimes be immense; but lifeguarding is also one of the most diverse and rewarding jobs available. There are innumerable opportunities to interact with the public, to gain special training, to learn leadership, to advance in the profession, to learn to manage people. Simply helping people can be a reward in and of itself. There is one very special reward though. How many people can go home after work with the satisfaction of knowing that they have performed the most important act of all—the saving of human life? Lifeguards have many opportunities to experience that very feeling, so long as they are prepared to respond professionally when the need arises.

Lifesaving is a family. There are lifeguards around the world performing much the same services, experiencing many of the same challenges. You will find, as a lifeguard, that when you meet lifeguards from other places, you have a common bond. It is a bond that will last a lifetime, providing friendship and hospitality wherever you travel. This spirit has been embodied in a phrase: *Lifeguards for Life*.

Chapter Summary

In this chapter, we have learned that lifeguards have a wide variety of responsibilities that extend well beyond water safety, but that they must ensure that public safety is never compromised, whatever they may be doing. We have learned that lifeguarding is a physically demanding job, with responsibilities similar to those of police or firefighters, and that lifeguards must work hard to maintain their readiness and to demonstrate their professionalism. As beach managers, lifeguards must be prepared to handle both safety and conflict. They must also behave ethically at all times. In performing to these expectations, lifeguards can expect lifelong rewards from their job that extend well beyond financial compensation.

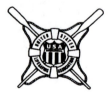

Discussion Points

- What is the difference between lifesaving and lifeguarding?
- What makes a lifeguard different from any other person who saves someone from drowning?
- How does the work of the lifeguard benefit society?
- What makes lifeguarding similar to police and firefighting work?
- What is a professional appearance and why is it important for lifeguards?
- Why is backup needed in managing safety?
- What are some ways to mediate conflicts among beach users?
- Why is there value in having a USLA Code of Ethics for lifeguards?
- What are some rewards you can expect from lifeguarding?

References

Branche C. M. & Stewart, S. (Eds.). (2001) *Lifeguard Effectiveness: A Report of the Working Group.* Atlanta, Georgia: Centers for Disease Control and Prevention, National Center for Injury Prevention and Control.

Mael, F., Seck, M., & Russell, D. (1998). *A Work Behavior-Oriented Job Analysis for Lifeguards.* Washington, D.C.: American Institutes for Research

Chapter 4

Open Water Lifeguard Qualifications and Training

In this chapter, you will learn that lifeguards work in a variety of environments. Open water lifeguards require specialized skills and training for the many different environments and circumstances in which they work. The USLA training system addresses these needs through a core curriculum, along with specialized training components. This chapter provides an overview of USLA recommended training standards for open water lifeguards and the various ways training can be provided. It explains how lifeguard agencies which adhere to these standards may become nationally certified under the USLA Lifeguard Agency Certification Program.

CHAPTER EXCERPT

USLA has set a minimum swimming proficiency standard of 500 meters in 10 minutes or less for open water lifeguards since 1980. USLA based this minimum standard on consensus input from representatives of the major aquatic safety organizations of the United States.

The USLA Lifeguard Training System

There are many different aquatic environments requiring lifeguard protection. USLA believes they fall into two general categories: (1) the controlled environment of pools and waterparks, and (2) the natural environment of open water. Because of the fundamental differences between these environments, we recognize two corresponding categories of lifeguards—pool/waterpark lifeguards and open water lifeguards.

In comparison to open water lifeguard training, pool and waterpark lifeguard training is highly standardized. Under existing training systems, if a candidate successfully completes training as a pool lifeguard in Michigan, for example, the training is likely to be accepted by a pool manager in Arizona as adequate for employment. This is possible because of the inherent similarity in the pool and waterpark environment regardless of where the facility may be located.

Conversely, the open water environment varies greatly from place to place, and open water is a more challenging environment for lifeguards. As well, open water lifeguards often have a more wide ranging array of responsibilities. For these reasons, open water lifesaving requires markedly differing physical conditioning, training, and skills, as compared to the controlled environment of pools and waterparks. So open water lifeguard training must be more intensive and adapted appropriately to local conditions. The following table provides some examples of the different challenges faced by these two types of lifeguards.

Comparison of Aquatic Environments

Condition	Pool/Waterpark	Open Water
Water Temperature	Can be controlled	Subject to natural conditions
Water Clarity	Can be controlled	Subject to natural conditions
Difficulty of Rescue	Accomplished by jumping into pool and wading, swimming or paddling a short distance	May require long distance swimming in adverse conditions
Natural Hazards	None	May be extensive and may not be readily apparent
Wave Action and Currents	None or fully controlled	Surf and currents may present the most significant source of swimmer distress and difficulty of rescue
Attendance Levels and Hours	Can be controlled	Generally not controllable
Weather Conditions	Little effect	Possible severe effect

Open water lifeguards must deal with a variety of natural hazards which cannot be controlled. Surf, currents, and underwater obstacles are examples. Rescues may take place far from shore. Open water lifeguards are sometimes stationed at locations distant from hospitals and ambulance services, so they must be prepared to support victims with medical problems for extended periods.

While open water lifeguard operations share many similarities with each other, they can differ in a variety of ways. A surf beach in Maine, for example, has a different climate, water conditions, and even a different type of visitor than a similar surf beach in Florida. An intensely populated surf beach on the urban Chicago lakeshore requires different lifeguarding approaches from a camp waterfront in rural Kentucky. The warm water conditions, large surf, and reefs on the North Shore of Oahu present markedly different challenges than the colder waters, sand bars, and longshore currents of the outer shore of Cape Cod.

In addition to variables in environmental conditions, open water lifeguards have varying responsibilities, organizational structures, authority, and lifesaving equipment. Some open water lifeguards are assigned responsibilities such as boat rescue, law enforcement, cliff rescue, flood rescue, marine firefighting, and scuba search and rescue. Open water lifeguards may be expected to operate emergency vehicles with lights and siren, rescue boats, and other technical equipment. Open water lifeguards may work for lifeguard departments, recreation departments, harbor departments, police departments, fire departments, state or national park systems, or private businesses, to name a few possibilities.

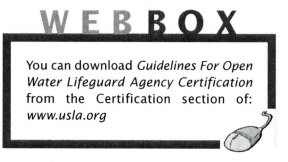

WEBBOX

You can download *Guidelines For Open Water Lifeguard Agency Certification* from the Certification section of: *www.usla.org*

To address these many variables, in developing this training text and training guidelines, USLA has taken into account the unique aspects of open water lifeguard operations across the country. The USLA publication entitled *Guidelines For Open Water Lifeguard Agency Certification* provides a training curriculum and recommended standards flexible enough to meet the training needs of all agencies employing open water lifeguards, while recognizing the many differences among them.

Under the USLA training system, open water lifeguard training in Colorado need not provide information on effecting surf rescues, for example. Similarly, a lifeguard training program for surf lifeguards in California need not discuss issues unique to rescues in reservoirs. With the time available for lifeguard training limited, this allows open water lifeguard training programs to focus on tasks specific to each local agency's geography and mission. Because of this specialization however, open water lifeguard training conducted under the USLA system is not interchangeable. Retraining is necessary if the lifeguard moves to an agency other than that which provided the training.

Despite the local training variables offered under the USLA system, central elements are consistent nationwide. This manual provides information both on the core aspects of open water lifeguarding in which all open water lifeguards should be skilled, as well as the specialized information needed to assist in training that is unique to particular geographic locations. It is the responsibility of agency

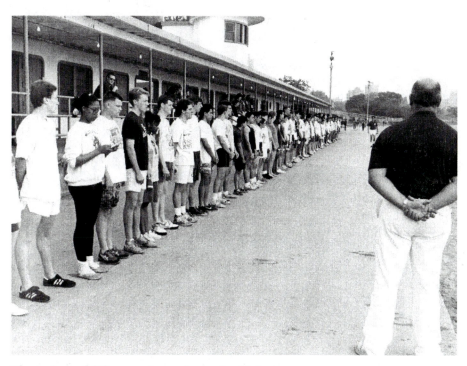

First day of lifeguard academy in Chicago.
Credit: Al Shorey

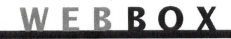

You can view a list of agencies currently certified by USLA in the Certification section at: *www.usla.org*

You can download *Training & Standards Of Aquatic Rescue Response Teams* from the Certification section at: *www.usla.org*

training officers to select portions of the text for trainees which are appropriate to the area where the trainee will work.

This text will be most effective when used to train lifeguards in a manner consistent with USLA's recommended curriculum for open water lifeguards. Lifeguard agencies which provide training and maintain standards in accordance with USLA's *Guidelines For Open Water Lifeguard Agency Certification* may achieve national certification under the USLA Lifeguard Agency Certification Program. Agencies which are certified by USLA have demonstrated their adherence to these guidelines and standards.

USLA also offers *Training & Standards Of Aquatic Rescue Response Teams* for the training of open water rescuers who are not lifeguards. These guidelines allow specialized aquatic rescue teams to achieve national certification under the USLA Aquatic Rescue Response Team certification program.

Training Modes

In promulgating guidelines for open water lifeguard training, USLA recognizes three major modes of training—prerequisite, pre-service, and in-service. The manner in which these types of training are used by an agency will impact the local training program.

Prerequisite Training

Employers in many fields of work require prospective employees to have a minimum level of training before they can apply for a job. This is sometimes true in lifeguarding. In the pool environment, for example, those seeking employment as lifeguards are often expected to have completed basic training prior to application. In the open water environment however, this is less typical.

Some open water lifeguard employers may require completion of a medical aid or CPR course, or both. Since USLA recommended standards include training in medical aid and CPR that is recognized by the Federal Government or the state government in the state of employment, nationally recognized courses like Department of Transportation First Responder or Emergency Medical Technician might be accepted as a prerequisite by an employer regardless of where the training was provided.

In May 2000, San Diego lifeguard Mike Clegg became the first in the United States to earn a college degree in open water lifeguarding. He earned his degree from Miramar College, where a college curriculum in lifeguarding was designed around the USLA recommended standards.

In some areas of the US, open water lifeguard agencies have joined with local colleges to develop open water lifeguard courses consistent with USLA recommended standards. Completion of these courses may be required as a prerequisite to application for local employment. For lifeguard training other than medical aid training, it is the view of USLA that currently available national training programs with a combined emphasis on the pool and inland beach environment lack the depth of training appropriate for open water lifeguards.

Some open water lifeguard employers require pool lifeguard training as a prerequisite to undergoing open water lifeguard training. While experience working as a pool lifeguard may well be of value for someone interested in working as an open water lifeguard, requiring pool lifeguard training as a prerequisite for open water lifeguard training is discouraged by USLA. There are fundamental differences between the training approaches for each environment that are, in some cases, contradictory. Thus, requiring pool lifeguard training prior to open water lifeguard training can create confusion and uncertainty.

Pre-Service Training

Pre-service training is that provided before assignment to lifeguard duties. It is a fundamental principle of USLA guidelines that no one should be assigned to the duties of an open water lifeguard prior to receiving the minimum training needed to perform the function assigned. This training may take place before or after hire.

The preferred method of pre-service training is to provide all training prior to assignment as a lifeguard. The USLA system allows an exception to this approach for agencies which elect to spread their training over a period of time. Under USLA guidelines, pre-service training, with the exception of medical aid and CPR training, may be integrated into the first 30 days of actual lifeguard beach work. This is permissible only if trainees work under the direct and immediate supervision (side-by-side in the same station or area) of a lifeguard with at least 1,000 hours of experience. The ratio of experienced

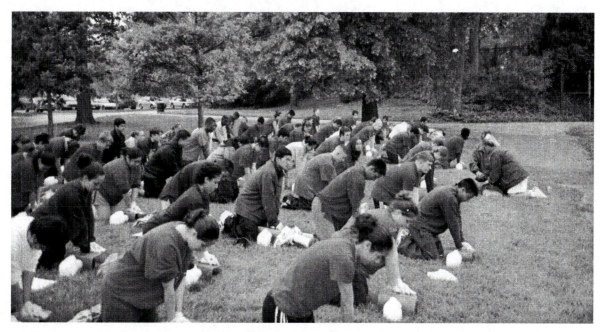

Lifeguards practice CPR during pre-service training.
Credit: Al Shorey

lifeguards to such trainees may be no greater than one to one. Minimum recommended pre-service training is detailed in the USLA *Guidelines For Open Water Lifeguard Agency Certification.*

In-Service Training

The third type of lifeguard training is in-service training. This is used to develop and maintain the skills and knowledge of lifeguards. Subsequent to their initial training, USLA guidelines call for lifeguard agencies to provide a minimum of 16 hours per year in formal training. As well, agencies are expected to provide daily opportunities, conditions permitting, for activities such as swimming, rescue board training, and running. This promotes physical fitness and hones lifeguard skills.

Required in-service training may include daily physical conditioning or regular reviews of rescue procedures. Drills, such as mock rescues and other simulated emergencies, are also encouraged. Programs to train and certify lifeguards in the operation of special rescue equipment, advanced rescue techniques, supervision, management, and other operational areas that lie outside the scope of basic lifeguard operations are highly recommended. Lifeguards may be encouraged or required to pursue higher levels of training in areas such as special equipment operation, emergency medical care, or law enforcement. For example, some agencies require lifeguards to acquire Emergency Medical Technician training after hire.

Lifeguard efforts to garner continuing education by taking courses and attending conferences aimed at improving their knowledge and skills should be both encouraged and supported by their employers. USLA includes an educational conference as part of each biannual Board of Directors meeting, and occasionally sponsors special conferences for open water lifesavers. These present excellent opportunities to garner nationally recognized training.

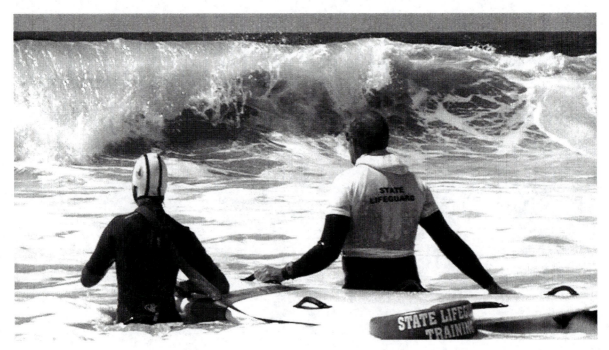

In-service rescue board training.

Credit: Ken Kramer

Minimum Recommended Standards

USLA has developed recommended standards to be met *and maintained*. In order for a lifeguard agency to be USLA certified its policies, equipment, training program, trainees, and lifeguards must meet these standards. USLA promulgates higher standards for agencies wishing to be certified as providing an advanced level of service. The USLA standards are detailed in the USLA booklet *Guidelines For Open Water Lifeguard Agency Certification.*

USLA guidelines establish *minimum* recommended standards only, whether at the regular or advanced level. To address local needs and conditions, lifeguard agencies are encouraged to establish standards that exceed them. The following is a brief synopsis of USLA training and employment standards current at the time of publishing this manual. (Equipment standards are discussed in the chapter *Lifeguard Facilities and Equipment.*) For the most recent information, visit the Certification section of USLA's website at *www.usla.org* where current standards and certification applications can be found.

USLA recognizes three classes of open water lifeguards: Open Water Lifeguard Trainee, Seasonal Open Water Lifeguard, and Full Time Open Water Lifeguard. USLA also sets recommended standards for Open Water Lifeguard Instructor. All USLA standards are subject to regular review and revision to address the most current needs in lifesaving.

- *Minimum Age—16 for Hourly Lifeguards and 18 for Full Time Lifeguards*—USLA recognizes that a lifeguard must be physically and mentally mature to handle the responsibilities of professional lifeguarding. Although age alone is not a perfect measure of maturity and competence, the consensus of opinion has long been that age 16 is an acceptable minimum age for an open water lifeguard. (McCloy & Dodson, 1981) Many professional open water lifeguard agencies have established higher minimum ages commensurate with more complex responsibilities. Full time lifeguards are typically assigned to broader responsibilities and may lead the work of hourly lifeguards. For this reason, USLA believes that 18 should be the minimum age for full time open water lifeguard employment.

- *Advanced Training in Emergency Medical Care*—USLA believes that all lifeguards should be trained at a level appropriate for professional providers of medical aid—that is, beyond training designed for the general public. This training, for lifeguards employed on an hourly basis, should be at least 21 hours in length, not including CPR training. For lifeguards employed full time, a course equivalent to U.S. Department of Transportation First Responder is the minimum recommended standard. USLA strongly encourages agencies to train all lifeguards employed on an hourly basis in a course

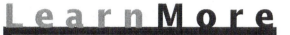

Learn More

To read about the national consensus conference which formed the basis for USLA's recommended standards, training, and certification program, visit the Lifeguard Library section of *www.usla.org* and select, *Guidelines For Establishing Open-Water Recreational Beach Standards—Proceedings of a Conference.*

WEBBOX

You can find the National Standard Curriculum for First Responder and Emergency Medical Technician on the Department of Transportation's website at: *www.dot.gov*

equivalent to First Responder, with Emergency Medical Technician highly recommended, especially for full time lifeguards.

- *Advanced Training in CPR*—Prolonged submersion results in respiratory distress and, ultimately, respiratory failure, leading to cardiac failure. Therefore, cardio-pulmonary resuscitation training is absolutely essential. USLA minimum recommended standards call for up-to-date successful completion of a course in providing one person adult, two person adult, child and infant CPR including obstructed airway training, accepted by the Federal Government or by the state government in the state of employment.

- *A Thorough Course In Open Water Lifesaving*—USLA recommended standards call for a course of not less than 40 hours, covering all curriculum elements delineated by USLA. This is *in addition to* training in first aid and CPR. More advanced agencies are expected to provide at least 48 hours of this training, as well as enhanced medical aid training.

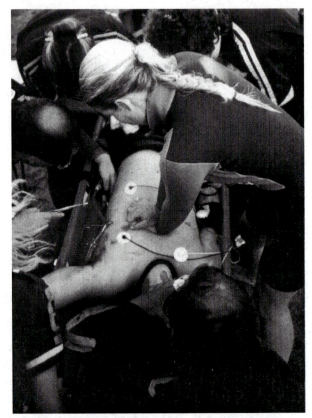

A lifeguard performs CPR on a drowning victim with the assistance of paramedics and a flight nurse.

Credit: B. Chris Brewster

- *Ability To Swim 500 Meters Over a Measured Course in Ten Minutes or Less*—Strong swimming skills are critical in open water lifesaving. While few rescues occur 250 meters offshore, the 500 meter (550 yard) timed swim is a well established minimum standard which should be met and maintained at all times by all open water lifeguards. It ensures that open water lifeguards will have adequate stamina to swim themselves and the victims they rescue to shore in adverse conditions, such as strong currents or surf. It also helps to ensure the stamina necessary to perform multiple rescues when necessary, as well as rescues of multiple victims. Agencies are encouraged to set higher standards for swimming proficiency to address local needs and conditions, so long as the minimum guideline is met. USLA has set a minimum swimming proficiency standard of 500 meters in 10 minutes or less for open water lifeguards since 1980. USLA based this minimum standard on consensus input from representatives of the major aquatic safety organizations of the United States. (McCloy & Dodson, 1981)

- *Health and Fitness Adequate for the Stresses of Lifesaving*—Open water lifeguards must possess adequate vision, hearing acuity, physical ability, and stamina to perform the duties of an open water lifeguard as documented by a medical or osteopathic physician.
- *Scuba Training*—Any open water lifeguard who will be required to utilize scuba in the course of employment must, at a minimum, be certified as a scuba diver at the basic level by a nationally recognized certifying organization. Higher levels of certification and training are encouraged. In addition to preparing lifeguards to use scuba, this training provides information regarding the physiology of scuba diving, which can be invaluable in treating victims of scuba related injuries.

Chapter Summary

In this chapter, we have learned that open water lifeguards require a higher level of training and preparedness than pool or waterpark lifeguards. This training must occur in the area where the lifeguard will be assigned, to address variables in local conditions. We have learned about three modes of training—prerequisite, pre-service, and in-service. We have learned that the minimum recommended standards for open water lifeguards include an age of 16 (18 for full time lifeguards), advanced training in emergency medical care and CPR, a course in lifesaving of at least 40 hours, and the ability to swim 500 meters in 10 minutes or less.

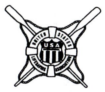

Discussion Points

- What are some challenges open water lifeguards could be expected to face that pool lifeguards would not?
- What are some ways that beaches you have visited differ from each other in ways that might be expected to require different training?
- What are some types of in-service training lifeguards might be expected to engage in?
- Why do open water lifeguards need to be mature individuals?
- Why do open water lifeguards need to be strong swimmers?
- What challenges might open water lifeguards face that would require strong medical aid skills?
- Why is advanced CPR training so important for lifeguards?

References

Brewster, B. C. (Ed.). (1996) *Training and Standards Of Aquatic Rescue Response Teams*. Huntington Beach, California: United States Lifesaving Association.

Brewster, B. C. (Ed.). (2001). *Guidelines for Open Water Lifeguard Agency Certification*. Huntington Beach, California: United States Lifesaving Association.

Emergency Medical Technician-Basic: National Standard Curriculum. Washington, D.C.: United States Department of Transportation, National Highway Traffic Safety Administration.

First Responder: National Standard Curriculum. Washington, D.C.: United States Department of Transportation, National Highway Traffic Safety Administration.

McCloy, J. D. & Dodson, J. A. (Eds.). (1981). *Guidelines For Establishing Open-Water Recreational Beach Standards—Proceedings of a Conference*. Galveston, Texas: Texas A&M Sea Grant College Program.

Chapter 5
The Surf Beach

In this chapter you will learn about the characteristics of surf beaches, including their attractions and dangers. We will explain how waves are formed in the open sea, how they change as they approach shore, and what causes them to become breaking waves. Here we describe rip currents, which cause lifeguards to provide the vast majority of rescues at surf beaches, and identify the various types of these currents. You will also learn about other aspects of surf beaches that pose hazards for beach users, including uprush, backrush, lateral currents, shorebreak, inshore holes, storm surge, and tsunamis.

CHAPTER EXCERPT

USLA has determined that rip currents are the primary source of distress in over 80% of swimmer rescues at surf beaches. This determination is based on annual reports from lifeguard agencies from throughout the United States. One may safely assume that rip currents are responsible for a comparable proportion of surf beach drownings in cases where lifeguards are not available.

At sea, powerful forces are continuously at work. The surf, calm at one moment, can quickly become rough and dangerous. Seemingly gently sloping beaches can hide deep channels that produce strong currents. Although calmer surf conditions may appear to allow lower lifeguard staffing levels than when surf is high, the unpredictable nature of surf necessitates consistent staffing levels aimed at reasonably anticipated conditions.

Lifeguards who have charge of surf beaches must be intimately familiar with waves and wave action, and prepared at all times to intervene when the power of the surf overwhelms swimmers, surfers, boaters, and others. USLA strongly recommends that all surf beach lifeguards spend extensive periods in activities such as board surfing, body surfing and paddling rescue boards, for example. Lifeguard employers should encourage and make time for this training. It allows lifeguards to learn to read waves, to know exactly when they will break, and to learn to use the same forces which endanger swimmers to quickly rescue them. It is only through intimate familiarity with the wide range of conditions at surf beaches that surf lifeguards can successfully effect rescues with necessary confidence and safety.

Waves

Waves are an extraordinary phenomenon of nature. They are a hypnotic, calming influence for those gazing seaward. They are an endless source of pleasure for all sorts of recreation. Surfing, whether through use of a surfboard, a bodyboard, or bodysurfing, attracts millions of people each year. Millions more who don't surf at all enjoy swimming in the surf. While it provides great pleasure, surf can be a powerful force capable of killing or injuring even experienced water users. Understanding the forces that create waves and surf is therefore of vital concern to every lifeguard assigned to a surf beach.

Wave Propagation

Waves are actually composed of cyclical forces of energy in the surface of the water. Each includes a crest and a trough. They can be measured in a number of ways such as:

- *Wave Period*—The time it takes two consecutive wave crests to pass a given point
- *Wave Length*—The horizontal distance between two wave crests (or troughs)
- *Wave Height*—The vertical distance between the crest and trough of a wave
- *Wave Velocity*—The speed at which the incoming set of waves advances

The most common type of open water waves are *surface waves,* also called *swells,* which are properly defined as such if they are moving in water deeper than one-half of their wave length (i.e. offshore). Surface waves move at speeds equal to three and a half times their wave period in seconds. (Bascom, 1980) For example, a wave with a period of ten seconds is traveling about thirty-five miles per hour.

Many people observing surface waves assume that the water in them moves forward at the speed of the wave itself. This is not the case. When offshore, these waves of energy simply cause the water surface to move up and down on a vertical plane, with hardly any forward movement, except in the most tempestuous conditions. Perhaps what confuses people in understanding wave energy is the end of the wave's life, as it breaks onshore, pushing water forward, up the beach. Offshore though, wave energy can be compared to a mouse running under a rug—the rug rises as the mouse runs along, but then falls back to the floor when the mouse has passed, moving forward little if at all.

With few exceptions, such as seismic activity (an earthquake), waves are formed by the force of wind on the water. Even the casual observer has seen ripples form on calm water as a breeze blows across it. Stronger, more continual winds create progressively larger ripples and ultimately form waves. Large waves can occasionally be created by strong local winds very near a beach, but most waves are formed by storms well offshore. These waves may travel across great expanses of water—sometimes thousands of miles of open sea—before the energy, initially created by the wind, is diffused as the waves strike the shoreline.

Three major factors contribute to the size and power of wind-generated waves according to Bascom (1980): (1) wind velocity at the generating point; (2) duration of the blow; and (3) the distance of open water over which the wind blows (*fetch*). Generally, increases in any of these factors produces

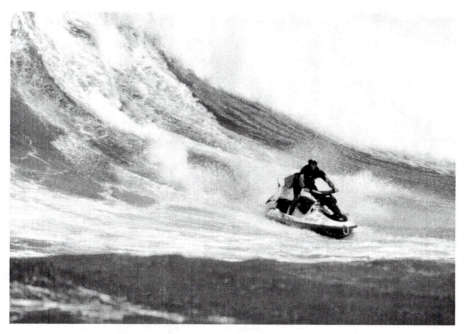

Lifeguards train in large surf.
Credit: Mike Waggoner

progressively larger waves. As waves form, moving out and away from the wind that creates them, their crests become more rounded and take on a similar period and height, becoming more regularized the farther they travel. A succession of waves from a single source, with a consistent direction is known as a *wave train*.

Set Waves

If all waves arriving at a beach came from a single wave train, the waves would tend to be quite similar in appearance and therefore of a fairly consistent period, length, height, and velocity. This is rarely, if ever the case because many different storms can contribute to the wave energy that ultimately arrives at a beach at any given point in time.

As two or more wave trains collide and intermingle, their behavior and appearance also changes. When waves from different wave trains merge trough to crest, they tend to cancel each other out and disperse the energy they carried, reducing wave height. On the other hand, when these waves match each other trough to trough, crest to crest, the ultimate height of the combined wave may be greatly increased over the individual height of the waves.

The intermingling of different wave trains often results in *set waves*. These are occasional groups of larger waves interspersed among a greater number of smaller waves. As the wave trains come into phase, matching each other's pattern, the waves increase in size. At other times when they are out of phase, the waves are smaller and irregular. Surfers will sometimes wait for long periods of time, well outside the surf break, for these larger set waves.

Rogue Waves

The same intermingling of wave trains which creates set waves, sometimes combined with open ocean currents, is believed to be responsible for what are known as *rogue waves*—waves that form suddenly in open water that are far higher than any other waves in the area. Bascom (1980) reports, for example on observations of the crew of the *Ramapo*, a 478 foot U.S. Navy tanker which survived a trip from Manila to San Diego despite encountering a surface wave estimated at 112 feet. Many ships encountering rogue waves, have not been so lucky. For example, the oil tanker *Cretan Star* disappeared with all hands shortly after the captain reported being hit by a huge wave in the Persian Gulf in 1976. In 1978, the German merchant navy ship München, en route to America, disappeared with all 27 hands, the likely victim of a rogue wave. All that was found was an empty lifeboat.

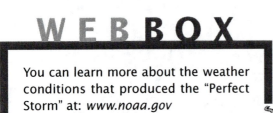

You can learn more about the weather conditions that produced the "Perfect Storm" at: *www.noaa.gov*

According to National Weather Service meteorologist Joe Sienkiewicz, "If you're facing average wave heights of 50 feet, it is possible that you'll see a wave as tall as 100 feet, or higher. Rogue waves can result if waves meet from different directions, or if they interact with currents, such as the Gulf Stream ... Either way, they are devastating." (NOAA, 2000) That was the case in the so-called *Perfect Storm*, which was the subject of a best selling book and popular movie that described events during a storm off New England in October 1991. Though it was not the most devastating storm on record, it produced peak waves recorded by at least one weather buoy (off Sable Island) of nearly 100 feet. (Drag, 2000)

Wave Characteristics

The character of waves can change predictably with the seasons. For example, in most areas, winter waves tend to be larger, more violent, and less regular. The prevailing direction of waves can also vary seasonally. For example, on the West Coast of the United States, predominant swell direction from late April to early October comes from storms as far south as 40 degrees latitude in the southern Pacific. From late October to mid-April, the swell direction changes and most waves originate in the Gulf of Alaska near the Aleutian Islands.

Depending on swell direction, some beaches are protected by the direction they face or by offshore islands. For example, according to Lascody (1998), "The southeast Florida coastline is protected from most long period swells. This is due to: 1) the north northeast to south southwest orientation of the shoreline, which prevents north swells from reaching the coast and 2) the shallow waters around the Bahama Islands which block most of the effects of northeast, east and southeast swells."

When standing at a beach and watching waves break, it often seems as though the waves are coming from a source directly perpendicular (or nearly so) to the beach. Actually, this is rarely the case. Instead, wave *refraction* causes wave trains to bend as they approach the shore. Refraction is an important concept for surfers because for them generally, the more acute the angle of approach of breaking waves the better. When waves strike a beach at a fully refracted, perpendicular angle they are difficult to surf and produce short rides. On the other hand, when waves strike a beach diagonally, the break moves laterally along the shoreline allowing long rides. Breaks caused by offshore reefs and peninsulas are often prized because the effects of refraction are muted and the break tends to peel off these geographic barriers.

Breaking Waves

As a wave approaches the shoreline it becomes a *shallow water wave*. Wavelength decreases, wave height increases, and velocity slows, but the period remains unchanged. As water depth lessens, the wave steepens, becoming higher and higher. Finally, upon reaching a depth approximately 1.3 times its height, the wave can no longer support itself and the crest falls forward, forming a *breaking wave*, which is commonly known as surf. (Bascom, 1980) Breaking waves cause an *uprush* of water, running up the slope of the beach. Once the uprush reaches its peak, gravity takes over and causes a *backrush* of water returning to the sea. Backrush, also known as *runback* or *backwash*, occurs wherever there is surf, but it is most powerful on steeply inclined beaches.

Bottom contour has a decisive influence on the manner in which a wave breaks. When a large swell is forced to expend its energy rapidly upon colliding with a steep underwater slope or reef, the crest of the wave tends to plunge or peak quickly, causing the water to mix with air and form foam or *whitewater*. A bottom that slopes gradually forms a wave that spills more gently, with the small froth of whitewater being pushed ahead of the broken wave on its journey up the beach. These gentle waves create less sound than plunging waves that spray into the sky as air and water are compressed together.

The experienced lifeguard knows how important the sound of waves in the darkness or in a fog can be to rescue work. Wave sounds can indicate to the lifeguard four vital conditions:

- The *type* of wave that is breaking
- The *power* of the surf
- The *location* of the main break in the surf
- The approximate *width* of the surf zone

Anyone who has sat by the shore and surveyed the sea understands that no two waves are ever alike—similar, but never identical. Breaking waves can however, be classified into three primary forms:

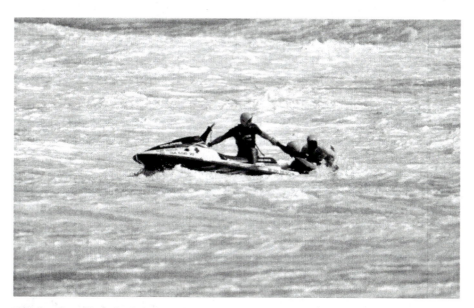

Victim loading in heavy whitewater.
Credit: Mike Waggoner

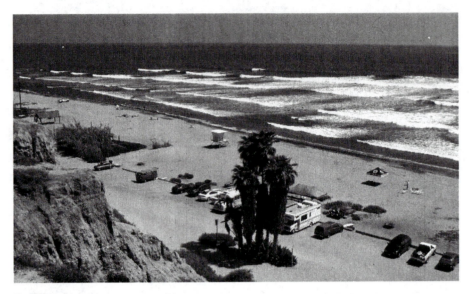

Spilling waves.

Credit: Ken Kramer

- *Spilling Waves*—Formed by swells as they move over a sea floor that ascends gradually beneath them, with the crest of the wave spilling onto the wave face until the wave itself is engulfed by foam
- *Plunging Waves*—Also known as *shorebreak,* they are formed when a swell suddenly strikes a shallow bottom, reef, or other obstacle and breaks with flying spray, both expending most of its energy and transforming it into a spilling wave for its remaining distance to shore
- *Surging Waves*—Created where water is deep adjacent to shoreline cliffs, reef, or steep beaches, with the waves keeping their rounded form until they crash against the shoreline barrier

Wave Measurement

Waves are measured in different ways for different purposes. The heights of waves are of vital interest to lifeguards, who use this information to assess the turbulence of the surf and its potential effect on those in, on, or near the water. The pioneering oceanographer Willard Bascom (1980) explained a simple procedure for this estimate: The observer stands on the beach at a point where the top of the breaking waves is visually in line with the horizon. The observer then notes the point on the beach at which the backrush curls back toward the sea. The height of the waves is the vertical distance from the observer's eye to the peak of the backrush. Bascom reports that the height of the backrush curl is equivalent to the average height of the sea surface.

Other methods of estimating surf size include measuring against a nearby structure of known size, or by comparison to the body of a surfer standing erect on a surfboard. Regardless of methodology, it is crucial that lifeguards learn to assess wave height consistently and objectively. This information is used to inform beach users about the relative hazard, to report observations to the media, and to cre-

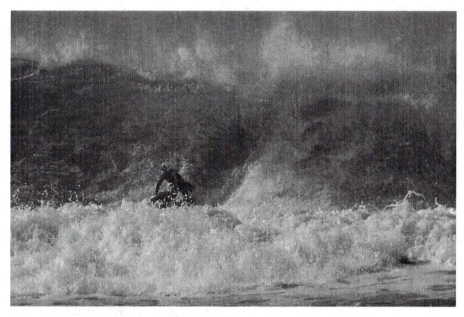

A training lifeguard can be used to estimate surf size.

Credit: Nick Steers

ate a historical record. If lifeguards report the same conditions differently, from day to day, credibility suffers and there is little value in the reporting.

Wave Hazards

Waves cause problems for beach visitors because of their tremendous power and energy. Many people underestimate this power and may be injured by the forward motion of the wave. As an example, consider an imaginary experiment in which one fills a gallon jug with water and tosses it to a friend. (A gallon of water weighs about eight pounds.) Most people would be concerned with such a weight being thrown to them. A single wave though, may represent the equivalent of thousands of such containers approaching at a similar velocity.

The downward motion of waves can violently thrust swimmers and surfers to the bottom, causing serious trauma to the head, neck, back, and other parts of the body. Uprush and backrush may knock visitors down and injure them. When surf is rough, backrush may be met by a second, forceful uprush, creating extensive turbulence at the meeting point that is particularly dangerous to young children and older people, who may lack the strength to maintain their footing.

The combined force of strong surf, uprush, and backrush is a particular hazard on steep beaches with shorebreak (plunging waves). On these beaches waves five to eight feet high or even higher have been known to break in knee deep water during heavy surf conditions. When this occurs, a vigorous suction is caused both by the breaking wave and by the backrush from previous waves. As a result of this seaward flow, a person can be knocked down and caught up in the next wave. Beachgoers can be injured and non-swimmers may actually drown under the sheer force of incoming waves. People caught off balance in such situations should push themselves under and toward the oncoming shorebreak, curl their bodies to withstand its force, and break out of this position on the other side of the wave. A tense,

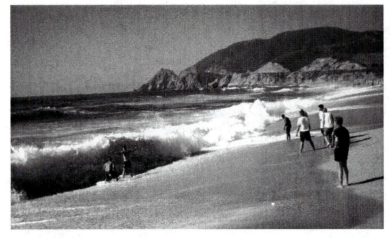

Shorebreak

Credit: Ken Kramer

extended body, if hit by the full force of these waves, can suffer serious injury to the back and neck and receive abrasions to the skin (important signs in evaluating the need to treat for spinal injury).

Very heavy surf may intimidate swimmers, keeping them close to shore, if not completely out of the water. Unfortunately, the relative calm period between set waves, known as a *lull,* can fool beachgoers. Inexperienced swimmers may go out during the lull and then be unexpectedly caught in the next group of set waves. Even pedestrians, particularly those observing larger than usual surf, are sometimes surprised and overcome by the uprush of set waves. This is one reason that it is wise to attempt to keep spectators well back in cases of large surf.

Shoreline Topography

The beach environment includes not only the exposed shoreline and water surface, but also the nearshore bottom of the sea. Beaches enlarge and contract in size based on many factors. The shoreline, combined with wave action, helps create forces that can both enthrall and endanger beachgoers.

Sandbars

Ridges of sand, called *sandbars,* exist off most, if not all surf beaches. They are normally submerged, but may emerge at low tide. They are created and modified by surf and related currents. Bascom (1980) reported that in 29 different beach surveys, each beach area surveyed had at least one sandbar and one beach had five. Typically there are one to three offshore sandbars.

Sandbars may run parallel to shore for many miles, one outside the other. They can also be quite irregular, depending upon surf conditions and currents. Usually, sandbars maintain regularity when surf size and direction are consistent, but as these influences change, so do the underlying sandbars.

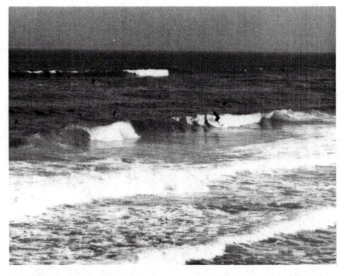

Spilling wave breaking on an offshore sandbar.

Credit: Mike Hensler

Winter storm surf typically moves sand from the beach offshore to sandbars. Calmer surf conditions, usually evident in summer, result in a sand transport from the sandbar to the beach. This is why many exposed surf beaches are wider in summer, narrower in winter. (Bascom, 1980) In areas that experience seasonal swell direction changes, the ocean bottom can become very uneven during these changes.

Sandbars can be attractive deceptions to poor swimmers. Seeing others standing in shallow water far offshore, poor swimmers may try to wade out, not realizing that deep water lies between them and their goal, and thus may quickly find themselves beyond their capacity to swim or to cope with currents. Another common scenario occurs when a poor swimmer wades successfully to the sandbar at a low tide, only to become entrapped by a rising tide and forced to attempt to swim ashore.

Serious, life-threatening orthopedic injuries can be caused when swimmers unfamiliar with a beach attempt a surface dive from a standing position, believing the water is deeper farther out. If the diver strikes the bottom, particularly headfirst, the head can be snapped back and the spinal cord compromised. Paraplegia and quadriplegia are possible results. Even persons who do not experience an immediate spinal cord injury may experience tingling in the extremities, short-term blackout, or simply neck pain. Lifeguards should take any complaint of pain following such an incident extremely seriously. The chapter on medical care in the aquatic environment explains proper treatment of these cases by the lifeguard.

These concerns notwithstanding however, the role of sandbars in creating and magnifying the effects of currents, is the greatest hazard they pose. This hazard is explained in detail later in this chapter.

Inshore Holes

Inshore holes are a hazard closely related to sandbars. These are depressions up to several yards in diameter dug into the sand by wave action and currents. Small children can easily step from ankle deep water into depths over their heads. They are also a significant hazard to lifeguards who can seriously injury a knee or ankle while running to make a rescue. Lifeguards at surf beaches tend to focus their attention toward the surf zone. Inshore holes can be killers and lifeguards must remember to scan the entire water area, both inshore and offshore.

Rocks, Reefs, and Other Obstacles

Underwater rocks, reefs, and other obstacles also pose hazards at surf beaches. Since they are usually hidden from beach visitors, they are difficult to avoid. They can cause surf to break unexpectedly, and swimmers may be thrown against them

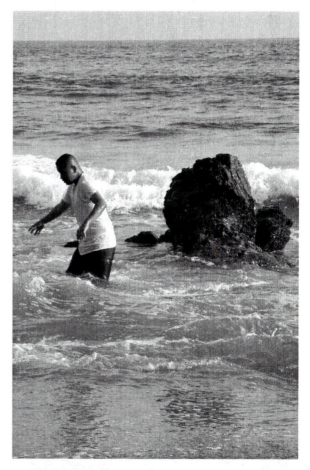

An inshore hole near a rock outcropping.
Credit: Ken Kramer

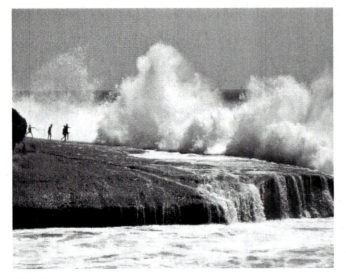

Children playing in a dangerous situation.

Credit: Ken Kramer

by the surf. Submerged objects in shallow water are particularly dangerous to surfers, body surfers, and bodyboarders, who are moving quickly through the surfline.

Above water, rock outcroppings, piers, groins, and cliffs can also present hazards. As is the case with underwater obstacles, a person forced upon them by waves and currents can suffer serious injury. Pedestrians may venture out onto these structures to be close to the water with no intention of swimming, perhaps to fish, for example. Waves can sweep them into the water, which is usually deeper than water just off the beach, or slippery surfaces may cause them to fall, sustaining trauma injuries. Rescues of such victims can be arduous and dangerous because the lifeguard may also be injured by the hard surface during the rescue attempt.

Cliffs and rock promontories often seem to invite people to dive, unaware of dangerously shallow water adjacent to the outcropping. Wave surges and tides alter water depth from one moment to the next and improper timing of a dive can then leave the diver in water shallow enough to cause serious injury.

It is not unusual for *flotsam* (seaborne debris) to appear at surf beaches, pushed ashore by waves and surf action. When feasible, dangerous pieces of flotsam should be removed immediately. One of the values of regular patrols by lifeguards is to check for the presence of beach and water hazards that can be removed or marked to protect beachgoers.

Rip Currents and Lateral Currents

Wave energy, combined with gravity, causes currents which can seriously threaten the safety of swimmers and other water users. Any body of water where waves of significant size are present, whether the ocean or a large lake, can experience these currents. The most serious of these by far are rip currents, but to best understand rip currents, one must first understand lateral currents.

Lateral Currents

A *lateral current*, also known as a longshore current or lateral drift, runs roughly parallel to the beach. These currents are often caused by waves coming from an angle diagonal to the beach, thus pushing water along the beach as the waves break. They may also be caused by tidal inflows and outflows from nearby entrances to harbors and bays. They can sweep swimmers along at a rapid rate. Most swimmers caught in a lateral current will naturally swim toward the safety of shore, and since this involves swimming across, rather than against the current they can normally reach shore relatively easily. Nonswimmers however, may be seriously endangered by a longshore current, and even strong swimmers may experience difficulty if the current pulls them off the end of a peninsula, for example. Many rescues on northerly reaches of the outer shore of Cape Cod, Massachusetts are caused by complications related to sand bars and longshore currents. A particularly hazardous role of a lateral current however, is to act as the feeder to a rip current, which can endanger the safety of even strong swimmers.

WEBBOX

Read more about rip currents and view rip current models in *Rip Currents—Rivers Through The Surf* on the United States Lifesaving Association website at: *www.usla.org*

Rip Currents

USLA has determined that *rip currents* are the primary source of distress in over 80% of swimmer rescues at surf beaches. This is based on annual reports provided by lifeguard agencies from throughout the United States. One may safely assume that rip currents are responsible for a comparable proportion of surf beach drownings in cases where lifeguards are not available. Rip currents are sometimes referred to as *the drowning machine* because of their almost mechanical ability to tire swimmers to the point of fatigue and, ultimately, death. According to Lascody (1998), "Rip currents, on average, result in more deaths in Florida than hurricanes, tropical storms, tornados, severe thunderstorms and lightning *combined.*" Nationally, there are more deaths from rip currents in an average year than from lightning, tornadoes, or hurricanes.

In some areas of the country, rip currents are referred to by colloquial, local terms. USLA encourages exclusive use of the term "rip current" because it helps to educate the public through consistent and scientifically recognized nomenclature. Use of other terms may confuse the public and thus adversely impact safety. The term *riptide* is sometimes used interchangeably with rip current, but this is incorrect. A riptide is a separate and distinct force, described later in this chapter.

The speed of a rip current can be very strong. One source cites current speeds as being as high as 4 knots. (Open University, 1989) In addition to speed, rip currents vary in size, width, depth, shape, and power. They are created primarily by the force of incoming waves, combined with the force of gravity. As previously described, once the force of uprush is expended, gravity creates a backrush of water to the sea. That backrush of water may be diffused fairly evenly along the shoreline, in which case currents will be minimal. When the backrushing water is channeled however, a concentrated current is created, which is properly known as a rip current. Some rip currents dissipate very close to shore, while others can continue for hundreds of yards.

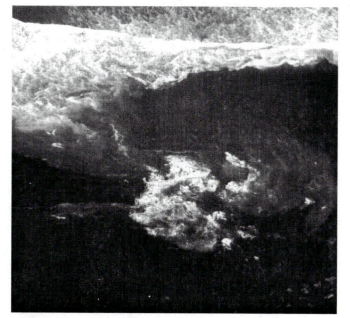

A large rip current.
Credit: Ken Kramer

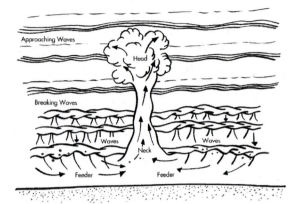

Multi-feeder

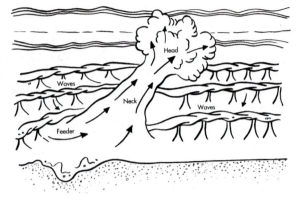

One Feeder

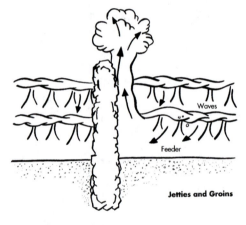

Jetties and Groins

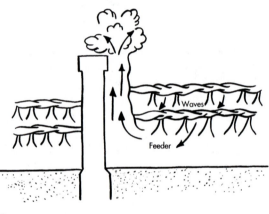

Piers

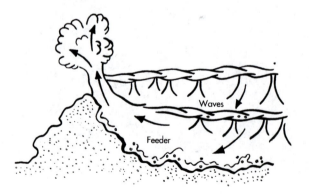

Rocky Points

Rip Currents Form in Different Ways

Components of Rip Currents

Rip currents have three major components:

- *Feeder*—This is the main source of supply for the rip. Water that has been pushed up the beach and is being pulled back by gravity follows the path of least resistance—the rip current channel. To get there, the water may have to travel laterally along the beach some distance. Once the water finds a channel or an obstacle in its lateral movement, it will turn seaward. A rip current may have one or two feeders. For example, waves breaking on both sides of a deeper water channel would create two feeders. Single feeder rip currents are however, much more common.

- *Neck*—This is the river of water running away from the beach. The neck can vary in width from a few yards to many tens of yards. The majority of both rescues and drownings occur in the neck. This is where the rip current has its strongest effect.

- *Head*—This is the area where the offshore current from the neck ends, dispersing broadly. The current's momentum, which was initially caused by waves pushing water up the slope of the beach and then by gravity pulling the water back from whence it came, has now been exhausted.

Types of Rip Currents

There are four types of rip currents:

- *Fixed Rip Currents*—These are found only on sand beaches. They pull offshore in one location because the depth directly underneath is greater then surrounding depths. These rips are usually created when the water transported by incoming surf "piles up" between the shore and offshore sandbars, as well as incoming surf. Eventually, the water returns to the sea, following the path of least resistance, which is normally a low point in the sandbar system. This return flow further erodes the underlying sand bottom, creating a rip current channel, which remains fixed in the same location so long as sand and surf conditions remain stable. (Bascom, 1980) When these surf conditions change, fixed rips may also change if wave action moves underlying sand. Therefore, a fixed rip may lie in a given spot for an extended period of hours, days, or even months, or change or even disappear within a matter of hours.

- *Permanent Rip Currents*—These rip currents are stationary year round, though they may vary in intensity. They are usually found on rocky coastlines and exist due to undulations in the bottom that do not change. The speed and power of these rips depend entirely on the size of the surf. Rock beach rip currents usually pull harder than sand beach rips because water moves more forcefully over solid, stationary obstacles and the excess flow of water may be more concentrated in pronounced, fixed rock channels. Piers, rock jetties, drain pipes, projecting points of land, and some beach contours may also force lateral currents to turn seaward, creating permanent rip currents. In many areas, permanent or fixed rips are given names that relate to nearby landmarks or streets. Such identification can be invaluable when lifeguard teams answer emergency calls because they pinpoint where assistance is needed.

- *Flash Rip Currents*—Temporary rips generated by increased volumes of water brought to shore from concentrated sets of waves are called flash rip currents. Flash rips do not typically accompany depressions in the bottom. Flash rips, like flash floods on land,

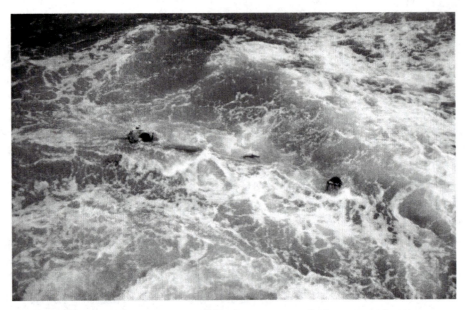

A lifeguard (right) tows a scuba diver toward shore against a strong rip current. The scuba diver holds a rescue buoy.

Credit: B. Chris Brewster

occur unexpectedly and without warning. When they strike an otherwise safe swimming area suddenly, part of the crowd can be quickly swept from shallow water. Since flash rips usually subside rapidly, many people caught in them can return to shore without assistance, but those who are non-swimmers or who have panicked require expeditious rescue. It is not easy to determine from the beach which of those pulled suddenly offshore is endangered due to lack of swimming ability, so rescue operations must begin immediately and usually several lifeguards are needed. In some cases, crowds of waders actually create an effect similar to that of a jetty or pier, obstructing the flow of a lateral current and causing it to turn seaward, forming a flash rip. In these cases, part of the group may be drawn seaward with the rip current.

- *Traveling Rip Currents*—Like other types of rip currents, traveling rip currents pull away from the beach, but these rip currents do not accompany depressions in sand or reef formations. They move along the beach pushed by the prevailing direction of the waves. Traveling rips usually occur in a strong, one-direction swell movement with long, well-defined periods. The wave action moves the rip away from the set of waves that feeds it. A traveling rip usually continues moving and pulling well into the lull period until the excess water has dissipated. The next set of waves starts the process all over again. Traveling rips can be pushed 200 or 300 yards and farther along the beach, depending on the size of the surf and/or the number of waves in a set. They are similar in all respects

WEBBOX

The National Weather Service maintains a website on rip currents at: *www.ripcurrents.noaa.gov/*

to flash rips except that their movement is predictable once their sequence has begun and the established pattern repeats itself. Like flash rip currents, traveling rips can wreak havoc on a swimming crowd as they move along the beach pulling large numbers of people offshore.

Characteristics of Rip Currents

Although rip currents can vary greatly in appearance, as a general rule they look somewhat different from the surrounding surf. A rip may seem especially rough or choppy, may have the dark color of deeper water, and may or may not have foam. Rips sometimes pick up debris, seaweed particles, or sand, giving the water a dirty or muddy quality. At other times the seaward current shows clear evidence that the water at the surface is running in the opposite direction from incoming waves—either flowing perpendicular to them or at another angle from the shore. Rips moving through calm, level surf are easily detected, but rips are harder to spot when the sea is rough and conditions are windy. Under most conditions, rips can be readily identified by a trained lifeguard.

Fixed and permanent rips typically pull harder when the tide recedes. Rip channels are more defined compared to the surrounding areas, which become progressively shallower. Consequently, the excess water is considerably more concentrated into the rip current channels while returning seaward. Of course, if a rip current channel is fully exposed by an outgoing tide, coming all the way out of the water, its effect will be negated by the tide. Rips may characteristically stop pulling at high tide, only to begin again as the tide recedes, although the reverse situation is also possible.

The power of rip currents typically relaxes when set waves arrive onshore, as the successive large waves create a damming effect between themselves and the shoreline. As soon as the set moves through however, the transient damming effect quickly subsides and rip currents can become particularly intense. Lifeguards observing set waves arrive should of course watch for distress that may be caused by the waves themselves, but as soon as they subside, great attention must be paid to the inevitable increase in the intensity of rip currents. The ever changing condition of rip currents is one reason lifeguards must constantly read the surf in order to safeguard the assigned area.

On steeper beaches, where shorebreak is present, rip currents tend to pull only a short distance offshore, but the combination of backrush and a rip current can both knock a beachgoer down and pull the person into deep water. For many years, the term *undertow* has been used, perhaps to describe this phenomenon. This term is a misnomer and should be used by lifeguards only to correct others.

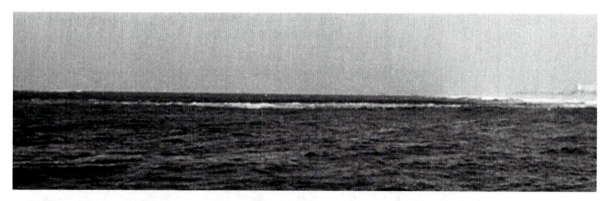

A 300 yard long rip current at Huntington State Beach, California.
Credit: Huntington State Beach

(Bascom, 1980) It suggests a condition which can actually suck a person under the water. Backrush, particularly on a steep beach, can knock a person down and, along with a rip, may pull a person off-shore, but it does not pull the victim underwater. Of course, if a non-swimmer or poor swimmer is carried into deep water, the person may submerge, but this is due to gravity and the loss of buoyancy, not a downward sucking action of current.

Although there are constant problems with rip currents at surf beaches in the United States, some areas report seasons when rips are particularly hazardous. For example, spring and early summer are the most hazardous times on the West Coast as the prevailing swell direction swings from its northerly origin to a southerly origin. This change of swell direction causes holes and channels in the sand that foster rip current formation. Other areas report more serious problems with rip currents in late summer, or at other particular times of the year.

Effects of Rip Currents

The hazard presented by rip currents is magnified by the fact that they often appear to be the calmest water area along the beach. This is because the underwater channels that can cause rip currents are deeper than areas on either side. Since waves break in a water depth of approximately 1.3 times their height, there are often breaking waves on both sides of a rip current channel, with little or no apparent wave activity in the rip current itself. In addition, the force of a rip current moving away from the beach tends to negate the power of incoming waves. Lack of surf often attracts unsuspecting beachgoers, who see the relatively flat water over a rip current channel and believe they are choosing the safest area for swimming. This can be a deadly error. (Bacscom, 1980)

Effects of rip currents on swimmers and surfers vary with water skills. Those caught in a rip current are pulled away from shore, which for non-swimmers can quickly be lethal. Persons with a basic ability to tread water may be able to stay afloat for a short time, but are likely to be quickly overcome by panic when pulled offshore by a rip.

The effect of a rip current on persons with moderate to strong water skills is different. These people may at first be completely unconcerned about being in water over their head and oblivious to any danger. Then they may attempt to swim directly toward shore, but notice that they are making no progress or going backwards. At this point, even good swimmers can panic. Once swimmers panic, their stroke becomes less effective and their energy is quickly expended. There is a marked desperation of persons in rip currents fed by their loss of control.

The simplest way for a swimmer to escape from the seaward pull of the neck is to swim perpendicular to the current. Since rip currents normally pull directly away from the beach or slightly diagonally, the best direction to swim is parallel to the beach. This will allow the swimmer to move across the current instead of against it. Once out of the rip current channel, the swimmer can turn and swim to shore, often aided by shoreward wave action which borders the rip current. This maneuver is relatively easy if the rip current is a stationary one, but if it is a traveling rip moving in the same direction as the swimmer, an attempt to escape the force by swimming to the side may be futile. Another danger is that swimmers may escape from the neck of the rip current and swim toward shore

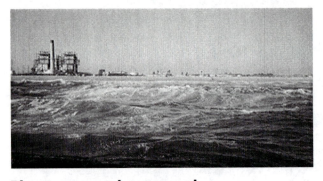

Rip current moving seaward.

Credit:Huntington State Beach

only to enter the broader feeder and be sucked back into the neck. Lifeguards sometimes refer to this as being recirculated by the rip.

Another way to escape from a rip current is to relax and allowing oneself to by carried to its outermost limit—the head—which is usually not far beyond the breaking surf. After judging the width of the rip current, the swimmer can then swim parallel to the beach in relatively calm water, reenter the surf, and swim safely to shore. This strategy is perhaps easier said than done. Even good swimmers with surf experience can become panicked when pulled away from the beach and some rip currents pull hundreds of yards offshore before expending their energy. It is therefore best to attempt to swim sideways to the rip current a significant distance and then to swim in.

Tides

Tides are rises and falls in the level of the ocean caused by gravitational attraction of the sun and moon. (While tides can occur in large lakes, their effect is virtually imperceptible.) Knowledge of tides, and a daily awareness of the times of the tides, is essential to effective lifesaving.

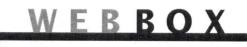

WEBBOX

You can access tide predictions for areas throughout the United States at the National Ocean Service website: *www.nos.noaa.gov*

Normally, there are two high tides and two low tides each day. Wave action, currents, boating traffic, and many other elements of the daily life of a beach are impacted by tides. One of the most obvious impacts on beach users is that there is more beach available at low tide. On beaches with significant tidal change, beach crowds can be pushed together by an incoming tide, sometimes causing interpersonal tension and making it more difficult for lifeguards to respond to emergencies.

As explained in the previous section, tides can exaggerate or minimize the effects of currents, depending on a variety of factors. Since tides can be reliably predicted through a variety of means, there is no need for complex calculations by lifeguards to predict tidal changes. Regional tide charts are widely available and should be kept at every lifeguard post.

Riptides

Unlike rip currents, which are primarily caused by wave energy, riptides are caused by tidal action. Riptides typically occur as water rushes through entrances to bays and estuaries during tidal changes. The Bay of Fundy's legendary tidal change, including currents up to eight knots, is an excellent example of a riptide.

One tragic example of the power of a riptide occurred in East Rockaway Inlet off New York City. In this inlet, tidal currents can reach 2.9 knots. (NOAA, 2001) On July 23, 2001, three girls wading off the beach were swept into deep water by the riptide and drowned.

Extraordinary Sea States

Waves and currents are normal sea states. They exist continually, thought their intensity may vary significantly. There are however, extraordinary ocean conditions which, while rare, can seriously endanger beachgoers.

Tidal Waves and Tsunamis

Most people have heard of a *tidal wave*, but what is it? First of all, the term "tidal wave" is considered by scientists to be a misnomer, since tides do not create these waves. Hence, *tsunami* is the favored term, although this Japanese word, meaning "harbor wave," is not much closer to a correct description of the phenomenon. Tsunamis are created by events that cause sudden shifts in the sea. The primary cause of tsunamis is earthquakes, but volcanoes, landslides, or even the unlikely crash of a meteorite into the sea can cause a tsunami.

To better understand the effect of a tsunami, consider this analogy: Most young swimmers have had the experience of themselves or others doing a "cannonball" dive into the water, by jumping into a pool while making their body into a ball. This causes a great splash and waves moving out in all directions. Imagine then, a similarly dramatic event on an exponentially larger scale in the ocean, or even in a lake. Unlike normal wind generated waves, this creates large, fast-moving waves that can quickly travel great distances and cause tremendous destruction.

Tsunamis can travel up to 500 miles per hour. Because of their very long wave length, they may be hardly noticed in the open sea, but upon striking land, can cause tremendous destruction, primarily by temporarily, but dramatically lifting the sea height. The threat of a tsunami is usually announced by disaster preparedness officials, but there is limited protection available, with the exception of evacuating to high ground.

Historically, some tsunamis have had devastating consequences. An 1896 tsunami killed some 27,000 people in Northern Japan. A 1946 tsunami which struck Hilo, Hawaii, caused 159 deaths and extensive destruction. In that case, it is said that many deaths occurred due to curious people noticing an initial drawdown of the water level in the harbor and walking out to observe, only to be inundated when the wave arrived, submerging them and the town itself.

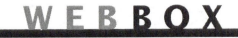

WEBBOX

Read a personal account of a resident of Kodiak, Alaska, who observed a tsunami hit her town in 1964 at: *www.kodiak.org/earthquake.html*

Learn more about tsunamis and view photos of the results online at the Pacific Tsunami Museum: *www.tsunami.org/*

Storm Surge

Storm surge occurs during violent storms near the shoreline, such as hurricanes. According to Brian Jarvinen of the National Hurricane Center, "The greatest potential for loss of life related to a hurricane is from the storm surge." (NOAA, 2003) Storm surge results when the wind within the storm pushes water toward shore, creating a *storm tide* (storm surge combined with tide) of 15 feet or more. The effect of storm surge is typically accentuated by high waves, caused by wind associated with the same weather conditions that create increased sea level. The fact that these storm waves come one after another mutes the normal backrush effect. Incoming waves then, continue to push water ahead of them. The result can be very serious coastal flooding.

Coastlines with flat terrain, many structures near sea level, and a gradual offshore drop-off toward the ocean are the most susceptible to the ravages of storm surge. Those with a steep drop-off and a more hilly coastline are less likely to sustain serious damage. According to the National Oceanic and Atmospheric Administration (2003), "Because much of the United States' densely populated Atlantic and Gulf Coast coastlines lie less than 10 feet above mean sea level, the danger from storm tides is tremendous."

LearnMore

Read about the devastating storm surge that inundated Galveston, Texas in the bestselling book: *Isaac's Storm: A Man, a Time, and the Deadliest Hurricane in History* (September 1999—Crown; ISBN: 0609602330)

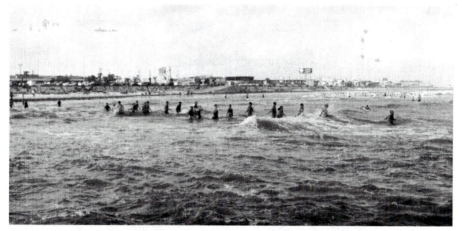

Lifeguards train along the Galveston, Texas coastline.
Credit: Peter Davis

One of the most disastrous examples of the effects of storm surge came in the Galveston, Texas flood of 1900. It is estimated that some 6,000 people drowned in storm tides of 8—15 feet. Lakes can be impacted by storm surge as well. In 1928, Florida's Lake Okeechobee was influenced by surge associated with a hurricane that caused 6—9 foot flooding and the deaths of over 1,800 people. Today, storm surge is better understood and predicted. Using estimates generated by sources such as the National Hurricane Center's Sea, Lake and Overland Surges from Hurricanes (SLOSH) computerized model, disaster preparedness officials typically arrange evacuations, sometimes of very broad areas.

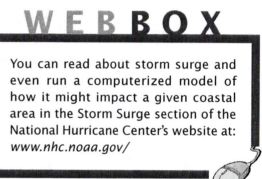

WEBBOX

You can read about storm surge and even run a computerized model of how it might impact a given coastal area in the Storm Surge section of the National Hurricane Center's website at: *www.nhc.noaa.gov/*

Chapter Summary

In this chapter, we have learned about how waves form and what factors impact their size, shape, and speed. We have learned what happens as surface waves approach a beach and become shallow water waves, then breaking waves. We have reviewed a variety of ways in which waves can provide enjoyment, fascination, and great danger to beach users. We have garnered an understanding of the manner in which shoreline topography both changes and is itself changed by the power of the surf.

This chapter has described the hazard presented by longshore currents and rip currents, and how rip currents are the primary cause of rescues and drownings at surf beaches. We have learned about the components, types, and characteristics of these currents. We have also learned about tides and the currents they produce, as well as the unusual and extraordinary threat to safety posed by tsunamis and storm surge.

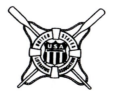

Discussion Points

- What sort of weather conditions produce waves?
- What three conditions in combination would produce the largest waves?
- Why is a mouse running under a carpet similar to a wave in the ocean?
- Why would waves on Pacific shores be expected, on average, to be more regular in size and period than those on Atlantic or Gulf Coast shores?
- When wave trains intermingle, what are the likely effects?
- What are some specific hazards created by set waves?
- Why do waves arriving at beaches seem to come from the same direction?
- Why is it important to ensure that estimates of wave height by lifeguards is consistent and accurate from lifeguard to lifeguard?
- What rare phenomenon (aside from a raging storm) was a particular threat to the safety of mariners during the "Perfect Storm"?
- If the width of many surf beaches in the U.S. is wider in summer, where does the sand go in winter?
- Why do sandbars help create rip currents?
- How do inshore holes threaten safety?
- Why is it important to remove or mark large flotsam?
- What factor limits the hazard of longshore currents?
- What factors help differentiate the four types of rip currents?
- How can set waves be expected to influence rip currents?
- What are some strategies to employ to extricate oneself from a rip current?
- What are key differences between rip currents and riptides?
- What steps might a lifeguard take to help safeguard the public if a tsunami is predicted?
- What steps might a lifeguard take to help safeguard the public if storm surge is predicted?

References

Bascom, W. (1980). *Waves and beaches*. New York: Anchor Books

Drag, W. (2000). A comparative retrospective on the Perfect Storm. Retrieved January 4, 2003 from the World Wide Web: *www.erh.noaa.gov/er/box/PS.htm*

Lascody, R. L. (1998). East central Florida rip current program. *National Weather Digest, 22,* 25–30.

National Oceanic and Atmospheric Administration (2000). NOAA meteorologists recall drama of forecasting "The Perfect Storm" [Article posted on the Web site *NOAA News*]. Retrieved January 4, 2003 from the World Wide Web: *www.noaanews.noaa.gov/stories/s451.htm*

National Oceanic and Atmospheric Administration (2001). Nautical chart #12352 (29th ed.). Ft. Lauderdale, FL: Bluewater Books and Charts.

National Oceanic and Atmospheric Administration (2003). Storm surge [Article posted on the National Hurricane Center Web site]. Retrieved January 6, 2003 from the World Wide Web: *www.nhc.noaa.gov/HAW/day1/storm_surge.htm*

Open University (1989). *Waves, tides, and shall-water processes*. Elmsford, New Jersey: Pergamon Press.

Chapter 6
The Flat Water Beach

In this chapter, you will learn about the unique features of flat water beaches and the special hazards they present. These can include lack of surf, reduced buoyancy, currents, drop-offs, plant life, and turbidity. You will learn about beach topography and an unusual condition called a seiche. A thorough understanding of these factors is critical to lifeguards seeking to maintain safety in flat water areas.

CHAPTER EXCERPT

At flat water beaches distress can develop immediately and unpredictably, requiring an instant reaction by the lifeguard prior to disappearance of the victim. This presents a major challenge for lifeguards.

Lack of Surf

Given a choice, many people select flat water beaches over surf beaches because they consider flat water to be safer, particularly for nonswimmers and those with weak swimming ability. Lack of surf seems to lessen fear of drowning. Parents may adopt a more relaxed approach, lowering their vigilance over children. Adults who are nonswimmers or weak swimmers may be lulled into a false sense of safety. Despite the absence of surf related hazards though, drownings and related accidents happen with surprising regularity at flat water beaches. A major contributing factor is that people underestimate the hazards, some of which lurk silently beneath the surface.

At surf beaches, most rescues develop as a result of observable surf and rip current conditions. Those venturing into the surf typically have moderate or even strong swimming abilities, enabling those in distress to maintain buoyancy for a time. Beach patrons at surf beaches with weak swimming ability are generally intimidated by surf and attempt to stay in shallow water, or stay out of the water altogether. These factors allow surf lifeguards to focus particular attention on known hazard areas. They also provide time for lifeguards to anticipate problems and react, because distress in the surf environment can often develop gradually. Not so in the flat water environment.

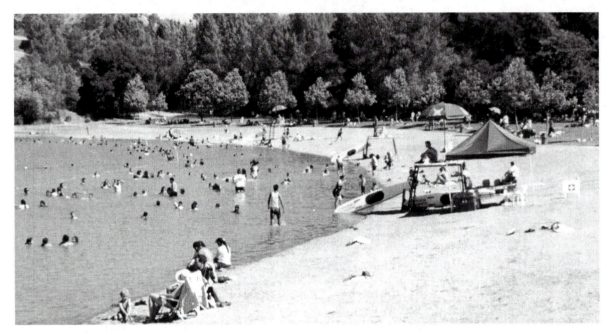

Credit: Dan McCormick

At flat water beaches distress can develop immediately and unpredictably, requiring an instant reaction by the lifeguard prior to disappearance of the victim. This presents a major challenge to lifeguards. A person standing in neck deep water playing with a ball, for example, may appear quite comfortable, but may be a complete nonswimmer. One step in the wrong direction can leave this person submerged and out of sight in the blink of an eye, with no observable sign of struggle. As a result, high levels of vigilance and the ability to quickly distinguish between play and struggle are essential for the flat water lifeguard. Constant scanning, timely and effective preventive actions, adequate breaks, and immediate, decisive action, when needed, are critical. A key preventive action is to work to counter the sense of overconfidence flat water may engender among beachgoers, helping them take prudent steps to avoid accidents.

Buoyancy and Resistance

Many flat water environments are fresh water, rather than saltwater. Because fresh water is less dense than saltwater, swimmers are less buoyant in fresh water. This lessened buoyancy affects people in several ways. Weak swimmers will tire more quickly in fresh water because they must expend more energy to stay afloat. Therefore, in fresh water people cannot stay afloat as long as they might in saltwater. If they sink, they will sink faster. The lifeguard will thus have less time to identify and respond to signs of distress. Buoyancy creates a different problem for waders by lessening the effect of gravity. That, combined with resistance of the water, limits the ability to maneuver while walking in deep water, particularly chest or neck deep. People walking on an uneven bottom or in a current, for example, can easily lose balance and may lack the ability to right themselves. Toddlers trying to walk in water can easily trip. Once face down, the water's buoyant effect, combined with lack of body control, can make it impossible for toddlers to right themselves. Thus, they can drown in very shallow water.

Flotation Devices

The nature of flat water beach design and public use patterns also has a significant effect on the lifeguard. One reason is use of flotation devices. Surf generally prevents poor swimmers with flotation devices from venturing out, but no such impediment is present at flat water beaches. Many people visiting flat water areas use inflatable rafts and similar devices to move offshore. These devices make it difficult or impossible for the lifeguard to assess swimming ability. Flat water beaches often have buoyed lines that mark the boundaries of the swimming area and provide separation from boating or other use areas. While there may be benefits to these lines, weak swimmers and nonswimmers sometimes cling to them as a means of staying afloat and venturing into deep water. Anchored diving platforms, rafts, buoys, boats and opposite shores also provide tempting deep water goals for the weak or non-swimmer to reach. The goal can be deceptively far due to the lack of visual reference over flat water.

The person using a flotation device may be an Olympic swimmer, or may be a nonswimmer, it's tough to tell. When poor swimmers and nonswimmers fall from rafts, slip from ropes, or overestimate their abilities and tire before reaching their goals, they may quickly disappear while a significant distance from shore, making effective rescue extremely difficult. This is one reason that some areas ban flotation devices and prohibit swimmers from clinging to the floating lines that mark the areas. In any case, prudent lifeguards assume that all people using flotation devices are nonswimmers, until they are able to ascertain otherwise.

Crowd Density

Crowd density presents another challenge for lifeguards. During heat spells or when large groups hit the beach, crowd density can skyrocket, particularly in the water. This increased level of activity not only makes it statistically more likely that trouble will arise, but crowd density can make it much more difficult for the lifeguard to spot trouble. During periods of high attendance, the sheer number of people engaged in water activity can make it very difficult for the lifeguard to adequately monitor everyone. One strategy, if possible, is to assign additional lifeguards when unusually high crowds deluge a beach area.

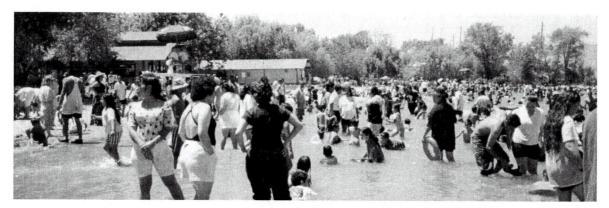

Credit: Dan McCormick

Currents

Although the water may appear calm, many flat water areas experience significant currents. In saltwater bays, tides can create inflow and outflow currents which are much stronger than rip currents. These are true riptides. People caught in such currents can rapidly be drawn to deep water, where serious problems can develop. (More information on riptides can be found in Chapter 5.) Wind and waves also create currents in flat water areas.

The currents of rivers can be far more dangerous than the rip currents caused by surf action, because river currents are relentless. There is no occasional lull between strong pulses, as is typical in the case of a rip. Strong river currents moving over obstacles in the river, including low dams, can create reverse currents just below them, trapping the victim in an inescapable cycle. Logs and other debris may form strainers, allowing water to move through, but not large objects, like people. Even a strong person caught in a strainer may be pinned underwater and drown. As well, river currents can carry weak or nonswimmers offshore, drive them into stationary objects, or pull them over falls. River currents are influenced by such factors as the width, grade, depth, upstream barriers, and water volume in the river channel. Currents in deeper water of rivers are often faster than in shallower water. In addition to rivers, currents are also prevalent at some lakes and reservoirs, particularly at areas close to inflows or outflows.

Many people caught in a current react by swimming against the current pulling them or try to swim toward a specific point on the other shore, taking an upstream *ferry angle* in an effort to make it to a particular area ashore. Little if any progress can be made with such an approach and the effort usually drains the energy and strength of the victim. Swimmers caught in flat water surface currents should normally be instructed to swim with and diagonally across the current toward the safety of shore.

It takes very little moving water to cause a strong current. When water appears calm, current speed and direction can be identified by watching for movement of the water, or of material in the water. Lifeguards working flat water areas with currents must be thoroughly familiar with the dynamics of the environment, both for the safety of those they protect and that of themselves.

Beach Topography

Currents, tides, natural configuration, and even human engineering can affect the topography of the beach at flat water areas. Where water is moving swiftly, the topography of the land under the water can change quickly and often. Drop-offs, where the bottom suddenly falls away to cause deep water

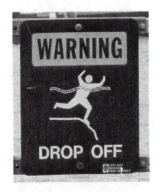

Warning sign indicating a drop-off.
Credit: Stephanie Korenstein

very close to relatively shallow water, are the greatest concern. They may be caused by currents, dredging, or other forces. The calm and even surface of the water hides this hazard from the unsuspecting wader, who may suddenly be in deep water without the skills necessary to deal with it. Nonswimmers who step into the drop-off may simply disappear, submerging instantly. At tidal areas, the distance from shore and depth of drop-offs can change markedly. A drop-off which threatens adults at high tide may be an equal threat to young children at a lower tide. The ideal beach design, particularly in a lake or similar aquatic environment, is a gradually sloping beach with no drop-off.

Rock outcroppings, cliffs, and rocky shores present safety hazards at flat water beaches. In many areas, the water just off a rocky shoreline can be quite deep. The unsuspecting person who jumps or falls into the water from shore may suddenly need immediate assistance. Outcroppings and cliffs also invite people to dive, even though the water may not be suitably deep for that purpose. Changing water conditions, reservoir heights, and tides may effect the water depth at popular diving spots, making them more hazardous. Submerged obstacles are a related problem, especially where water bodies and beaches have been created by planned flooding, such as in reservoirs. Tree stumps, rocks, and other objects can lie hidden below the water's surface. Other submerged objects may be washed in with currents and deposited beneath swimming areas.

The greatest hazard posed by submerged objects involves diving. Serious injury can result from diving into unknown waters. The unexpected striking of an underwater hazard or shallow bottom is a prime cause of the most tragic of non-lethal injuries—paralysis from permanent spinal cord damage. There is another hazard posed by submerged objects. Nonswimmers may stand on them, then step off into deep water, resulting in problems similar to drop-off.

Where feasible, extraordinary hazards which are not normal features of the area should be removed or marked. This is not to suggest that every stump or outcropping of rock must be signed or eliminated, but such action is appropriate for those hazards which are of an unusual nature or easily removed. The

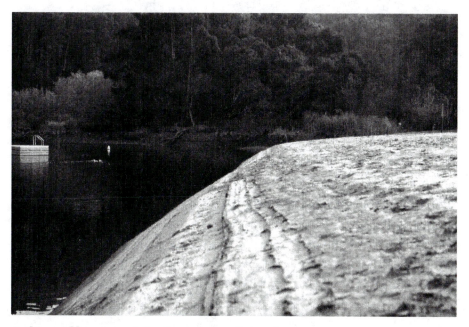

A drop-off exposed during water draw-down.
Credit: Lucy Woolshlager

most obvious examples are logs and other floating debris that wash up on a beach. Regular patrols to check for beach hazards are appropriate, particularly during and after storms.

Weeds and Plant Life

Calm water areas can experience problems with weeds and other plant life that flourish in the absence of currents. While the obvious problem may seem that people will become entangled in weeds, this is very rare. Instead, the fear of becoming entangled in weeds may cause a panic that is more dangerous. When some swimmers come in contact with an unseen substance, they panic and require assistance, though they may not actually be endangered. While swimming through heavy plant life, slow deliberate movements should prevent entanglement. If entanglement does occur, slow shaking motions as the swimmer moves away should cause the plant to slide off. When feasible, swimmers should be kept out of areas with heavy plant life.

Turbidity

Water clarity can cause problems at flat water beaches. Currents, where they exist, may churn up debris. In areas with no current, sediment may build up on the bottom, only to be disturbed when people enter the water, causing it to become cloudy. This becomes a particular problem during missing person incidents or an underwater search procedure. Depth perception is eliminated when the water is turbid, while drop-offs and other underwater hazards are obscured.

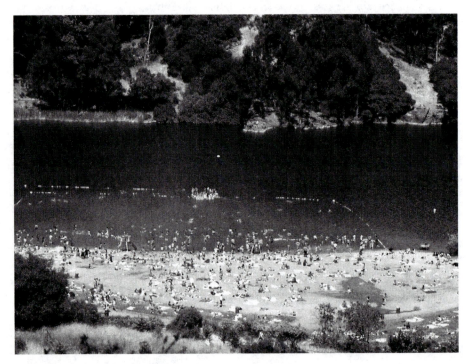

Swimmers cause turbid water.
Credit: Lucy Woolshlager

Seiches

A seiche (pronounced say-sh) is a rare condition that typically occurs in a landlocked body of water, though seiches also occur in bays and harbors. It involves oscillation of the water surface. A seiche can be created by the same events as a tsunami (see Chapter 5), such as seismic activity, but may also be created, for example, if a very strong wind blows

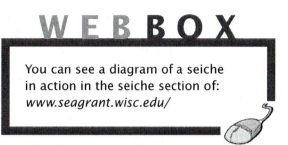

WEB**BOX**

You can see a diagram of a seiche in action in the seiche section of: *www.seagrant.wisc.edu/*

across a lake pushing water on the surface to one side, then subsides. You can simulate a seiche in a bucket of water by placing it on a flat surface and shoving it. The water sloshes back and forth until the water surface eventually flattens again. In a similar manner, water in a lake or bay may move alternately higher and lower on either side until well after the forces that created the seiche subside. It is believed by some scientists that the 1946 Hilo, Hawaii tsunami was actually magnified by a seiche condition in the bay.

Flat Water Lifeguard Strategies

The unique elements of flat water beaches require adaptations by lifeguards working them. Swimming areas at flat water beaches are often smaller than those at surf beaches, and may be defined by a buoyed boundary. This helps keep weaker swimmers closer to shore, and the protection of lifeguards. In absence of surf, and perhaps tides, flat water lifeguard towers can be placed nearer the water's edge, allowing closer supervision and faster response to persons in distress. In the flat water environment, zones of responsibility for lifeguards are often smaller, with multiple towers having specifically defined overlap. In some

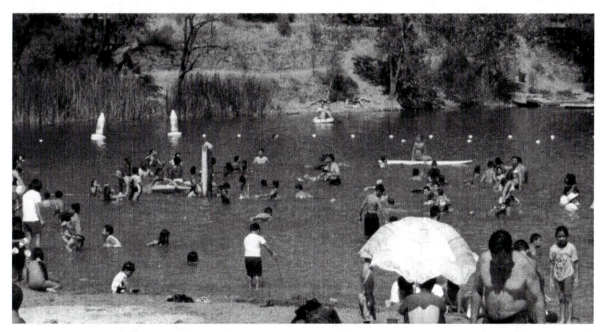

Deep water rescue board patrol.
Credit: Dan McCormick

areas, lifeguards rotate among stations, to help reduce boredom. Backup lifeguards are typically positioned closer to the swim area. Preventive actions, like keeping weak swimmers and persons on flotation devices in shallow water, are critical. Shoreline walking and deep-water rescue board patrols are often employed to keep lifeguards alert and positioned near crowds of swimmers. The rescue board, originally designed for the surf environment, is an excellent tool for making deep water rescues.

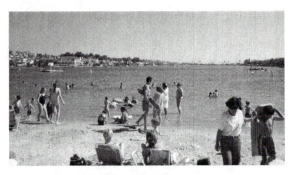

Shoreline walking patrol
Credit: Lake Mission Viejo Lifeguards

Chapter Summary

In this chapter, we have learned that flat water presents unique challenges for the lifeguard. The lack of surf creates an inviting environment for weak swimmers to visit. The tranquility though, can be deceptive as it may hide many hazards and lull people into a false sense of security. We have learned that flat water attracts a very wide range of swimming ability, making even calm conditions a serious threat to some. In fresh water, decreased buoyancy can shorten the length of time the lifeguard has to recognize and respond to distressed swimmers.

We have also learned that dense swimming crowds and the misuse of flotation devices can make it extremely difficult for the lifeguard to spot a victim in distress before submersion. Currents can be relentless and sweep swimmers from safety. Beach topography creates a variety of hazards. Rock outcroppings, cliffs and rocky shores may also attract diving that is unsafe due to submerged objects lying hidden below the surface. Changing water levels from tides or other causes can expose hazardous areas, such as drop-offs. Swimmer contact with underwater plant life can cause panic, though the risk of entanglement is low. Each of these factors contribute to the need for flat water lifeguards to develop specific observation and response procedures to keep their beaches safe.

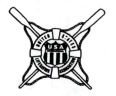

Discussion Points

- What are some hazards to be expected at a flat water beach that may not be present at a surf beach?
- What are some hazards shared by surf and flat water beaches?
- If one could design the safest possible underwater bottom to a flat water swimming area, what would it be like?
- What impacts might the lessened buoyancy in fresh water have on lifeguards?
- Why do underwater objects pose a safety hazard?
- Why might a flat water swim area decide to ban the use of inflatable rafts?
- What problems might turbidity cause for a lifeguard?
- What factors might cause a seiche condition?

Chapter 7
Aquatic Life and Related Hazards

In this chapter, you will learn about various types of aquatic life, as well as the impact of humans on the aquatic environment. Aquatic life includes organisms (plants and animals) that live totally or partially in water. Some aquatic life threatens the safety of water users, but other aquatic life may simply provoke their interest or fear. You will learn that sharks are an ominous, but statistically minimal threat. You will also learn about a wide variety of other aquatic life, including barracuda, schooling fish, venomous fish, stingrays, jellyfish, marine mammals, urchins, mollusks, leeches, turtles, snakes, and plants. Since aquatic life differs widely between saltwater (marine) and freshwater environments, it will be discussed separately for those two areas. Treatment of injuries associated with aquatic life is discussed in the chapter *Medical Care in the Aquatic Environment*.

CHAPTER EXCERPT

Shark attack is viewed by many as the most feared risk associated with swimming in the ocean. In fact, the danger of shark attacks is statistically miniscule—many times less than the chance of being struck by lightning.

Marine Life

One of the keys to understanding the dynamics of ocean beaches lies in the fact that they represent components of large and complex marine ecosystems. A host of highly adapted organisms, many of which can injure or be injured by humans, live in these ecosystems. Aquatic injuries associated with marine life typically include bites, stings, lacerations and abrasions. Death can result, but is very rare.

Usually when one thinks of dangerous marine life, such notorious animals as sharks, barracuda, and Portuguese man-of-war come to mind, but even seemingly non-threatening organisms such as

LearnMore

You can learn more about dangerous marine animals in the book, *Venomous and Poisonous Marine Animals: A Medical and Biological Handbook,* edited by Williamson, Fenner, Burnett, & Rifkin.

barnacles and kelp can cause injury. Conducting a complete inventory of all hazardous marine life inhabiting American coastal waters is beyond the scope of this text. We will therefore discuss some of the most common.

From a lifeguard's perspective, the initial consideration when dealing with any form of potentially dangerous marine life is early, accurate identification. Complicating this, some dangerous marine animals can be confused with those not generally considered dangerous. For example, in Florida waters, several kinds of large fish and mammals may be confused with sharks. Proper identification is essential, because clearing the water due to presence of a non-threatening species may cause panic and later non-compliance when a real danger exists. To prevent this, some agencies use a key—a small sheet with pictures—to help lifeguards make correct identifications.

Sharks

Shark attack is viewed by many as the most feared risk associated with swimming in the ocean. In fact, the danger of shark attacks is statistically miniscule—many times less than the chance of being struck by lightning. Administrators of the International Shark Attack File, maintained by the American Elasmobranch Society and the Florida Museum of Natural History, were able to confirm less than 75 shark bite incidents per year *worldwide* during the 1990s, with 10 or fewer deaths each year. (International Shark Attack File, 2003a) They report that, "In the United States the annual risk of death from lightning is 30 times greater than that from shark attack." (International Shark Attack File, 2003b) In Florida from 1959—1990 there were 313 fatalities attributed to lightning and only four attributed to sharks, a ratio of 78:1. (Brewster, Burgess, Gallagher, Gould, Hensler, & Wernicki, 2002)

In recent years, the primary activities associated with shark attacks have been surfing, scuba diving, and swimming, in that order of frequency. In fact, a surfer was three to four times as likely to be attacked as was a swimmer in the 1980s and 1990s. While the incidence of documented, unprovoked shark attack has increased over the years, it coincides with population increase and popularity of ocean recreation. (International Shark Attack File, 2003a)

Historically, the US states with the highest numbers of documented, unprovoked shark attacks through 2001 were Florida (474), California (111), and Hawaii (101), but outcome of these attacks has varied significantly. Approximately 20% of shark attacks in Hawaii have resulted in death, whereas in California the proportion is roughly 9%, and less than 5% were fatal in Florida. (International Shark Attack File, 2003a)

Australia, through 2001, had reported fewer confirmed, unprovoked shark attacks (323) than Florida, but almost 50% (152) of the reported Australian attacks had resulted in death. Historically, this is more than twice the number of unprovoked shark fatalities reported in the entire United States (67). South Africa's experience, in terms of the percentage of reported attacks that prove fatal, is comparable to that of Hawaii—roughly 20%. It should be noted however, that both Australia and South Africa employ shark deterrent procedures, such as netting, without which the number of attacks would undoubtedly be higher. Interestingly, the fictional setting of the famous movie *Jaws* (New York) has never had a confirmed, unprovoked, fatal shark attack. (International Shark Attack File, 2003a)

Experts recognize over 200 species of sharks; but only a few are considered a serious threat to people. Three shark species are the most frequent attackers of humans. These are the white shark (known as the great white shark), the tiger shark, and the bull shark, in that order. More than 50% of fatal attacks are attributed to the white shark. (International Shark Attack File, 2003a)

Most shark attacks occur in nearshore areas. This includes the area between sandbars, where sharks are sometimes trapped at low tide, and in areas with steep drop-offs. Sharks are drawn to such areas because their natural prey can be found there. Attacks occur more commonly when waters are murky. This condition increases the chance of a shark making a prey identification mistake.

WEB BOX

You can view statistics on shark attacks and other information about sharks in the International Shark Attack File at: *www.flmnh.ufl.edu/fish/Sharks/ISAF/ISAF.htm*

A prey identification mistake occurs when the shark accidentally attacks something other than its natural prey. It is generally believed that most shark attacks occur for this reason, rather than an intention on the part of the shark to attack or eat a human. Differing sizes and types of shark prey in various areas of the world may help explain variations in the likelihood of an attack being fatal to a human.

In Florida, the predominant food items of sharks are fish. In this area, shark bites seem to occur when sharks confuse the splashing of surfers and swimmers in murky nearshore waters as being from schooling fish. Most attacks in Florida result in a single bite or slash, with no repeat passes at the victim. (Burgess, 1994)

Along the California coast, the threat to humans engaged in aquatic recreation is essentially confined to one species: white sharks. Attacks in this area are believed to occur when the shark confuses the size, shape, and actions of a person with a seal or sea lion—a major indigenous food item. (Burgess, 1994) Great whites attack this prey with a ferocity intended to maim or kill an animal of that size.

In Hawaii, attacks largely involve the tiger shark. Like the white shark, this species is known to attack humans and life-threatening injuries can result. Surfers are the most likely victims. A favorite haunt of the tiger shark is the area where the surf breaks over reefs, which is also an area where surfers congregate. (International Shark Attack File, 2003a)

Dolphin and porpoise are often mistaken for sharks, but are normally harmless to swimmers. These small whales have a horizontal tail fin, so they usually expose only their dorsal fin when swimming near the surface. Dolphin, particularly the common bottlenose dolphin, regularly swim in groups, continually surfacing and submerging in forward arcs. Sharks, on the other hand, have a vertical tail fin. When swimming along the surface, the dorsal fin cuts through the water, while the tail fin moves back and forth. Sharks do not swim in an arcing motion. Instead, when swimming along the surface, they cruise at a fairly consistent depth, with their fins exposed for longer periods than porpoises. Such observations are extremely rare on the West Coast, but occasionally seen on the Gulf Coast and East Coast, particularly in Florida.

Periods that shark attack is more likely along the West Coast include times of heavy seal and sea lion activity, especially during the annual birthing period. Under these conditions, white sharks are more likely to move into the surf zone. Along the East Coast and Gulf Coast, where shark bites are sometimes sustained near schooling fish, it may be prudent to warn swimmers away from heavy concentrations of fish—often indicated by sea bird diving. In addition, periods of onshore winds along the east coast of Florida can result in concentrations of fish and sharks in poor visibility water—a bad combination when humans are added to the mix. In Hawaii, surfers and swimmers should avoid dawn and dusk periods when tiger sharks are particularly active and the areas around the mouths of rivers, especially after heavy rains, where tiger sharks may scavenge. (Burgess, 1994)

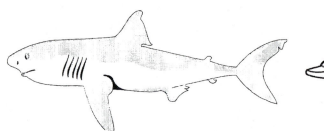

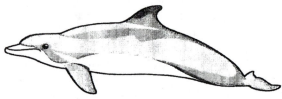

This drawing of a shark shows the vertical tail fin.

Porpoises have a horizontal tail fin.

For further information on preventing, treating, and responding to shark bite incidents, please refer to the chapters on *Preventive Lifeguarding, Medical Care in the Aquatic Environment,* and *Special Rescues.* Lifeguards are strongly encouraged to report shark attacks to the International Shark Attack File, so that information can be gathered for future reference. For information on reporting, see the organization's website at: *www.flmnh.ufl.edu/fish/Sharks/ISAF/ISAF.htm.*

Barracuda

Barracuda are large, streamlined predator fish usually found in tropical and sub-tropical waters. Biologists classify at least 20 species of barracuda. Only one of these species, the Great Barracuda, is considered dangerous to people. Although attacks are rare, there have been authenticated reports. Most of these attacks are associated with blood in the water; either from an injured fish or a human. There are also reports which suggest that bites may result from swimmers wearing bright and shiny objects during times of poor water visibility. When a barracuda, especially a large one, is observed near a swimming area, it should be monitored carefully. Some agencies will establish a barracuda sighting as criteria for the water to be cleared of swimmers, especially if it appears that there are also baitfish in the area.

Schooling Fish

Most schooling fish do not represent a problem because they are not equipped with the physical anatomy to injure a swimmer. A few species, under certain circumstances, can inflict injury. Some of these include jacks, tarpon, mackerel, and bluefish. During migrations and feeding frenzies, these

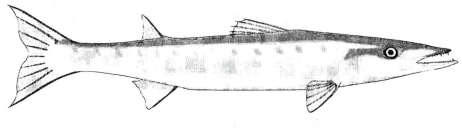

Barracuda

species have been known to brush against a swimmer causing lacerations and abrasions. Schools of blue-fish have been reported nipping at swimmers' hands and feet, causing numerous bites. Schooling fish can also attract larger predatory fish (e.g., sharks and barracuda). Whenever schools of large fish are observed, they should be carefully monitored. Some lifeguard agencies clear the water of swimmers immediately. This is an agency by agency decision based on past experience.

Stingray

Only a few members of the ray family are considered dangerous. The most common is the stingray, whose tail has a venomous barb or barbs. Stingrays are not aggressive animals and are easily frightened; but they often bury themselves in the sand in shallow water. If accidentally stepped on by a hapless wader or otherwise struck, stingrays reflexively flip their tail. This flip of the tail can result in the barb or barbs lacerating the skin and venom entering the victim's body. A recommended method for avoiding the sting of a stingray is to do the "stingray shuffle." In areas where stingrays are common, by shuffling your feet instead of leaping forward in shallow water, you may lessen the chance of surprising a stingray, stepping on it, and being stung.

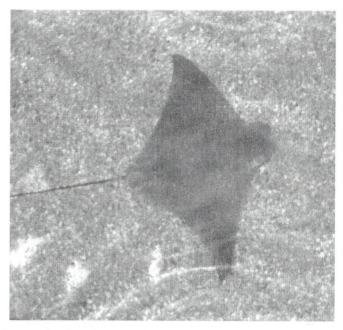

A ray in shallow water.

Credit: Dave Foxwell

Serious bleeding can result in these cases and deaths have been caused from exsanguination (massive blood loss), but the most noticeable result is typically intense, sharp, shooting pain in the affected area. (Knight, 1989) (Liggins, 1939) If left untreated, the pain may intensify for up to 90 minutes, then slowly subside. Besides pain, the victim may experience rapidly declining blood pressure, vomiting, diarrhea, sweating, arrhythmia, and muscular paralysis leading to death in some cases. Wounds to the chest or abdomen are particularly serious and have resulted in death. The usual site of a sting from a stingray however, is the foot or ankle, and the most serious immediate result is usually severe pain, minimized by methods explained in the chapter *Medical Care in the Aquatic Environment*.

Jellyfish

Most jellyfish are free swimming, colorless, and range in size from a few inches to three feet in diameter. Their appearance on surf beaches tends to be seasonal—spring and summer is when they are most common. Jellyfish feed on small marine animals caught in dangling jellyfish tentacles and stung by nematocysts in those tentacles. Humans are stung in the same way when they come into contact with the tentacles.

Although there are hundreds of species of jellyfish, only a few are considered to pose a serious danger. Perhaps the best known is the box jellyfish, which can cause death to a human within a few minutes after contact. (Fenner & Williamson, 1996) This species, seen most commonly in Australia, is extremely rare in the United States, with only one reported death. (Bengston, Nichols, Schnadig, & Ellis, 1991) There are a wide variety of remedies employed around the world for jellyfish stings. The only treatment recommended by USLA can be found in the chapter on *Medical Care in the Aquatic Environment*.

Portuguese Man-of-War

The Portuguese man-of-war is sometimes confused with the jellyfish, to which it is related. It is a colony of animals called hydroids, which appear to be a single animal. Portuguese man-of-war are found in many warm water areas, but also drift north with warm currents to cooler zones. In marine waters of the United States, they are found most often in the Gulf Stream of the northern Atlantic Ocean.

The Portuguese man-of-war is most readily identified in water by a brilliant blue, pink, or violet float, usually floating on the surface, which is gas filled and bladder-like. The float is typically about two to eight inches in length. Atop the float is a crest which functions somewhat like a sail, allowing the man-of-war to move with the wind. Hanging below are tentacles which serve the same function as in jellyfish, and which have a similar stinging effect on humans.

Marine Mammals

Marine mammals are common visitors to nearshore waters, usually on a seasonal basis. Marine mammals living in coastal waters of the United States include whales, manatees, dolphins, porpoises, seals, sea lions, and sea otters, among others. Under normal conditions, these mammals are not dangerous. When sick, injured, or stressed however, some can present a considerable danger. Consequently, whenever a marine mammal is observed behaving abnormally or is hauled out on a beach, people should be kept at a distance. Many areas have local marine mammal stranding networks capable of responding to a sick or injured animal.

Various federal and state laws protect marine mammals from harm or harassment. The most notable is the Marine Mammal Protection Act, which became law in 1972 and has been amended since.

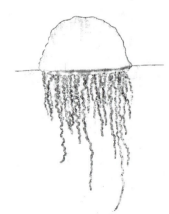

Portuguese Man-of-War

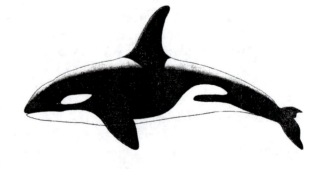

Killer Whale

According to the act, it is unlawful, "… to harass, hunt, capture, or kill, or attempt to harass, hunt, capture or kill any marine mammal." The term "harassment" is defined as any act of pursuit, torment, or even annoyance that has the potential to disturb or injure a marine mammal in the wild.

Lifeguards are sometimes called upon to protect marine mammals being harassed. While local protocols consistent with federal law should be followed, it is generally best to keep the public away from marine mammals and to consult authorities with expertise in handling marine mammal incidents. This will most typically involve agents of the National Marine Fisheries Service, along with state fish and wildlife officers.

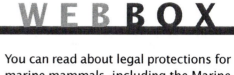

WEBBOX

You can read about legal protections for marine mammals, including the Marine Mammal Protection Act, on the website of the National Marine Fisheries Service website at: *www.nmfs.noaa.gov/*

Venomous Fish

Venomous fish are classified in the family *Scorpaenidae*. There are hundreds of species in the family widely distributed along both coasts of the United States. Most biologists divide these fish into two groups: scorpionfish and stonefish. Stonefish are not found in US waters. Some of the common names for members of the two groups include: lionfish, rockfish, turkeyfish, and sculpin.

These fish are usually bottom feeders. Many are found in or around coral reefs or kelp beds, in which they blend quite well due to their protective coloration. Some species prefer sandy bottom habitats and often lie motionless on the bottom for long periods of time.

The venom of the scorpionfish is stored in special sacs located in hypodermic-like dorsal spines. When a swimmer steps on these fish, venom is injected into the wound. The result is intense, sharp, and shooting pain. Besides pain, the victim may suffer convulsions and nervous disturbances. Although there have been reports of deaths from the scorpionfish sting, none have been confirmed. A few deaths have been confirmed for stonefish. (Williamson, Fenner, Burnett, & Rifkin, 1996)

Other Marine Life and Hazards

There are a host of other marine organisms capable of inflicting injury to humans. Some of these include barnacles, crabs, marine worms, coral, sea urchins, marine shells, eels, catfish, and sea turtles. Due to the limited distribution of many of these animals and the limited danger they represent, only a few are covered here.

Coral

Coral can cause cuts, abrasions, welts, pain, and itching. Severe reactions are unusual.

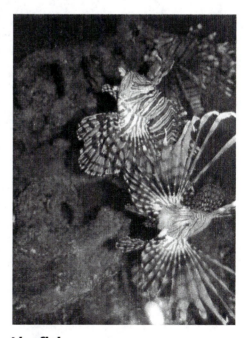

Lionfish
Credit: Dave Foxwell

Sea Urchins

Sea urchins are spiny marine invertebrates, found in rocky crevices in the intertidal area. Urchin wounds are usually sustained when people step on urchin spines. The spines from these creatures are equipped with multiple venom organs. They can penetrate the skin, even through protective clothing, to cause a wound with intense burning sensations followed by redness, swelling, and aching. More severe reactions to urchin wounds include weakness, loss of body sensation, facial swelling, and irregular pulse. Rare cases involving paralysis and respiratory distress have occurred.

Mollusks

Barnacles, mussels, oysters, and other mollusks can cause lacerations that are easily infected.

Sea Snakes

Certain species of sea snakes can bite. Toxic signs, appearing within twenty minutes, can include malaise, anxiety, euphoria, muscle spasm, respiratory problems, convulsions, unconsciousness, and all signs of shock.

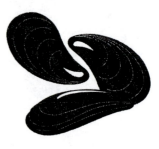

Mussel

Kelp

Kelp is a leafy seaweed, which can grow in water as deep as 60 feet and beyond. Kelp attaches itself to rocks on the bottom and grows upward to the surface. It is common in some areas of California. Kelp is home to many species of marine life and attracts scuba divers. The hazard posed by kelp is entanglement, particularly of scuba divers whose protruding equipment may become wrapped in the kelp. A panicked diver may drown or abandon underwater breathing apparatus and shoot for the surface, producing diving related injuries. The best way to avoid this outcome is good dive training, use of the buddy system while diving, and a dive knife. Treatment of scuba related injury is addressed in the chapter on *Scuba Related Illness and Treatment*.

Non-Native Marine Plants

A variety of problems are created in saltwater areas of the United States by non-native plants. The problems they present can be quite serious. For example, *Caulerpa taxifolia* is a weed native to tropical waters which became popular with people keeping home aquariums. According to Woodfield (2002), it was released into the Mediterranean Sea and within a decade covered over 11,000 acres of water. This weed was discovered in Southern California in 2000 and a major eradication effort was commenced, out of concern that the weed could quickly overwhelm natural aquatic species and prevent recreational activities. Examples such as this one are a result of problems throughout the world when species are transported from one area to another, sometimes with disastrous effects. Lifeguards can be a key defense by noting and reporting sightings to the proper authorities for eradication.

Freshwater Life

Although the number of animal species capable of inflicting harm on swimmers is much larger in saltwater than in freshwater, lifeguards at lakes, rivers, and ponds should take the time during their training to become familiar with local species and assess the possible risks to visitors. Some of the types of potentially dangerous freshwater aquatic life are listed here.

Leeches

Leeches are bloodsucking worms. They typically have a flattened, segmented body with a sucker at both ends, used to bore into flesh and draw out blood. Leeches are found in many freshwater bodies throughout the United States. Although leeches are not life threatening, the presence of a leech on a person usually evokes a strong emotional response and requests for assistance.

Snapping Turtles

Several species of turtles frequent the freshwater bodies of the United States. Most pose no danger whatsoever. One type of turtle that may present limited concern is the snapping turtle. These turtles have a rough shell and powerful jaws. Although most are not particularly dangerous, some species have been known to deliver painful bites to people who knowingly or unintentionally corner or trap them. Lifeguards should become familiar with the turtles specific to their area and which, if any, display aggressive behavior. Lifeguards can then work to minimize possible confrontations between them and humans. With this knowledge, lifeguards can also reassure those who may become needlessly concerned.

Mussels

Freshwater mussels are bivalve mollusks found in many areas of the United States. These mussels usually have a dark, elongated shell and dwell on the bottom in the mud. The edges of their shells can be very sharp and lacerate the feet of beach visitors. This is particularly likely in the case of half-shells from dead mussels.

Zebra Mussels

An unusual problem in the Great Lakes, as well as the Mississippi River and its tributaries, is posed by zebra mussels. While not a serious health hazard, aside from lacerations, zebra mussels propagate at a high rate and are said to pose a multi-billion dollar threat to drinking water supplies, native species, and shipping. These barnacle-like mussels are the only freshwater mollusks that attach themselves to solid objects.

According to the US Geological Survey, zebra mussels originated in the Balkans, Poland, and the former Soviet Union. They are believed to have been introduced into the US through ballast water in ships. Zebra mussels look like small clams with a yellowish and/or brownish D shaped, striped shell. They can grow up to two inches long, but most are under an inch in length. Sightings of zebra mussels should be reported to state fish and wildlife departments.

Fish

Although many species of fish are found throughout freshwater bodies of the United States, few pose any threat to swimmers. Some areas report problems with different species of catfish due to their tactile barbs, but injuries involving fish usually occur when people fishing remove them from the hook.

Snakes

Some types of water snakes or snakes that travel on water can be dangerous or poisonous, particularly in warmer climates. Snake problems are regional in nature and should be addressed through local training programs.

Other Reptiles

Some species of reptiles can prove dangerous to beach visitors, particularly in the South. Alligators, for example, can be extremely dangerous in a freshwater body that also includes a swimming beach.

Semi-Aquatic Animals

Semi-aquatic animals are animals that, while not adapted to living underwater, spend a great portion of their time in the water environment. Examples of semi-aquatic animals include beavers, otters, muskrats, and various species of waterfowl.

Most of these animals will pose no threat to swimmers at freshwater beaches, as they usually actively avoid contact with humans. There may be situations, however, when a semi-aquatic animal approaches or even enters a swim area unsuspectingly. Waterfowl may be drawn into a swim area when visitors attempt to feed them. While waterfowl are not usually dangerous, they may be hosts to various parasites that can cause conditions in visitors like *swimmer's itch*. This occurs when water with the parasites that infest waterfowl dries on the skin of humans. It can cause an allergic reaction that primarily involves itching and redness. The best avoidance measures are to keep swimmers away from waterfowl and to encourage those who swim in such areas to wash themselves thoroughly immediately upon leaving the water.

Non-Native Freshwater Plants

As is the case in the marine environment, non-native weeds have been introduced into the freshwater environment, sometimes causing serious environmental impacts that may close aquatic areas to recreation. One of these, *Hydrilla vericillata* has infested aquatic areas throughout the United States. Like *Caulerpa taxifolia,* it was apparently spread through use in aquariums, water from which may have been dumped into lakes. Lifeguards are a frontline resource in identifying the presence of these weeds, reporting them, and discouraging the dumping of aquaria into the waters they protect.

People

In closing this overview of aquatic life, some mention must be made of the impact of people. While people are visitors to the aquatic environment rather than part of it, the presence of people can create or intensify environmental problems. For example, people may litter, discharge wastes into the water, leave fires burning on the beach, or bury hot coals in the sand. They may annoy, provoke, or injure wildlife. They may underestimate environmental conditions and place themselves or other people in danger through actions like placing a beach umbrella in the sand on a windy day.

Lifeguards are seen by many as aquatic park rangers, whether or not they have actual enforcement authority. This image should be used to help educate beachgoers about the aquatic environment and to encourage them to leave it as they have found it so that others may enjoy it too. Some beach areas employ a maxim worth repeating to beach users throughout the world: "Leave Only Footprints."

Chapter Summary

In this chapter, we have learned that a wide variety of aquatic life can impact humans, just as humans can impact aquatic life. We have learned that the danger of sharks, though they are greatly feared, is minimal. We have also learned about the types of sharks involved in shark bites and the areas where different types of sharks are more common. In addition to sharks, we have learned about the many

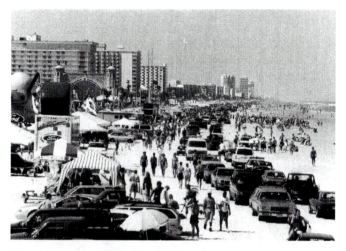

Cars are permitted on Daytona Beach in Florida.
Credit: Mike Hensler

types of other fish, mammals, mollusks, reptiles, and jellyfish that can injure humans, most in a minor way that is easily treated. We have learned about the problem of infestations, both of plants and animals, transported to the U.S. from other areas of the world. And we have learned about the impact people can have on the beach environment.

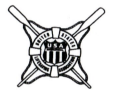

Discussion Points

- What types of sharks frequent beach areas with which you are familiar?
- Why do reports of shark attacks, though very infrequent, provoke so much public interest?
- Why would great white shark bites be more likely to cause death than some other shark bites?
- What advice could you provide to beach users about avoiding envenomation by a stingray?
- What part of the jellyfish causes stinging?
- Why do you think certain types of marine mammals are protected by federal law?
- What are some ways to protect from infestations caused by non-native aquatic plants?
- What are some actions of humans you have observed that negatively impacted the beach environment?

References

Bengston K., Nichols M. M., Schnadig, V., & Ellis, M. D. (1991). Sudden death in a child following jelly-fish envenomation by Chiropsalmus quadrumanus: case report and autopsy findings. *Journal of the American Medical Association, 266,* 1404–1406.

Brewster, B. C., Burgess, G. H., Gallagher, T., Gould, R., Hensler, M., & Wernicki, M. D., P. (2002). United States Lifesaving Association position statement—shark bite prevention and response. Huntington Beach, California: United States Lifesaving Association.

Burgess, G. H. (1994). Personal correspondence with the editor.

Fenner P. J., Williamson J. A., & Skinner R. A. 1989. Fatal and non-fatal stingray envenomation. *Medical Journal of Australia, 151,* 621–625.

Fenner P. J. & Williamson J. A. (1996) Worldwide deaths and severe envenomation from jellyfish stings. *Medical Journal of Australia, 165,* 658–661.

International Shark Attack File (2003a). Retrieved January 16, 2003 from the World Wide Web: *www.flmnh.ufl.edu/fish/Sharks/ISAF/ISAF.htm*

International Shark Attack File (2003b). Shark attacks in perspective. Retrieved January 16, 2003 from the World Wide Web: *www.flmnh.ufl.edu/fish/Sharks/Attacks/perspect.htm*

Knight J. (1989). Obituary: Andonis Neofitou, better known as Anthony Newly. *South Pacific Underwater Medicine Society Journal, 19,* 197–198

Liggins J. B. (1939). An unusual bathing fatality. *New Zealand Medical Journal, 38,* 27–29

Rathjen W. F. & Halstead B. W. (1969). Report on two fatalities due to stingrays. *Toxicon, 6,* 301–302.

Williamson J. A., Fenner P. J., Burnett J., & Rifkin J. (Eds.). (1996). *Venomous and poisonous marine animals: a medical and biological handbook.* Sydney, Australia. New South Whales University Press.

Woodfield, Rachel (2002). Noxious seaweed found in Southern California coastal waters. San Diego, California: Merkel and Associates.

Chapter 8
Weather

In this chapter, you will learn about weather. While weather produces wind and surf, as explained in the chapter on *The Surf Beach*, it produces a number of other threats to public safety as well, including storms, lightning, waterspouts, fog, wind, floods, and temperature variations. The sun itself creates a hazard. In this chapter you will learn how to anticipate adverse weather conditions and to protect beach users from their impacts.

CHAPTER EXCERPT

Lifeguards should be aware of the weather forecast for the coming day and for the next week. When will the rain end? How rough will the waves be? What time tonight will a cold front drive thunderstorms to the coast? Will the wind be a problem? What time is fog likely to form? The answers are not only valuable to public safety, but also to provide information to beachgoers.

Trouble from the sky! The beach is a unique boundary between land and water. Severe weather can strike suddenly and may have devastating consequences. This threat is exacerbated by the fact that people in a recreational setting sometimes ignore obvious signs of threatening weather until it is too late. At that point, panic and injury may occur when people run for cover or are injured by lightning, high winds, and the like. Prudent lifeguards take steps to anticipate adverse weather conditions, so that they can protect beachgoers, and they develop action plans for reasonably anticipated problems related to weather.

The National Weather Service (NWS) exists to predict weather, providing forecasts throughout the United States. These forecasts are disseminated through the news media, over the Internet, and via a variety of other means. Lifeguards should be aware of the weather forecast for the coming day and for the next week. When will the rain end? How rough will the waves be? What time tonight will a cold front drive thunderstorms to the coast? Will the wind be a problem? What time is fog likely to form? The answers are not only valuable to public safety, but also to provide information to beachgoers.

LearnMore

You can quickly acquire a broad understanding of weather by reading, *The Weather Book,* a richly illustrated text by Jack Williams, published by Vintage Books (2nd Revision July 1997)

In addition to forecast information, it is useful to be familiar with the local climate—for your sake as well as for visitors who will ask you questions. How hot does it usually get around here? What is the usual water temperature? Which month is the most threatening for hurricanes or tornados or waterspouts? During the day, when does the sea breeze usually begin or end? People will want to know.

Weather predictions are just that—predictions. There is no certainty these predictions will prove accurate. NWS maintains a system of mechanical and human monitoring systems for real-time feedback. Those reports, in addition to updated weather predictions, are broadcast on the National Oceanic and Atmospheric Administration's *NOAA Weather Radio System.* This system can electronically trigger properly equipped weather radios to sound an alarm when NWS issues *severe weather warnings.* A weather radio doesn't cost much, and it pays for itself many times over.

The most direct source of information on local weather conditions comes not from the prognostications of meteorologists, but from you, the lifeguard. By monitoring conditions closely, lifeguards can learn to anticipate likely weather outcomes. Certain cloud formations may portend imminent lightning, for example. Simple weather monitoring can be accomplished with visual observation and use of a barometer. Keep an eye to the sky. As public safety professionals, lifeguard reports to NWS of unusual weather are extremely valuable. Contact your local NWS office to schedule training on local weather conditions and severe weather reporting. Your observations, quickly communicated to NWS, and via NWS to the general public, can be critical to the safety of thousands.

To help beach visitors avoid injury from storms lifeguards can:

- Keep abreast of current weather predictions
- Use a weather radio for updated information
- Monitor weather conditions to help anticipate storms
- Warn beach visitors of impending storms
- Advise and assist visitors in reacting to approaching storms

Frontal Storms

The atmosphere flows across the planet in waves of colder and warmer air, with varying concentrations of water vapor (humidity). When a wave of colder air invades, the leading edge is called a *cold front,* a term first used in weather at the time of World War I. As with clashing armies, the most dramatic results often occur near the advancing front. One result may be lines of thunderstorms as tall as 50,000 feet with updrafts of 100 MPH and freezing temperatures at high altitude. Warm front behavior is similar, but usually a warm southern surge carries more moisture, and the transition is slower and wetter—the "takeover" weather is not as violent.

The dangers of storms associated with fronts are obvious to anyone who has experienced them. Sudden torrential rain and sometimes hail, lightning, severe downburst winds, tornadoes and waterspouts can occur. In many cases, frontal storms appear unexpectedly, taking beach visitors by surprise. The lifeguard, however, must be aware and ready.

Other Storms

While frontal storms often blow through an area in less than 3 hours, weather associated with large low pressure systems (atmospheric whirlpools of varying intensity) can settle in for a longer period. These events are usually well forecast and will affect beach operations mostly by keeping people away. However, the beach itself may be impacted by rain and wind causing heavy surf, rip currents, high water, beach erosion, and possible storm surge flooding.

A hurricane is a powerful atmospheric whirlpool (low pressure system) that forms to exhaust the heat of the summer tropical ocean skyward. If NWS issues a hurricane watch or warning for the coast, beaches are normally

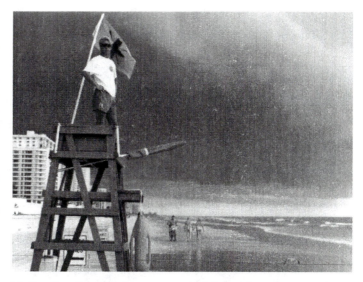

Lightning threatens as a storm approaches.
Credit: Mike Hensler

closed, contingency plans go into effect, and everyone waits with anticipation to learn the result. However, a distant hurricane may also be dangerous. Although the storm may be 1000 miles off the coast with no change in the local weather, long period waves generated by the storm arrive on storm-facing beaches, causing dangerous rip currents and powerful surf. These conditions may surprise beach visitors expecting water conditions to reflect the local weather. Surfers and swimmers may be overcome by the unexpected power of the waves, and pedestrians may be swept into the water.

Lightning

Lightning is a giant, violent electric spark from a thunderstorm that instantly heats the air in its path to about 50,000 degrees Fahrenheit, which is hotter than the surface of the sun. The spark makes the first noise heard close to the strike. Thunder, which can be heard at a greater distance, is the sound of the exploding superheated air in lightning's path. It is estimated that 15 to 40 million lightning strokes hit the ground each year in the United States.

Lightning is the fourth leading cause of death from severe weather incidents. During the 10 year period ending in 2001, an average 52 fatalities per year were attributed to lightning. (National Weather Service, 2002a) Most people killed by lightning are outside in open areas, such as beaches. Florida leads the nation in lightning caused deaths with about 10 a year—almost twice as many as any other state. Conversely, Hawaii and California average less than one lightning-related death per year. More than two-thirds of lightning caused deaths occur in June, July, and August. (Baker, O'Neill, Ginsburg, & Li, 1992)

Cumulonimbus clouds, commonly known as thunderheads are the tall and sometimes anvil shaped clouds that produce thunder and lightning, as well as heavy rain, strong wind and sometimes hail and tornadoes. Their formation near the beach

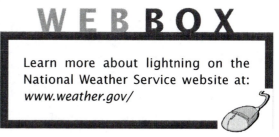

WEBBOX

Learn more about lightning on the National Weather Service website at: *www.weather.gov/*

Thunder Rule: Remember, if you can hear thunder, you can be hit by lightning, even if the storm is not overhead.

should be monitored closely. If you see lightning, the distance between you and the lightning strike can be estimated by timing the interval between the flash and the arrival of thunder. Sound travels through the air at about 1000 ft/second or about one mile every five seconds, but light travels almost instantaneously. The National Weather Service recommends the *30/30 Rule:* When you see lightning, count the time in seconds until you hear thunder. If it is 30 seconds or less, the storm is within six miles. Take shelter. (Franklin, 2002) As the time between observed lightning and audible thunder narrows, the storm is approaching. If only four seconds pass, the strike was 4000 feet distant—less than a mile away. The next strike could be on your beach. Once shelter is taken, under the 30/30 Rule NWS recommends that people remain sheltered until 30 minutes after the last observation of lightning. "Don't be fooled by sunshine or a blue sky!" (Franklin, 2002)

Lifeguards in areas heavily impacted by lightning strikes, particularly Florida lifeguards, should develop contingency plans for responding to lightning storms. Since lightning tends to strike the highest point in an open area, during these storms lifeguards should descend from towers or stands which are not built to protect occupants from lightning. Swimmers and beachgoers may be advised to leave the beach and seek shelter in automobiles or buildings. Static charge precedes a lightning strike. According to the National Weather Service (2002b), "If you feel your skin tingle or your hair stands on end, squat low to the ground on the balls of your feet. Place your hands on your knees with your head between them. Make yourself the smallest target possible, and be sure to minimize your contact with the ground!"

Devices to automatically detect lightning strikes were first developed in the 1970s. Information from antennae that detect radio frequency pulses of lightning and vector the locations, can be sent to computers and even hand-held devices. Satellites also track lightning strikes. Many areas, particularly in areas of high lightning activity, have policies whereby outdoor activities will be terminated in case of lightning strikes detected within a certain radius, particularly if the strikes are moving toward the affected location.

Waterspouts

Waterspouts are tornadoes over water. Near the beach they may form during violent thunderstorm events, but a less violent form of waterspout may develop on still, sunny summer mornings, off the beach over warm water, similar to dust devils over deserts. Waterspouts pose a direct threat to boats and aircraft, and they may come ashore and threaten beach users. The primary danger is flying debris, so shelter and protection should be sought if it appears that a waterspout may come ashore. Lifeguards should report sightings immediately to the local National Weather Service office so that appropriate advisories can be issued.

Fog

Fog is cloudiness that forms near the earth's surface. Fog can result from several situations that cause humid air to cool to its dew point, so that water vapor condenses into tiny droplets. In fog, visibility is lost, leaving the lifeguard without the most basic tool for identifying persons in distress. Swimmers

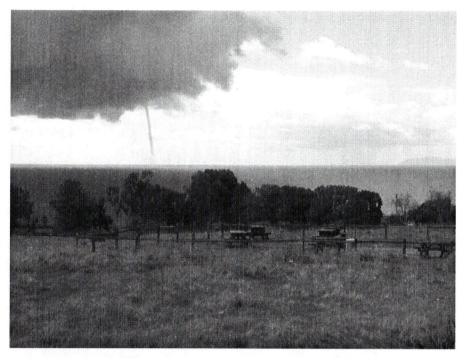

A waterspout offshore.

Credit: Ken Kramer

and surfers may become disoriented and panic. Boaters may inadvertently run aground, threatening those aboard and any swimmers in the area.

Like some other weather conditions, fog may not be a major management problem, simply because it will keep people away from the beach; but in some areas, fog will not dissuade surfers and other beach enthusiasts from water recreation. It may also arrive suddenly and unexpectedly, surprising those in the water.

The drowning prevention work of lifeguards depends upon the ability of lifeguards to become aware of victims in distress and to respond to that distress. When fog conditions prevent surveillance, some lifeguard agencies close the beach and remove people from the water. Others employ patrol procedures along the shoreline in vehicles or on foot, listening for distress cries. This is a particularly important procedure in areas with high boating traffic. Without regular fog patrols, serious accidents can occur in close proximity to lifeguard stations with lifeguard personnel left totally unaware.

Wind

Wind plays an important role in the generation of waves at all types of beaches, inland and coastal; but wind also affects beach operation in other ways. Strong winds may blow beach sand, causing discomfort and injuries to visitors. Wind, particularly sudden gusts of wind, can blow beach umbrellas over, which occasionally results in surprisingly serious injuries. Wind can blow balls and other floating objects away from swimmers, causing them to chase these objects into deeper water, from which they are unable to return. Offshore winds can literally blow people on flotation devices away from the beach.

Temperature

Air temperature at the beach may place even healthy visitors at risk of heat-related illness, especially when there is little shade. Extreme heat is the number one severe weather related killer in the United States, with 219 deaths per year from 1992–2001. (National Weather Service, 2002a) Although heat-related illness is a particular problem in high temperature conditions, it is also common at resort areas where visitors are not acclimated to local weather. Heat cramps, heat exhaustion, and heat stroke are possible outcomes that lifeguards may be required to treat. Heat also affects lifeguards, who should protect themselves from the sun and keep weil hydrated.

Cold and hypothermia are another danger. Cold water removes heat from the body 25 times faster than cold air. Local climate, water depth, and prevailing ocean currents can keep water very cold. Although hypothermia is generally thought to be a problem only at beaches in the northern latitudes, water under 70 degrees Fahrenheit is considered by some medical experts to be cold water. Many lakes, rivers, bays, and surf beaches in warmer climates have water temperatures below this temperature. Several factors will determine the extent of the effects of cold water on swimmers, including immersion time, relative air temperature, and wind.

The immediate effects of sudden immersion in water below 60°F can be a debilitating, short duration (approximately 2–3 min), reflex response called *cold shock*. This response includes life-threatening respiratory and cardiovascular effects. The respiratory effect involves quick onset (<30 seconds) uncontrollable rapid breathing, which impairs breath holding and facilitates aspiration of water (which can lead to drowning). The cardiovascular response involves an immediate constriction (closure) of the blood vessels near the surface of the body, an increase in heart rate, and a surge in blood pressure. These factors may lead to incapacitation from a cardiovascular accident, such as heart attack or stroke, or death from drowning following aspiration. (Golden & Tipton, 2002)

After about three minutes, the initial effects of sudden cold-water immersion decline. Thereafter, in those whose airway is clear of the water, progressive whole body cooling occurs, leading to a gradual fall in deep body temperature (hypothermia). Before a significant level of hypothermia develops however, there is a progressive cooling of the muscles and joints in the exposed limbs through shivering and stiffening. This impairs locomotion and thus swimming performance, which is likely to lead to drowning before a life-threatening level of hypothermia develops, unless the victim is wearing a life-jacket (PFD) capable of keeping the airway clear of the water. (Tipton M.J., Eglin C., Gennser M., & Golden F., 1999) This impairment of locomotion also impedes the victim's ability to assist in the rescue effort.

One very rare complication of contact with cold water is *cold urticaria*. This condition is an allergy-like reaction to contact with cold water, as well as other sources of cold (Bentley, 1993). Within minutes, the skin may become itchy, red, and swollen. Fainting, very low blood pressure, and shock-like symptoms can present.

Cold temperatures can also produce ice. While most open water lifeguards are not on duty during periods that ice is present, one of the most challenging types of open water rescue involves the rescue of persons who have fallen through the ice. The chapter on *Special Rescues* includes information on ice rescue.

Floods

Floods, particularly flash floods, come second after heat as extreme weather killers in the U.S. From 1972 to 2001 there were an average 127 deaths per year from flooding. (National Weather Service, 2002b) While flooding is not typically a threat to beach areas, lifeguards are often called upon to assist in flood rescues due to their aquatic skills and rescue equipment. Some lifeguard swiftwater rescue teams, such as the San Diego Lifeguard River Rescue Team, are essential components of local flood disaster response.

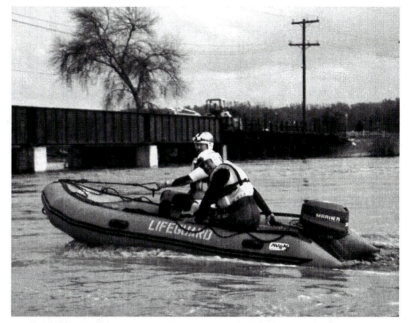

People are most often caught in flood waters when they try to cross apparent low points in vehicles or on foot. They may become stranded or swept downstream. Floodwaters are extremely hazardous, perhaps even more so than heavy surf conditions because flood waters are relentless—there's no lull between sets of waves—and the water level may rise dramatically in a very short period of time.

Credit: Ken Kramer

Rescuers are also seriously endangered by floodwaters. Each year, rescuers are killed in attempts to effect rescues in swiftwater flood conditions. Lifeguards who lack special training in swiftwater rescue should make every effort to avoid making a rescue that requires use of a boat or actual entry into the swiftwater environment. Instead, methods which allow rescuers to remain onshore should be utilized. For a further discussion of flood rescue considerations and basic techniques, please refer to the chapter entitled, *Special Rescues*.

Sun

Long term exposure to the sun has been demonstrated to cause accelerated aging of the skin and is believed to enhance the potential for contracting skin cancer. The most immediate danger from the sun comes from overexposure, which affects both beach visitors and lifeguards. Sunburns can range from minor redness of the skin to serious burns, requiring medical care. Any significant exposure to the sun results in some degree of damage that is cumulative. Problems with overexposure to the sun are not restricted to the more southern latitudes. Anywhere the sun is shining, there is the potential for injury from overexposure.

The problem of overexposure is compounded by the belief of some that a sunburn is a normal part of the beach recreation experience and that one or two episodes of overexposure each beach season will not be harmful. Indeed, some visitors accept and even look forward to a sunburn as tangible evidence that they enjoyed themselves at the beach. Lifeguards should monitor their beach crowd for persons who appear to be overexposed, paying particular attention

WEBBOX

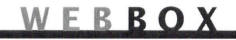

You can read about the value of sunscreen on the website of the U.S. Food and Drug Administration at: *www.fda.gov*

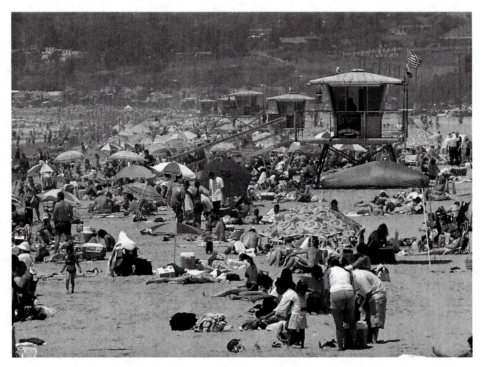

Credit: Nick Steers

to people with light skin, along with small children and babies who must rely on their parents to protect them. Dermatologists have found that sunburns, particularly when sustained by young children, can greatly increase the potential for contracting skin cancer later in life. Lifeguards can recommend use of sunscreen, shade, and protective clothing, for example.

Lifeguards are particularly susceptible to sun related injury. For a full discussion of this issue, please refer to the chapter entitled, *Lifeguard Health and Safety*.

Chapter Summary

In this chapter, we have learned about storms and how they form. We have learned about the hazard presented by lightning, and how lifeguards can protect themselves and beach users. We have learned about waterspouts, fog, wind, temperature variations, and flooding. We have also learned about the impacts of the sun itself. With a better understanding of weather, we are better prepared for our role as lifeguards.

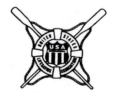

Discussion Points

- What types of frontal storms occur in beach areas you have visited?
- What are some examples of shelters from lightning?
- What outcomes might be expected when fog obscures the water?
- How might wind, associated with storms or waterspouts, impact the safety of beach users?
- How might lifeguards be affected by hot temperatures or cold water?
- What factors make flooding particularly dangerous?
- How can lifeguards protect themselves and beachgoers from the effects of the sun?

References

Baker, S. P., O'Neill, B., Ginsburg, M. J., & Li, Guohua (1992). *The Injury Fact Book* (second edition). New York: Oxford University Press

Bentley II, Burton (1993). Cold-induced urticaria and angioedema: diagnosis and management. *American Journal of Emergency Medicine, 11,* 1: 43–46.

Franklin, Donna (2002). Lightning, the underrated killer. National Weather Service. Retrieved March 5, 2003 from the World Wide Web: *www.lightningsafety.noaa.gov/overview.htm*

Golden & Tipton (2002). *Essentials of sea survival.* Champaign, IL: Human Kinetics.

National Weather Service (2002a). 62-year list of severe weather fatalities. Retrieved January 19, 2003 from the World Wide Web: *weather.gov/om/severe_weather/62yrstat.pdf*

National Weather Service (2002b). Lightning—the underrated killer. Retrieved January 20, 2003 from the World Wide Web: *www.crh.noaa.gov/fsd/lightning.htm*

Tipton M. J., Eglin C., Gennser M., & Golden F. (1999). Immersion deaths and deterioration in swimming performance in cold water. *Lancet, 354,* 626–629.

Chapter 9
Drowning

In this chapter, you will learn about death resulting from drowning, which lifesavers throughout the world seek to prevent. We will provide statistics related to populations at high risk of drowning, as well as activities that are more likely to result in drowning. You will learn about the stages of drowning and the pathophysiology of drowning.

CHAPTER EXCERPT

Studies have demonstrated that the actions of lifeguards in rescue and resuscitation of drowning victims are the most important link in the chain of survival. In fact, the outcome of drowning patients is usually more dependent upon the timeliness and effectiveness of the initial rescue and resuscitation efforts than on the quality of hospital care.

Drowning is a leading cause of accidental death, both in the United States and worldwide. In the year 2000, over 3,400 people were reported to have died in the U.S. as a result of drowning, which made it the fourth leading cause of accidental death for all age groups. (Miniño, Arias, Kochanek, Murphy, & Smith, 2002) Many more people died due to complications related to drowning, long after the initial accident. Moreover, death from drowning is only the tip of the iceberg. It has been demonstrated that for every 10 children who die by drowning, 140 are treated in emergency rooms and 36 are admitted for further treatment in hospitals. (Wintemute, Kraus, Teret, & Wright, 1988) Those who survive drowning incidents are sometimes left with permanent disabilities of grave severity, including paralysis and irreparable brain damage. In addition to great psychological trauma, both to victims and their families, there are significant costs. Mael, Seck, and Russell estimated the average cost of supporting a person who survives, but is incapacitated by a drowning incident at more than $5 million. (1998)

What is drowning? The word *drowning* can be used to refer to a past event (e.g., she died by drowning) or an action in progress (e.g., he's drowning.) Experts at the World Congress on Drowning 2002 developed the following definition: "Drowning is the process of experiencing respiratory impairment from submersion/immersion in liquid." Drowning is an event that may result in death, or may be interrupted by timely rescue or effective medical care.

WEBBOX

A variety of information lifeguards can use to inform the public about drowning avoidance measures can be found in the Public Education section of: *www.usla.org*

Drowning takes place in a wide variety of environments. Wherever there is liquid, there is the danger of drowning. In fact, infants have died by drowning in buckets. In a study of people under age 20, in cases where a site was listed, it was found that 47% of drowning deaths occurred in freshwater (rivers, lakes, ponds, etc.), 32% in pools, 9% in the home (bathtubs, etc.), and 4% in seawater. According to the study, "Infants were most likely to drown in bathtubs, young children in swimming pools, and older children and adolescents in natural bodies of freshwater." (Brenner, Trumble, Smith, Kessler, & Overpeck, 2001)

Previous chapters of this text have described several environmental hazards that contribute to drowning; but not all drownings can be attributed solely to environmental hazards. Human factors such as swimming skill, aquatic safety knowledge, poor judgment, social pressures, trauma, inexperience, pre-existing illness, and intoxication are substantial contributors. Lifeguards may believe that they have little control over these factors, but that is not the case.

The primary role of lifeguards is drowning prevention. This should be viewed in the broadest sense. If lifeguards wait until people visit the aquatic area for which they are responsible, significant preventive opportunities are lost. If, on the other hand, lifeguards work in their communities to promote water safety, drowning prevention can be addressed well before patrons visit an aquatic area, whether or not lifeguards are present. The chapter entitled *Preventive Lifeguarding* provides extensive recommendations on prevention strategies. Of course, effective supervision of aquatic areas by lifeguards, preventive actions at the site, timely rescue, and, where needed, effective resuscitation are key measures in the prevention of death by drowning. This is why USLA promotes the provision of lifeguards at aquatic recreation areas and encourages people to *swim near a lifeguard.*

Activities Associated with Drowning

Most deaths from drowning occur in the open water environment. (Dietz & Baker, 1974) They may be associated with a variety of activities. This section covers some of the most common.

Swimming

Non-environmental factors that contribute to swimming deaths include poor swimming ability, alcohol and drugs, peer pressure (taking a dare, impressing friends), and carelessness or lack of good judgment. Environmental factors include currents, waves, drop-offs, and a variety of other contributors. Another factor is acts of attempted rescue, where would-be rescuers reacting to the imminent death of others drown in the rescue attempt. Hyperventilating and trying to swim underwater can lead to shallow water blackout.

Boating

Boating is a very popular pastime in the US, with over 12 million registered boats and thousands of others that are not required to be registered. (U.S. Department of Transportation, 1998) With the popularity of boating comes boating accidents, which occur in the thousands each year. Hundreds of these result in fatalities, 85% of which involve boats that are less than 26 feet in length. (U.S. Department of Transportation, 1998) Approximately 70% of recreational boating deaths are due to drowning, representing close to 20% of all drownings in the US. (U.S. Department of Transportation, 1998) The two primary types of fatal boating accidents are falls overboard and capsizing of the vessel, in that order, not collisions. (U.S. Department of Transportation, 1998) Alcohol use has been determined to be a significant contributing factor in boating accidents, not only due to the possibility that the boat operator will make misjudgments leading to an accident, but also because intoxicated occupants fall overboard and drown. In fact, one study found that 46% of boating fatalities associated with falling overboard occurred when the boat was stationary. (Smith, Keyl, Hadley, Bartley, Foss, Tolbert, & McKnight, 2001) This is why the wearing of a personal flotation device (life jacket) is considered so important as a drowning prevention measure for boaters.

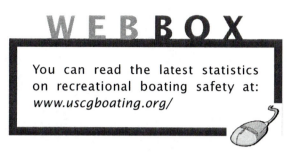

WEBBOX

You can read the latest statistics on recreational boating safety at: *www.uscgboating.org/*

The typical boat operator involved in a boating accident has no formal boating instruction and 40% or more have no more than 100 hours of experience in operation of a boat. Overall, about 90% of all boating fatalities occur on boats where the operator has not completed a boating safety course.

> The United States Lifesaving Association encourages all boaters to take a course in safe boating and encourages the wearing of personal flotation devices by all aboard.

Diving

People who dive and strike the bottom or underwater objects can sustain injuries that incapacitate them, leading to drowning. Trauma may result directly to the victim's head, causing a concussion, fractured skull, or brain hemorrhage. There are an estimated 675 spinal injuries, including deaths, sustained each year in the United States by people who dive from heights or even surface dive into shallow water, striking the bottom or a submerged object. (Think First Foundation, 2000) Over 80% of the victims of spinal cord injury are male and the highest per capita rate of injury occurs between the ages of 16 and 30. (Think First Foundation, 2000) Often, consumption of alcoholic beverages is involved as it inhibits natural fear. Body surfing injuries are similar to diving injuries when the body surfer surfs down the face of the wave and strikes the bottom. A major problem in diving injuries is that the victim may be quickly removed from the water by friends unaware of the spinal injury or lacking training for proper spinal injury management. Information on treating spinal injuries can be found in the chapter *Medical Care in the Aquatic Environment*.

Learn More

Hoag Hospital in Newport Beach, California, offers extensive information about spinal injuries from diving at: *www.hoag.org/projectwipout/ projectwipout.html*

Alcohol Consumption

According to the Centers for Disease Control and Prevention (2002), "Alcohol use is involved in about 25-50% of adolescent and adult deaths associated with water recreation. It is a major contributing factor in up to 50% of drownings among adolescent boys."

Scuba Diving

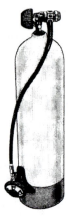

In recent years about 90 recreational scuba diving deaths per year have been reported to the Divers Alert Network. (Divers Alert Network, 1999) Most of these occurred within the United States, but they include some deaths of US citizens traveling abroad. Using 1997 as an example, an additional 17 diving deaths were reported that involved working divers on the job. (Divers Alert Network, 1999)

Most scuba fatalities result from drowning due to panic, entanglement, running out of air, or a heart attack. Typically the diver runs out of air and is unable to surface in time. Florida and California have the highest diver populations and the highest numbers of associated deaths. Well over 900 cases of non-fatal decompression illness are sustained each year among US scuba divers. (Divers Alert Network, 1999) For more information, please see the chapter on *Scuba Related Illness and Treatment.*

Higher Risk Populations

People of all races, ethnicities, and ages, both male and female, are susceptible to drowning. No one is immune. There are however, statistical data indicating that some are more likely to drown than others. These are broad-based statistics though, and no average is true of all members of an identified group. The following are based on studies covering the United States.

Youth

In 2000, drowning was the second leading cause of accidental death for those under 15 years of age and the third leading cause for those 15–35. (Miniño, et al., 2002) On average, 350 small children drown

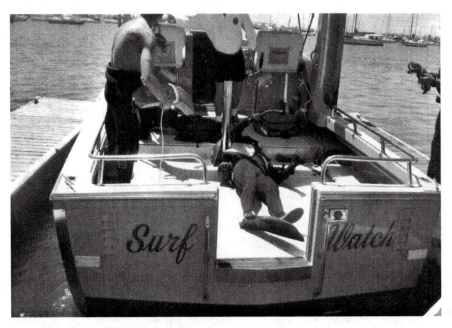

A scuba diving fatality.
Credit: Ken Kramer

each year in swimming pools. Most of these are backyard (residential) swimming pools. Another 2,600 are treated annually in emergency rooms for drowning related problems. (Whitfield, 2000) These drownings typically result from failure to adequately fence off pools and particularly from inadequate supervision by adult guardians. While open water lifeguards have little opportunity to directly intervene in backyard pool drownings, unless they simply happen to be there when the emergency occurs, lifeguards can help raise public awareness of the problem, and thereby help prevent drownings. Back-

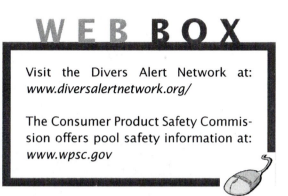

WEB BOX

Visit the Divers Alert Network at: *www.diversalertnetwork.org/*

The Consumer Product Safety Commission offers pool safety information at: *www.wpsc.gov*

yard pools should be surrounded by fences at least four feet high which are enclosed by locking, self-closing gates. If doors from the home enter into the pool area, they should have alarms. Power safety covers are recommended, as well as lifesaving equipment and CPR training for all child guardians. Young children, particularly those unable to swim, should never, ever be left alone anywhere near a pool.

Males

Males drown at a significantly higher rate than females. The ratio of male to female drownings is about 4 to 1. (Centers for Disease Control and Prevention, 2002) Adolescent males, in particular, are highly physically active and known to be relatively frequent risk takers. It is often said that teenage males act as though they are immortal. For example, they are the most likely people at a beach to recklessly dive from significant heights into unknown water or to enter obviously hazardous waters.

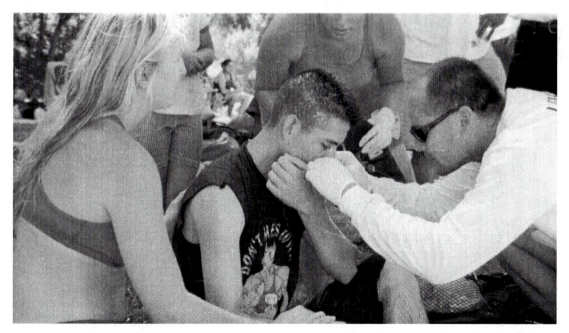

A rescue victim receiving care.
Credit: Dan McCormick

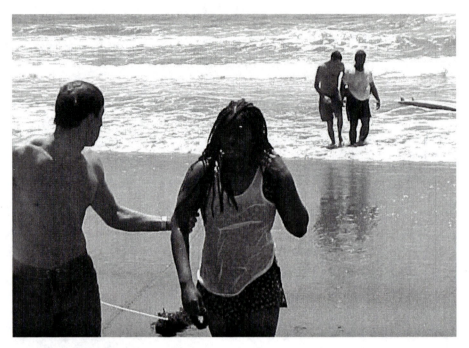

Rescued swimmers.

Credit: Mark Norman

Affluence

Statistics indicate that drowning rates vary inversely with income in the area of residence of drowning victims. (Baker, O'Neill, Ginsburg, & Li, 1992) In other words, people from lower income areas are more frequent drowning victims. This may well be attributable to lack of access to learn-to-swim programs and other aquatic recreation opportunities. Paradoxically however, affluence can also have a negative impact on aquatic safety, as is evidenced by the fact that the small children of backyard pool owners are at relatively high risk of drowning. The CDC reports, "Black children ages 1 through 4 years had a lower drowning rate than white children, largely because drownings in that age group typically occur in residential swimming pools, which are not as accessible to minority children in the United States." (2002)

Race and Ethnicity

A variety of statistical studies have found ethnic and racial differences in drowning rates. Native Americans have the highest rate of drowning in the U.S. Asian Americans and whites have the lowest. (Baker et al., 1992) Nationally, according to the Centers for Disease Control and Prevention (2002), "In 1998, the overall age-adjusted drowning rate for blacks was 1.6 times higher than for whites. Black children ages 5 through 19 years drowned at 2.5 times the rate of whites." In a study to determine why black military recruits were, on average, less capable swimmers than white recruits, Mael (1995) postulated that less access to pools, and particularly the opportunity to learn to swim at a young age, was a major contributing factor. He also noted, with regard to swimming skills, that "This has a number of negative consequences, ranging from lost recreational and employment opportunities to increased risk of drowning."

USLA strongly encourages the greatest possible access to public learn-to-swim programs for purposes of drowning avoidance and equal access to aquatic related employment, including lifeguarding. Barriers to public swimming programs can have both lethal and economic consequences that disproportionately affect segments of the U.S. population.

Epileptics

People with epilepsy are disproportionately likely to drown. Epileptic seizures usually leave victims without control over their motor functions—a deadly circumstance in the water. People with epilepsy should be cautioned to advise lifeguards before swimming and to *wear personal flotation devices* during any activities in or around the water. (Ryan, 1993)

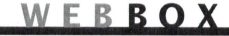

WEBBOX

You can learn more about epilepsy at: *www.epilepsyfoundation.org/*

Drowning Stages

In the open water environment, the drowning process involves three distinct stages which can be interrupted through timely intervention:

1. Distress
2. Panic
3. Submersion

This process is usually progressive, but not always. Either of the two initial stages may be skipped completely depending upon a variety of factors.

Distress

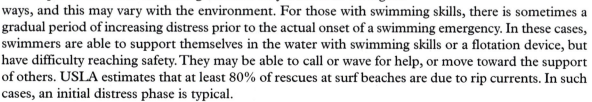

Drowning can occur for a number of reasons. A nonswimmer who is wading may suddenly step into water that is overhead (a drop-off), or may fall from a boat or dock. A poor swimmer may swim off-shore to retrieve a ball or help another person, only to tire and be unable to return to shore. Even a strong swimmer may be overpowered by a rip current or river current. These are just a few examples.

People of different swimming abilities may behave in divergent ways, and this may vary with the environment. For those with swimming skills, there is sometimes a gradual period of increasing distress prior to the actual onset of a swimming emergency. In these cases, swimmers are able to support themselves in the water with swimming skills or a flotation device, but have difficulty reaching safety. They may be able to call or wave for help, or move toward the support of others. USLA estimates that at least 80% of rescues at surf beaches are due to rip currents. In such cases, an initial distress phase is typical.

Some distressed swimmers may not immediately recognize their predicament and may swim against a current without realizing they are making no progress. A distress presentation may last a few seconds or can go on for an extended period of time. As the strength of the swimmer ebbs, the distress presentation will digress to panic if the victim is not rescued or cannot make it to safety. Alert lifeguards on a properly staffed beach are usually able to intervene during the distress phase of the drowning process. In fact, it is not unusual for some victims to protest that they need no assistance because they have yet to feel they are in distress, though it may be clear to the lifeguard that they are in jeopardy.

In-water distress is serious, but this phase of the drowning process does not always occur. For example, some nonswimmers may be completely unable to keep themselves afloat and simply submerge, or a medical condition may render the person immobile. In any case, rapid intervention can ensure that the victim suffers no ill effects and goes on to enjoy the rest of the day.

Panic

A poor swimmer who falls off a flotation device or steps off a drop-off into water that is overhead may immediately enter the panic stage, with no initial distress presentation. Alternatively, the panic stage of the drowning process may progress from the distress stage, as a swimmer loses strength and feels a sense of desperation. In the panic stage, the victim is unable to adequately maintain buoyancy due to fatigue, complete lack of swimming skills, or a physical problem (e.g., cramps).

Nonswimmers in the panic stage have an ineffective kick. The head and face are low in the water, with the chin usually extended to keep the mouth above the surface. Arms flail at the side in a desperate effort to stay afloat. The victim focuses all energy on grabbing breaths of air. In a film depicting actual drowning victims at a tidal, non-surf beach, Pia (1970) branded this the *instinctive drowning*

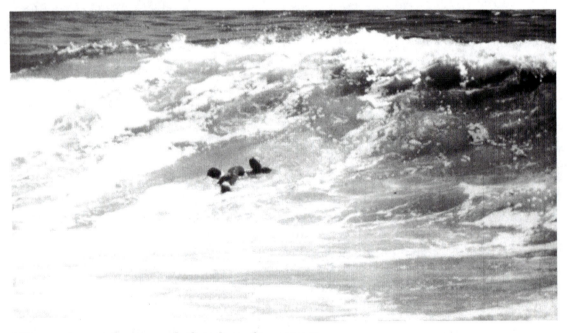

Lifeguard rescuing two victims in a rip current.

Credit: Laguna Beach Lifeguards

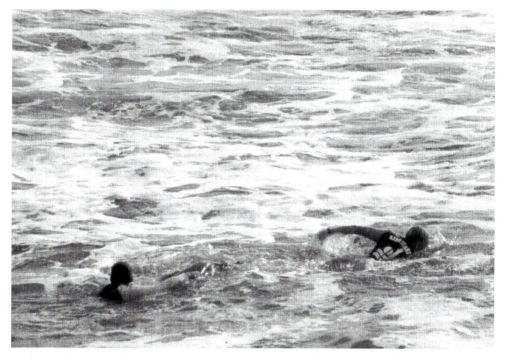

Rescue from a rip current.

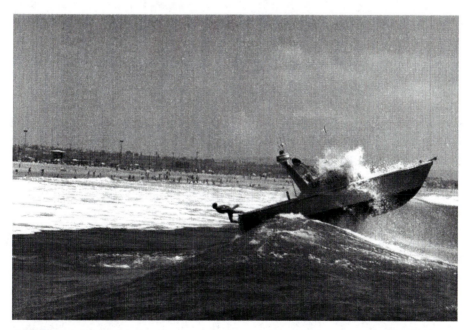

A lifeguard jumps to the rescue from the stern of a rescue boat.
Credit: Ken Kramer

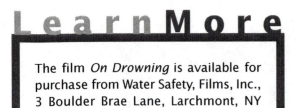

The film *On Drowning* is available for purchase from Water Safety, Films, Inc., 3 Boulder Brae Lane, Larchmont, NY 10538.

response. Persons experiencing this level of distress are unlikely to call for help and nearby swimmers often don't notice them, so alert lifeguards are essential to their safety.

Panicked victims with limited swimming abilities, particularly in a current, may use an ineffective stroke similar to a dog paddle. Lifeguards refer to the appearance of victims in this stage as "climbing out of the hole" or "climbing the ladder." The panic stage rarely lasts long because the victim's actions are largely ineffective and consume great amounts of energy. This is the stage where a victim may grab a nearby swimmer in an effort to stay on the surface and breathe, possibly leading to multiple victims. Some studies have suggested that this stage typically lasts between 10 and 60 seconds; but it can progress almost immediately to submersion unless a rescue is performed, so the lifeguard must react very rapidly.

Submersion

Contrary to common belief, most drowning incidents do not result in a person floating face-down in the water. Even in the enhanced buoyancy provided by seawater, most people without a flotation device who lose their ability to maintain buoyancy, rapidly submerge and sink to the bottom. Aspiration of water, which replaces some of the air in the lungs, contributes to this lack of buoyancy. In freshwater, which provides less buoyancy than sea-

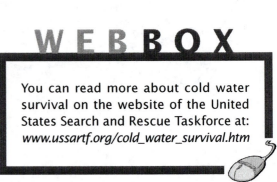

You can read more about cold water survival on the website of the United States Search and Rescue Taskforce at: *www.ussartf.org/cold_water_survival.htm*

water, submersion can be expected to occur more rapidly. Submersion in and of itself is not fatal if the victim is recovered in time and resuscitation is applied as needed, but this can be a tremendously difficult task. Unlike the clear water of the pool environment, open water is often murky and water visibility may be as low as zero. Currents and surf action can move the body a significant distance from the point of initial submersion. Once submersion occurs, the chance of a successful rescue declines dramatically. This is what makes intervention at the distress or panic phase crucial.

Based on the experience of professional open water lifeguards, USLA believes there is a *two minute window* of enhanced opportunity for successful recovery and resuscitation of submerged victims. Thereafter, the chances of successful recovery decline very quickly. In colder waters, successful recoveries have been documented after up to an hour or more of submersion, but these are extremely rare cases and dependent upon the rapid onset of hypothermia.

Pathophysiology of Drowning

In a drowning, breathing typically occurs in fitful gasps on the surface, when possible, and there may be coughing and sputtering as water is inadvertently drawn in with a breath. The inhalation of water into the lungs is known as *water aspiration*, while the swallowing of water into the stomach is *water ingestion*. Both of these usually occur. Victims may attempt to hold their breath to avoid water aspiration. If water gets into their mouth, which is usually unavoidable, they typically swallow it. A significant quantity of water is often ingested and may be vomited later, particularly in case of resuscitation efforts.

Once the victim's airway is underwater, the victim may inhale water, but the larynx will sometimes close reflexively, preventing all but a small amount of water from being aspirated. As is the case on the surface, the victim may swallow significant amounts of water instead. As the victim loses consciousness due to lack of oxygen in the tissues of the body (*hypoxia*), the larynx may relax, allowing more water to enter the lungs. Vomiting may occur secondary to cerebral hypoxia or gastric distension. Without freshly oxygenated blood, the heart will cease functioning. Brain death usually begins in three to six minutes after adequately oxygenated blood stops circulating, although in some very unusual cold water drownings, this may be greatly delayed. In these cold water cases, significant hypothermia occurs which decreases the cerebral requirement for oxygen.

Some believe that in 10-15% of cases, the larynx closes upon initial contact with water and never relaxes, thus preventing water from ever entering the lungs. This has been referred to as *dry drowning*. A review of the research upon which this theory is based however, concluded that there may be no such thing as a dry drowning. Thus, whenever a corpse is recovered from the water, and there is no evidence of water aspiration at autopsy, other causes of acute death must be considered. (Modell, Bellefleur, & Davis, 1999) In any case, treatment of a recovered drowning victim by the lifeguard is the same, whether water has been aspirated or not. If no water was aspirated, and resuscitation is successful, it is likely that the submersion time was less than two minutes, and extensive post resuscitation care is usually not necessary. (Modell, 2003)

Drowning is not simply a case of suffocation. In most cases the lungs are traumatized by aspiration of water. Even if the victim is rescued and revived, this trauma will make it difficult for the lungs to transfer oxygen to the bloodstream and tissues. In addition, the drowning process produces a frothy liquid (pulmonary edema) in the airways. When a drowning victim is recovered, the person is typically experiencing severe hypoxia. Immediate resuscitation efforts are therefore needed, ideally with administration of 100% oxygen and, if possible, positive pressure ventilation. (Orlowski & Szpilman, 2001) For more information on resuscitation, please refer to the chapter on *Medical Care in the Aquatic Environment*.

The effects of freshwater and seawater drowning differ somewhat. In freshwater drowning, water quickly enters the bloodstream through the lungs. If sufficient quantities are aspirated, this can result in dilution of serum electrolyte concentrations. Changes to a level which require specific therapy though, are seen in less than 15% of victims. (Modell, 2003) Spasm or constriction takes place in the bronchi and the tiny sacs known as alveoli, which form the direct link for exchange between air in the lungs and the bloodstream, become unstable or collapse. In seawater drowning, the aspirated seawater is *hypertonic* and can actually draw fluid from the bloodstream into the lungs. On the part of the lifeguard, treatment is the same for both cases.

Studies have demonstrated that the actions of lifeguards in rescue and resuscitation of drowning victims are the most important link in the chain of survival. In fact, the outcome of drowning patients is usually more dependent upon the timeliness and effectiveness of the initial rescue and resuscitation efforts than on the quality of hospital care. (Plueckhahn, 1979)

Automatic external defibrillators (AED) are becoming a common tool of lifeguards. They are primarily intended to correct problems associated with sudden cardiac arrest. AEDs can sometimes stop *ventricular fibrillation*, an uncoordinated beating of the heart. Ventricular fibrillation is rare in submersion victims. (Orlowski & Szpilman, 2001) (Morley, 2002) Most drowning victims have healthy hearts that simply cease to function due to hypoxia. The best approach in treating drowning victims is to prioritize immediate CPR measures, ideally with high flow oxygen. If available, an AED should be used,

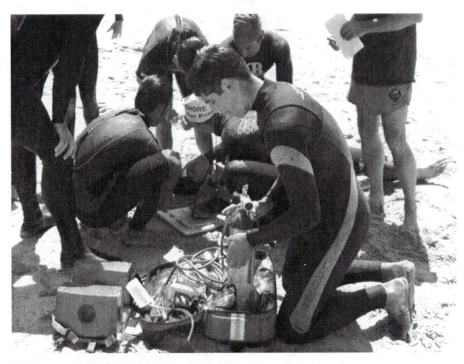

Lifeguards training with oxygen.

Credit: Ken Kramer

in accordance with the manufacturer's instructions, in the relatively unlikely case the victim is experiencing ventricular fibrillation.

Abdominal thrusts (the Heimlich maneuver) should not be used in resuscitation of drowning victims, except in cases that repeated repositioning of the airway suggests a foreign body obstruction (other than water). This maneuver will not remove significant amounts of water from the lungs. It may cause regurgitation and aspiration of stomach contents and other serious complications to resuscitation and recovery of the victim. (American Heart Association, 2000) (Orlowski & Szpilman, 2001)

Sudden Submersion Syndrome

In some cases, people in water are rendered unconscious, disabled, or dead due to situations that may include heart attacks, cardiovascular accidents (strokes), epileptic seizures, head or neck injury, severe trauma, alcohol or drug overdose, cold shock, and other conditions. A victim on the surface suddenly submerges, usually without a struggle. We define this as *sudden submersion syndrome.* Sudden submersion syndrome is particularly difficult to prevent because it typically happens so quickly. The victim may have shown no prior indication of problems and be in a water area with no obvious hazards. The tremendous difficulty involved in spotting a victim of sudden submersion syndrome, particularly with a large beach crowd under observation, makes the importance of effective surveillance all the greater. Even so, sudden submersion syndrome presents a tremendous challenge to the lifeguard because it is not preceded by a distress or panic phase. A type of sudden submersion syndrome that is even more difficult to detect results from *shallow water blackout*. In this case, a person hyperventilates on the sur-

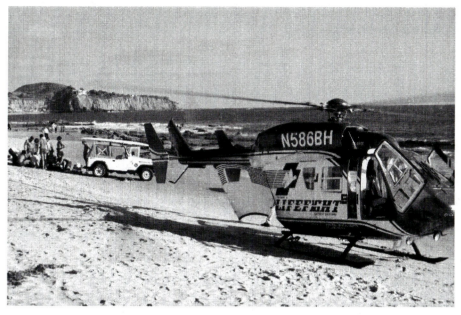

Credit: Ken Kramer

face in an effort to stay underwater for an extended period of time and intentionally submerges, but stays underwater too long and loses consciousness due to cerebral hypoxia. Some drowning victims are first observed when their body is found immobile in the water and, therefore, no history of the preceding events is known.

Delayed Effects

Part of the drowning process involves water aspiration. People who are rescued from drowning (or who rescue themselves) may initially appear to be healthy, but if they have aspirated water or vomitus, they may later suffer serious complications. This is typically due to damage to the lungs and their oxygen exchange capabilities. One possibility is adult respiratory distress syndrome (which can also affect children). ARDS can have a rapid onset and cause death hours or days after the drowning event.

Victims who have been rescued from drowning are often in a state of denial or embarrassed and simply want to walk away. It is very important to carefully evaluate those who appear to have aspirated water for signs and symptoms of water aspiration. Specific guidelines for treatment of drowning victims and for determining whether they should be sent to the hospital for further care can be found in the chapter *Medical Care in the Aquatic Environment.*

Chapter Summary

In this chapter, we have learned about some of the most common activities associated with drowning, including swimming, boating, scuba diving, diving from heights, and consumption of alcohol. We have learned about populations at higher risk of drowning, which include young people in general, males, less affluent people (generally), some members of racial/ethnic groups, and epileptics. We have learned about the classic stages of drowning: distress, panic, and submersion. We have also had an overview of the pathophysiology of drowning.

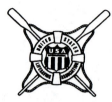

Discussion Points

- Why are some activities more likely than others to result in drowning?
- What factors are likely to cause young males to have a significantly higher drowning rate than young females?
- Why might affluence play a part in drowning?
- What value do you see in understanding the stages of the drowning process?
- How does the pathophysiology of drowning impact appropriate medical aid procedures?
- Why is it important to provide high flow oxygen to a drowning victim?
- What might cause sudden submersion syndrome?

References

American Heart Association (2000). Guidelines 2000 for Cardiopulmonary Resuscitation and Emergency Cardiovascular Care. *Circulation, 102,* 8.

Baker, S. P., O'Neill, B., Ginsburg, M. J., & Li, Guohua (1992). *The Injury Fact Book* (second edition). New York: Oxford University Press.

Brenner, R. A., Trumble, A. C., Smith, G. S., Kessler, E. P., & Overpeck, M. D. (2001). Where children drown, United States 1995. *Pediatrics, 108,* 1: 85–89.

Centers for Disease Control and Prevention (2002). Drowning prevention. Retrieved January 20, 2003 from the World Wide Web: www.cdc.gov/ncipc/factsheets/drown.htm

Dietz, P. E. & Baker, S. P. (1974). Drowning: epidemiology and prevention. *American Journal of Public Health, 64,* 303–312.

Divers Alert Network (1999). *Report on decompression illness and diving fatalities.* Durham, North Carolina: DAN.

International Life Saving Federation Medical Commission (2000). *Who needs further help after rescue from the water.* Leuven, Belgium: International Life Saving Federation.

Mael, F. (1995). Staying afloat: within-group swimming proficiency for whites and blacks. *Journal of Applied Psychology, 80,* 4: 479–490

Miniño, A., Arias, E., Kochanek, K., Murphy, S., & Smith, B. (2002). Deaths: final data for 2000. *National Vital Statistics Reports, 50,* 15. Atlanta, Georgia: Centers for Disease Control and Prevention.

Modell, J. H. (2003). Personal communication with the editor—January 29, 2003.

Modell, J. H., Bellefleur, M., & Davis, J. H. (1999). Drowning without aspiration: is this an appropriate diagnosis? *Journal of Forensic Sciences, 44,* 6:1119–1123.

Morley, P. (2002). Unusual rescue circumstances and considerations. *World Congress on Drowning 2002.* Amsterdam, The Netherlands.

Orlowski, J. P. & Szpilman, D. (2001). Drowning, resuscitation, and reanimation. *Pediatric Clinics of North America, 48,* 3.

Pia, F. (1970). *On Drowning.* Larchmont, New York: Water Safety Films, Inc.

Plueckhahn, V. D., (1979). Drowning: community aspects. *Medical Journal of Australia, 2,* 226–228.

Ryan, C. A. (1993). Drowning deaths in people with epilepsy. *Canadian Medical Association Journal, 148(5),* 781–784.

Smith, G. S., Keyl, P. M., Hadley, J. A., Bartley, C. L., Foss, R. D., Tolbert, W. G., & McKnight, J. (2001). Drinking and recreational boating fatalities. *Journal of the American Medical Association, 286,* 23: 2974–2980.

Think First Foundation (2002). Spinal cord injury. Retrieved January 20, 2003 from the World Wide Web: *www.thinkfirst.org/news/spinalcord.html*

US Department of Transportation (1998). *Boating Statistics—1998.* COMTPUB P16754.12

Whitfield, T. W. (2000). An evaluation of swimming pool alarms. Consumer Product Safety Commission. Retrieved January 20, 2003 from the World Wide Web: *www.cpsc.gov/library/alarm.pdf*

Wintemute, G. J., Kraus, J. F., Teret S. P., & Wright, M. A. (1988). The epidemiology of drowning in adulthood: implications for prevention. *American Journal of Preventive Medicine, 4,* 343–348.

Chapter 10
Preventive Lifeguarding

In this chapter you will learn about the importance of the lifeguard's primary role—prevention. You will learn that there are a wide variety of tools that can be employed to prevent drowning and other accidents from happening. These include public education, rules and regulations, signs and flags, identification of pre-events, taking on-site preventive actions, special operation modes, extended shifts, after hours and post season response plans, maintenance, and even facility design.

CHAPTER EXCERPT

Lifeguards, more than any other providers of public safety, have an ongoing responsibility for accident prevention.

The primary role of many providers of public safety is one of responding to emergencies after they have developed. For example, the primary role of firefighters is often defined as fire suppression. That is, the fire has started and firefighters respond to extinguish it. Responding to emergencies is also an important role of lifeguards, but lifeguards, more than any other providers of public safety, have an ongoing responsibility for accident *prevention*. In fact, prevention is the primary role of lifeguards. This is critical because the worst outcome of water emergencies is death by drowning and the drowning process can be very rapid. There are also many other types of injuries that can occur at the beach which can be prevented by timely and appropriate action by lifeguards.

Public Education

If lifeguards wait until people arrive at their beach to provide information about its hazards and about ways to safely enjoy the beach, important opportunities are lost. Most days, lifeguards cannot possibly individually meet each arriving visitor to personally educate them. Even if this were possible, it would be very inefficient and distract the lifeguard from more immediate duties, like water surveillance.

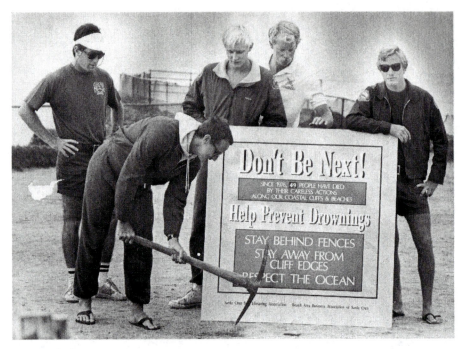

Credit: Rick Gould

Beach users arriving when lifeguards are off-duty or at beaches with no lifeguards, receive no benefit from this approach. For these reasons, a comprehensive and effective drowning prevention program involves efforts to reach beach users well before they arrive at the beach.

Public education programs include activities and materials developed to teach people about the hazards that exist in the aquatic environment and how they may avoid or escape some of those hazards. Public education programs also promote better understanding of lifeguard services and procedures, along with support for and patronage of areas protected by lifeguards. USLA produces many educational publications available nationally and through local chapters.

Educational Materials

Printed educational information includes posters, bumper stickers, handouts, brochures, coloring books, and similar material designed to convey a message of safety or environmental awareness to the public. Some agencies develop special brochures on local beach facilities, along with explanations of warning signals and tips for safe swimming. All of this material can be provided to local schools, hotels, clubs, restaurants, and any place where potential beach users may be. Many lifeguard agencies will also post these materials at beach bulletin boards or in window displays and will provide visitors with handout materials on request.

The Internet is another useful method to offer public education materials. Safety information can be placed on agency websites with links to organizations like USLA. As people research and plan activities for their beach visit, they can also receive

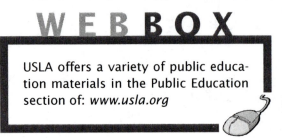

WEBBOX

USLA offers a variety of public education materials in the Public Education section of: *www.usla.org*

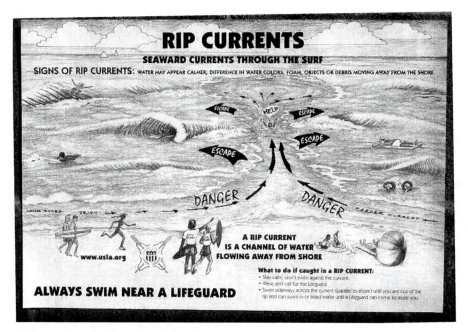

Credit: Sandra McCormick

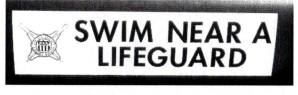

Credit: Sandra McCormick

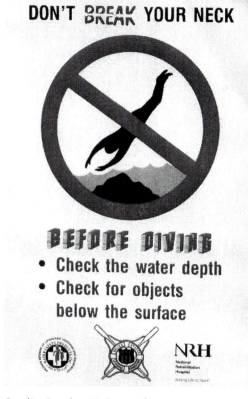

Credit: Sandra McCormick

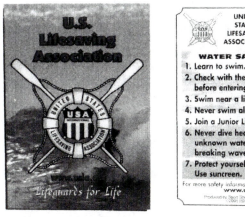

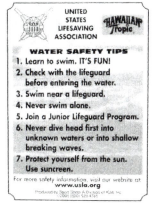

Credit: Sandra McCormick

information on how to make their visit safer and more enjoyable. In fact, by posting brochures on websites and making them printable, lifeguard providers ensure a wide dissemination of materials at low cost. A wise strategy is to include how-to information integrated with safety information. For example, including a map of nearby parking lots with the nearest lifeguard posts and the USLA slogan *swim near a lifeguard* may encourage people to park near and swim in guarded areas.

Kiosks

At some parks and beaches, brochures are offered to provide further information to interested visitors. This may be of value, but brochures can quickly become litter in a beach environment. An alternative is an informational kiosk with more detailed explanations of various rules and local phenomena, including natural hazards. This way, persons interested in educating themselves have an opportunity to do so and litter is minimized. Often, the people who take the time to view such kiosks subsequently advise others in their party about what they have learned.

Recorded Information Lines

Special telephone lines with regularly updated, recorded information on local beach conditions are a popular and inexpensive way to provide water safety information. Using this approach, lifeguards will update the recorded information throughout the day, with the latest water and weather conditions. These recordings can include safety tips, as well as information on lifeguard hours of protection and locations. In case of closures due to water contamination or severe weather, this information can be included as well. An important audience for recorded beach information lines is employees in the tourism industry, who may wish to provide their guests with the latest information. Boaters, scuba divers, and surfers may also find the service valuable. As with brochures, interweaving information that interests these users (e.g., surf reports) with safety messages helps get the message out. An added benefit of recorded information lines is that they reduce the number of individual phone calls that must be fielded for routine questions about current conditions.

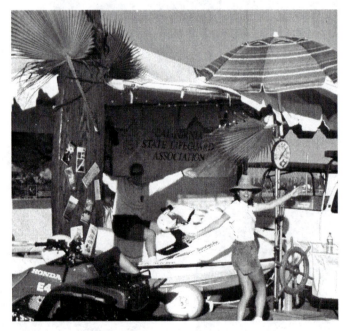

Credit: Ken Kramer

Public Appearances

One of the most effective ways to provide public information is to have lifeguards attend special events and deliver lectures to school and civic groups. In these cases, the investment of a few hours of time may provide concentrated delivery of the safety message to large numbers of people. These events also result in "pass-along" education, as the attendees tell friends and family about what they've learned.

Providing local employees who are likely to come in contact with tourists with basic aquatic safety information is also of great value. Front desk personnel at hotels are good examples, but so are police, cab drivers, and bellhops. These employees, though rarely experts in aquatic safety, may often be asked for water safety information, such as, "Where's the safest place to swim?" They need to be prepared to provide good advice or know how to refer those inquiring to more authoritative sources of information.

It is a good practice to produce a slide show, computer-based presentation, or video in preparation for these events. The next step is to contact school principals, the leaders of local civic organizations, hotel owners, and others to offer services. In seasonal areas, it is best to schedule presentations just before the season begins, so that information is timely. Public appearances can continue throughout the beach season, either at the beach or in parks, campgrounds, or other recreation areas.

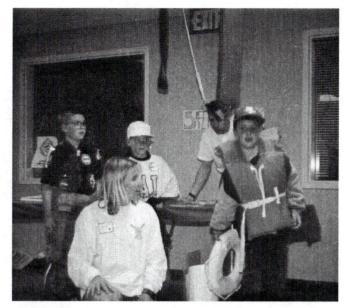

School visit.
Credit: Lucy Woolshlager

Mass Media

Television, newspapers, radio, and other mass media are an excellent way to disseminate public safety messages. There are a variety of ways this can be accomplished. By establishing a rapport with a newspaper or television station, lifeguards may be interviewed about current topics. The media can be invited to cover interesting events, like a lifeguard training program, special holiday preparations, or the employment of new lifesaving equipment. In case of a special event that might be considered newsworthy, some lifeguard agencies issue a *news release* with pertinent details and deliver the release in person or by fax. A particularly effective strategy is developing public service announcements, both for radio and television, that can be aired during periods that the stations offer public access. Working with a local college's production lab may allow this to be developed at low cost.

Special Events

Lifeguard agencies sometimes work with local schools to sponsor poster contests, essay contests, and beach field trips relating to water safety. In some areas, lifeguard agencies tie in sponsorship of other special events, including concerts, fundraising events, fairs, and sporting events, like footraces or triathlons. These special events often include opportunities for spreading information on water safety and for generating support of lifeguard services.

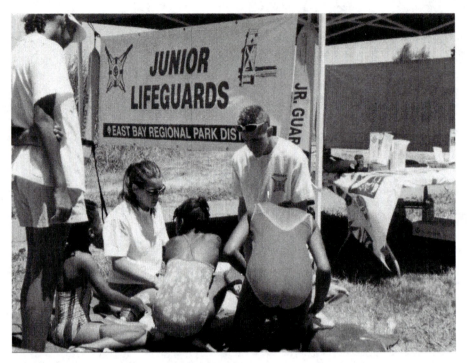

Water safety booth at a special event.

Credit: Dan McCormick

Each year, just prior to the beginning of summer, USLA sponsors *National Beach Safety Week* in an effort to remind beachgoers to use caution in the aquatic environment. National Beach Safety Week begins the Monday before Memorial Day (the last Monday in May) and ends seven (7) days later on Memorial Day. The USLA Public Education Committee is responsible for coordinating National Beach Safety Week through direct efforts and through the eight USLA regions.

USLA regions, local chapters, and lifeguard agencies can assist in promoting National Beach Safety Week by requesting that their local and state political leaders issue a proclamations declaring National Beach Safety Week and by sponsoring press conferences to inform the public. These activities can help draw media attention at a time when water safety education is very important to the beach-going public. To encourage political leaders to declare National Beach Safety Week, it is best to send a letter to the political leader, along with a sample proclamation. It is recommended that letters be sent no later than March 1. A sample letter and proclamation are available in the Public Education section of *www.usla.org*.

Lifeguard competitions also serve as public education events at many beaches throughout the United States. These events combine motivation for

WEBBOX

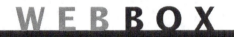

Information on National Beach Safety Week, including a sample resolution for local political bodies, is available in the Public Education section of: *www.usla.org*

Information on pending lifeguard events can be posted in the Events section of: *www.usla.org*

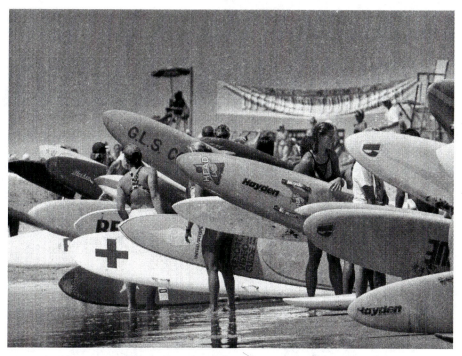

Competitors line-up at the start line of a rescue board race.
Credit: National Park Service

physical fitness among lifeguards, a fostering of interagency relationships, a demonstration of the physical demands placed on open water lifeguards, and an appreciation for the challenges inherent in the beach environment. USLA-sanctioned lifeguard competitions take place across the country, culminating each year at the USLA National Lifeguard Championships.

Special Programs

In addition to special events, many lifeguard agencies sponsor or assist ongoing programs to develop water skills and water safety awareness. Although open water lifeguards are not swimming instructors during work hours, many lifeguard agencies assist with learn-to-swim programs. Other instruction programs sponsored or assisted by lifeguard agencies may include skin and scuba diving courses, surfing instruction, and lifesaving training. Basic information on lifesaving may be provided to local police and firefighters. One of the most effective programs of this nature is the junior lifeguard program. For more information on these programs, see the chapter on *Junior Lifeguard Programs*.

Rules and Regulations

Most jurisdictions overseeing a beach area establish rules and regulations to help prevent accidents and injuries, as well as to ensure that all beach visitors can enjoy the beach experience without being unduly bothered by others. These regulations may address a number of issues. Examples include banning littering, regulating pets, and requiring that lifeguard directions be followed. In addition to local beach rules and local ordinances, many beach areas are protected by national, state, or regional laws which regulate boat or aircraft traffic, or which are intended to protect the environment.

Separating Incompatible Activities

There are a wide variety of activities practiced at aquatic areas. These activities are sometimes incompatible. Conflicts can arise which cause disputes and can threaten public safety. An effective practice in promoting beach and water safety is taking steps to separate incompatible activities. An obvious example of incompatible activities is motorboating and swimming. A swimmer can easily be injured or killed by a motorboat, so it is important to try to keep motorboats away from swimmers. Another example is surfing and swimming. On the beach, keeping ballgames away from sunbathing activities could be expected to reduce conflict and injury. Rules and regulations may also establish special procedures for participating in particular water or beach activities. Permits may be necessary for surfing or scuba diving and those activities may be restricted to established time periods. Evaluating these issues in advance and taking proactive steps to separate incompatible use can reduce the potential for injury, while enhancing the enjoyment of everyone.

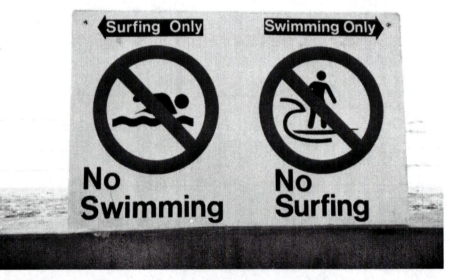

Signs divide swimming and surfing areas.
Credit: B. Chris Brewster

Enforcement

Lifeguards are usually provided with some degree of authority to enforce regulations. Without lawful authority to enforce rules and regulations, it can be very difficult to manage a beach area, because recalcitrant violators will quickly learn that lifeguard warnings will not be enforced and ignore them. Lifeguard enforcement authority may be limited to issuing warnings which, if disobeyed, will ultimately be enforced by police officers summoned to the scene. Even if police are readily available, this can become very time consuming. As well, police are sometimes reluctant to become involved in disputes over beach regulations they may consider of minor importance. For this reason, in some areas lifeguards are appointed as peace officers or law enforcement officers and authorized to enforce local or regional laws to the point of citation or arrest. In cases where lifeguards lack ultimate enforcement authority, it is important that they establish a good rapport with the primary enforcing authority in order to help assure support when requested. In either case, good public contact skills are invaluable in gaining voluntary compliance whenever possible.

Lifeguards should become conversant with the regulations that pertain to the beach area under their supervision. Enforcement often involves lengthy discussions with people who want a detailed explanation of the rules. Lifeguards need to be in a position to fully explain what is and what is not permissible.

Enforcement of beach regulations requires tact and patience. Persons coming to the beach are in a recreational mode. Often they have driven long distances and had a difficult time finding parking. Perhaps they have had a very stressful work week. People coming to the beach want to play. They may therefore be understandably unhappy if told that the form of recreation they want to practice must be modified or terminated.

In enforcement of minor beach regulations, lifeguards should normally approach in a friendly manner, perhaps first making conversation over unrelated issues. Whenever possible, this should be done by a lifeguard whose primary assignment is to patrol the beach or provide backup to tower lifeguards. This way, surveillance of the area is not compromised during the contact.

It is often helpful to remove sunglasses, and if the person is sitting or lying, to squat or kneel down, so as to be at the level of the person which whom you are speaking. A negative reaction is less likely if the subject first sees the lifeguard as a polite person. The lifeguard should explain the regulation and, if possible, the basic reason for it. It is important that the person understand why the lifeguard is taking the time to enforce the regulation. At the same time, it is not the lifeguard's responsibility to justify regulations in great detail. After all, the lifeguard is rarely responsible for having created the regulation. Rather, the lifeguard usually has some level of responsibility for seeing that it is followed.

As an example, many beach areas prohibit glass containers because of the possibility of breakage and resultant injury to barefoot beachgoers. Unfortunately, beachgoers sometimes arrive unknowingly with all of their drinks in bottles. If the lifeguard approaches and simply states that bottles are not permitted, the beach patron may immediately consider the regulation unreasonable and react negatively. On the other hand, if the lifeguard explains that the intent is to prevent injury, most people will respond in an understanding manner.

In any enforcement contact, it is important to clearly explain the action the person must take to come into compliance. For example, in the case of the bottle, after explaining the regulation the lifeguard might direct the person to immediately remove the bottle from the beach to a nearby car. The person now knows what the regulation is, the reason for it, and what must be done to achieve compliance.

Another excellent technique in enforcement of regulations is to *provide alternatives*. The beachgoer told that football is impermissible on the beach may be very upset. Perhaps this was the primary reason to visit the beach. Is there a nearby park where football is permitted that this person could visit instead? Is there an unused portion of the beach where football could be tolerated? Providing options shows concern for the person's needs and a desire to help.

An excellent technique in enforcement of regulations is to *provide alternatives.*

The professional lifeguard maintains a calm disposition throughout an enforcement contact. It may be very frustrating to observe a person acting in an inappropriate manner, but the lifeguard should avoid making judgments about the person's motivations. The lifeguard should be positive, polite and avoid becoming confrontational, while listening attentively to the beach patron's feedback. An even temperament, even in face of abusive language, is almost always the best approach. Regulation enforcement should never become a personal issue. Avoid complicated discussions and reasoning. The lifeguard's approach can simply be "These regulations exist for your safety and the safety of others." If resistance to compliance persists, attempt to reduce tension by expressing understanding of the individual's frustration and offer information about where they can pursue their concern further. Lifeguard conduct should always reflect positively on the employing agency and the lifeguard profession. If compliance is completely resisted, the next step depends upon agency policy and the level of authority provided to the lifeguard.

Beach disputes sometimes arise between two beach users or groups of users. In these cases, the lifeguard may have to assume the role of referee. A valuable tool in helping defuse confrontations between people is to separate them. This is done by asking to speak with each party individually, but out of earshot of the other, to get their side of the story. If both parties are assured that they will be heard in full, this technique prevents one from interrupting the other or becoming more hostile based on what is said to the lifeguard. As well, many people are desirous of telling someone in a position of authority why they feel that they have been wronged. The lifeguard can often perform this role quite effectively. After considerately hearing both sides, listening thoroughly without interrupting, and carefully considering the issue, the lifeguard may be able to propose a resolution with which both parties can agree. This is the ideal outcome. If not, informing each party of the decision quietly and individually may reduce resistance.

Signs and Flags

Regardless of how effective a lifeguard agency may be in providing local public education about the beach, many beach visitors are tourists, some from areas of the country or world with no beach. Others are simply unaware of local regulations or hazards, or oblivious to adverse conditions. Signs and flags can help.

Signs can help gain voluntary compliance to regulations. Most people who are aware of regulations will follow them. By posting signs explaining regulations at beach accesses, compliance will typically improve greatly. It is generally wise to attempt to phrase the information in a positive manner, as opposed to a purely negative one. For example, a sign banning glass containers at the beach could state, "No Glass Containers," or it could state, "For Your Protection, Glass Containers Prohibited." The first is a purely regulatory message. The second indicates that the regulation exists for the benefit of the beachgoer. Informational signs should include pictograms as well as language, so that those who do not read English can understand the message. In addition to rules and regulations, signs can be used to convey safety information. Some lifeguard agencies also fly flags for this purpose.

Signs and flags, though a valuable component of a comprehensive prevention strategy, are limited in their effectiveness. Studies have demonstrated that a surprisingly small percentage of people pay attention to signs and warning flags. Others may not understand them or worse, may misunderstand their meaning. Of course, signs and flags cannot rescue people in distress. They are therefore no substitute for the staffing of properly trained and equipped lifeguards. Rather, they are one element of a comprehensive prevention strategy.

Warning Flag Guidelines

For decades, lifeguard agencies in the United States and around the world have employed warning flags to notify swimmers of conditions, to warn of hazards, to identify safer areas for swimming, and to notify beach users about regulated areas. Unfortunately, inconsistent use of flags limited their effectiveness. For this reason, in 2002 USLA developed national guidelines for warning flags. By following these warning flag guidelines, lifeguard agencies can help ensure a universal understanding of their meaning and thus improve their effectiveness.

To be fully effective, the use of warning flags to notify the public of current hazard levels should be based on measurable criteria that can be logged, tracked, and changed with conditions. Flying flags that indicate a heightened level of hazard when conditions are relatively calm is analogous to crying wolf and likely to cause people to ignore the flags on days when they carry a pertinent message. It is therefore important that they be handled consistently in accordance with conditions.

One of the greatest challenges to the effectiveness of warning flags is the message they convey. A green flag may be intended to convey calmer conditions, but drownings occur even in flat water with no surf, so a green flag may cause complacency. As well, conditions that may warrant great concern for the average swimmer may be relatively harmless for strong swimmers. These factors underline the need for consistent use of flags based on objective, measurable criteria employed by trained persons, along with good public education efforts to explain the meaning of the flags flown.

Ocean conditions vary throughout the United States. Conditions that may be considered relatively mild in some areas, may be seen as a significant safety threat in others. Therefore, in each area where warning flags are employed, USLA recommends that specific local criteria be developed that provide objective, measurable criteria for posting the flags, and that the public be clearly notified of those criteria. USLA recommended warning flag guidelines are intended to provide general levels of hazard to be further defined locally. The first four flags (see table) are intended to provide general notification of overall conditions for a beach area. That is, if it is decided that water conditions present a "moderate hazard" on a given beach, it should cover the entire beach, not a portion or area of beach. This does not prevent use of additional flags of the same warning level to accentuate the notification, but a single beach should not fly a green flag in one area and a red flag in another.

Some or all of the flags listed may be employed. It may be decided, for example, to adopt the first three, but none of the others. This is a local decision. However, USLA strongly discourages use of flags of similar colors that conflict with the meaning of those listed. This would negate the value of national consistency and confuse the public. In any case, with the exception of the double red, which indicates a closed beach, the first three should never be flown simultaneously. Where warning flags are flown, the public should be notified of their meaning via signs placed at multiple, conveniently located places. Examples might include beach access-ways, ramps, lifeguard towers, parking lots, and the flagpoles themselves.

Flag Color	Condition
Green	Low Hazard (small surf, light currents, and clean water)
Yellow	Moderate Hazard (moderate surf and/or strong currents)
Red	High Hazard (high surf and/or very strong currents and/or contaminated water advisory)
Red over Red	Water is closed to public contact. (One red flag flown above a second red flag.)
Purple	Marine pests present (e.g.: jellyfish, stingrays, Portuguese man-o-war) - Note: This is not intended to be used to notify of the presence of sharks. If water is closed or hazardous due to the presence of sharks, use red flag(s).
Yellow with Black Ball	Surfing prohibited - Note: According to local regulation, this may include a variety of defined surfriding devices.
Black	Surfing permitted
Checkered	Use Area Boundary (example: boundary of a swimming and surfing area)
Red over Yellow	Protected Area Boundary (end of lifeguard protection)

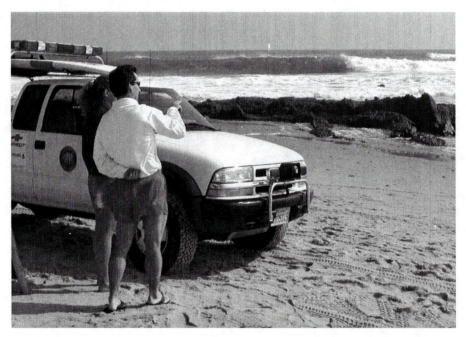

Credit: Ken Kramer

Identifying Pre-Events

Before an accident occurs, any accident, there is a pre-event. For example, a person driving a car may spill hot coffee on themselves, causing them to swerve and collide with another car. Driving with hot coffee is the pre-event that ultimately resulted in the accident. The same is true of the beach environment. If lifeguards can identify pre-events, and effectively intervene, they may be able to prevent the accident from occurring. Identifying typical pre-events also helps lifeguards key in on activity that is more likely to lead to injury or death and provides greater lead time in preparing to respond to an emergency.

Every beach area has unique hazards. Every beach area also shares similar hazards with other beach areas. A pre-event to an accident at just about any beach might be a game of football in close proximity to other beachgoers. A lifeguard can easily imagine the possible outcome of a player going for a pass and knocking into another beachgoer. At a surf beach, the pre-event might involve a person walking into a rip current. At a flat water beach, the pre-event might be a ball being blown offshore, that the owner may then try to retrieve.

By identifying pre-events likely to result in accidents at a beach, lifeguards can better prepare to intervene or, if unable to do so, to respond to the event. One way to identify pre-events is through a review of past accidents. What were the pre-events? Once that is known, lifeguards can be instructed to watch for them occurring in the future. Another way is to simply survey the environment. Is there an area that is always slippery at low tide? Are there rocks with shellfish attached that people swim near? By cataloging these, lifeguards may be able to better focus their attention and to more effectively prevent accidents.

On-Site Preventive Actions

For every rescue effected, most lifeguards log tens, if not hundreds of preventive actions. Not all accidents can be avoided by preventive actions and repeated warnings can become tiresome to both lifeguards and beach patrons. In fact, being overly preventive may unreasonably restrict recreational opportunities. In many cases though, timely preventive actions can reduce the number of rescues and injuries at a beach to manageable levels. They can be critical in the avoidance of injury, death, and property loss.

Preventive work starts when the lifeguard comes on duty. In includes a visual survey of the beach for anything unusual, identifying hazards and taking steps to mitigate them, posting daily information signs, and informing other lifeguards of notable observations. As the day progresses, preventive actions may include directing visitors away from a rip current area, counseling poor swimmers to move to

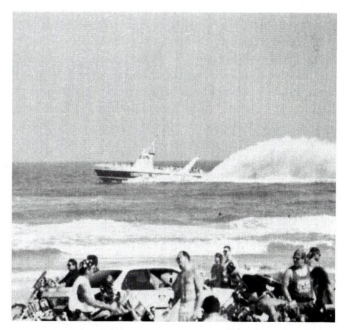

A motorboat buzzes a swim area.

Credit: Mike Hensler

Priority Activity of United States Lifeguards

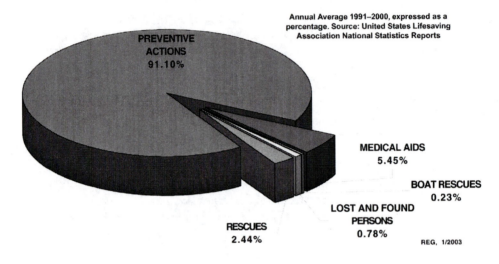

Annual Average 1991–2000, expressed as a percentage. Source: United States Lifesaving Association National Statistics Reports

PREVENTIVE ACTIONS
91.10%

MEDICAL AIDS
5.45%

BOAT RESCUES
0.23%

LOST AND FOUND PERSONS
0.78%

RESCUES
2.44%

REG. 1/2003

Credit: Rick Gould

shallow water, or discouraging people with flotation devices from entering deep water. All preventive actions, should be noted in the lifeguard tower log since they are a critical, if often unnoticed aspect of lifeguard duties. Each preventive action logged indicates that a lifeguard identified a safety concern, or that a potentially hazardous situation was developing and mitigating action was taken.

The use of recreational equipment often fosters a need for preventive actions. Boats and other water vehicles can be major problems, especially large powerboats. Inexperienced boaters and sailors can intrude on a swimming area, presenting hazards to people in the water. Other types of equipment that can pose danger are surfboards, bodyboards, flotation devices, and a wide variety of beach and water toys. Keeping them separated from those whom they might injury is an important element of accident prevention.

Although preventive actions are important in averting possible accidents and injuries, lifeguards must use good judgment in determining when an activity becomes too dangerous to permit. It is sometimes difficult to determine what activities should be considered unusually dangerous, since occasional injuries are an inherent part of physical recreation. For example, throwing a football may be viewed as an innocent act of recreation or may be seen as a potentially dangerous activity which could lead to the injury of someone in the immediate vicinity. One good rule to follow is that whenever the recreational activity of one person significantly threatens the safety of another, it should be stopped or modified. A high speed boat in the vicinity of swimmers is an example of an unusually dangerous activity.

Lifeguards who overuse preventive actions can create problems for themselves and their agencies. Constant warning and overly intensive supervision can lead to unnecessary confrontations, repeated complaints, or active non-compliance with requests. Each agency, according to its own philosophy of preventive lifeguarding, should establish guidelines for the use of preventive actions by lifeguards. Once an agency's preventive action guidelines are established, lifeguards should receive ongoing in-service training on their implementation.

Since the lifeguard is an expert in recognizing hazardous situations that the public often doesn't, the lifeguard is obligated to take preventive actions when appropriate. Fulfilling this obligation not only improves safety by reducing hazards, but often has the added benefit of increasing lifeguard attentiveness by broadening the sense of responsibility. Nevertheless, the primary goal must always be toward preventing the most serious outcomes—death and injury. Therefore, an effort to terminate a beach game that poses a minor hazard may have to be delayed for a time if it would compromise drowning prevention.

> Whenever the recreational activity of one person significantly threatens the safety of another, it should be stopped or modified.

Special Operation Modes

Natural hazards can be intensified during periods of high surf, wind, fog, and other weather conditions. Unusually high attendance can also make safety more difficult to maintain. During these periods, many agencies initiate special operation modes. These may involve modified operations, actual beach closings, or beach advisories.

Modified Operations

Certain water, weather, or crowd conditions may lead lifeguard supervisors to modify operations. This may include suspension of certain activities. For example, extremely high surf may lead to suspension of surfing to help prevent possible injuries. High offshore winds may lead to restrictions on the use of flotation devices to prevent users from being blown far from the beach. Beach activities that take up a large amount of space may be curtailed or restricted during periods of heavy beach congestion. In most agencies, the authority to suspend or restrict activities is granted in the agency's established rules and regulations.

Modified operations may also take the form of special lifeguard procedures initiated by the area supervisor. When rescue volume increases dramatically or weather draws unusually high crowds, lifeguard management must be prepared with plans to handle increased beach activity or hazards. Regular staffing levels may otherwise be completely overwhelmed in case of a heat wave.

The growing number and popularity of open water swims and triathlons also call for modified lifeguard operations. Lifeguard management must integrate preventive measures into event logistics when planning with the organizers. Clear criteria should be established for environmental conditions that would cause the event to be modified or cancelled. A maximum number of competitors and heat size may need to be determined. Adequate lifeguard surveillance is critical and is usually best done with some combination of powered and non-powered rescue craft. Specific action plans should be established in the event of rescue, medical, or search emergencies.

Beach Closings

Some conditions necessitate closing a beach area to swimming and other water activities. Examples include water contamination and lightning. Decisions to close beaches to swimming call for careful judgment, and are usually made only by area supervisors following specific, predetermined criteria. Once these criteria have been met, patrol lifeguards are informed and warning signs or flags may be erected to inform beach visitors. Public address system announcements may also be broadcast regularly during such periods. In case of urgent, pending threats, care must be taken to avoid causing panic. This is best done by conveying the message calmly, while emphasizing the need to evacuate in an orderly manner. It may be helpful to have a police presence in cases that a reluctance to leave is anticipated. When conditions allow reopening of the beach, lifeguards are notified and warning signs and flags are removed.

Advisories

Lifeguard agencies lacking the authority to close beaches may instead initiate special advisories. Advisories are also utilized by agencies with closure authority when it is believed that outright closure is unjustified, but strong caution should be urged. When criteria for advisories are met, lifeguards are notified and warning flags or notices may be erected to inform the public. Regular lifeguard operations continue, but lifeguards may be required to approach visitors entering the water to verbally warn them against participation in certain activities. When conditions stabilize, lifeguards are notified of the suspension of the advisory and warnings are removed.

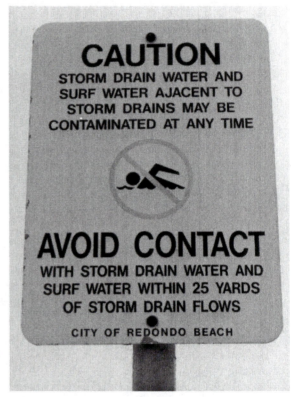

Credit: Rob McGowan

Shark Sightings

The fear of sharks creates great concern on the part of beachgoers, but as explained in the chapter on *Aquatic Life and Related Hazards,* the statistical chance of being injured (or even seeing) a shark is miniscule. Nevertheless, in some areas, shark encounters are more likely than in others. In 2002, USLA developed *Shark Bite Prevention and Response Guidelines* to assist lifeguard agencies in dealing with shark sightings and shark bite incidents (Brewster, Burgess, Gallagher, Gould, Hensler, & Wernicki) This section is based on those guidelines. The most recent version of the guidelines can be found at *www.usla.org.*

Lifeguards should be trained to recognize sharks common to their area of responsibility and shark behavior that may be considered threatening. When behavior of a shark or sharks appears to present an unusual hazard to swimmers, an evaluation should be made as to whether it is appropriate to warn those involved in aquatic activity or to advise them to leave the water.

In areas where shark bites are known to occur with greater frequency than normal, posted signs may be appropriate to warn of the elevated hazard. If a shark bite occurs, people in the water in the area should be advised and encouraged to leave the water until such time as the immediate threat appears to have abated. Lifeguards in adjacent areas should be notified and advised to maintain heightened vigilance. Local ordinances may require that the water be closed. Since shark behavior is unpredictable, this may involve a fixed period of time or observed criteria, such as the absence of schooling fish that may have attracted shark activity. In the case of a shark attack, wherein the shark repeatedly bites or pursues a human, the water in the immediate area should be cleared of all swimmers and kept clear until it can be determined that the immediate threat is over.

In beach areas where shark bites have historically occurred with a frequency that is significantly higher than normal, specific policies appropriate to local conditions are recommended. These policies should be based, in part, on consultation with shark experts and local emergency medical authorities.

Extended Shifts

In some areas of the U.S., daily lifeguard hours of operation have traditionally been from mid-morning until dusk, while in other areas, they have traditionally terminated at five or six p.m. These patterns developed in response to the time periods that beaches were most heavily used. Changing demographics and lifestyles in recent years however, have resulted in increased beach use in early morning and evening hours.

One way that lifeguard agencies have found to extend coverage into early morning and late evening hours is by use of staggered shifts. Under this approach, part of the staff arrives early and part arrives later in the day, with an overlap mid-day. In this manner, while morning and evening staff may be lower, mid-day staff remains at peak levels. Since beach attendance levels in morning and evening are typically lower than at mid-day, this approach generally ensures that lifeguard staffing levels mirror daily variations in attendance levels, while broadening safety protection. Administrators must be careful not to violate minimum staffing and equipment regulations in jurisdictions where such legislation has been enacted.

After Hours and Post Season Prevention

Aquatic emergencies don't happen during daylight hours alone. They also happen at night. Perhaps someone decides to go for an evening swim and becomes distressed, or a pedestrian slips and falls into the water, or a boater encounters problems. In any of these cases, lifeguards may be able to provide essential lifesaving assistance, if they can be quickly responded to the scene.

In much of California, Florida, and Hawaii year-round open water lifeguard coverage is typical, with staffing levels varying in accordance with anticipated beach use. Other areas of the country may have coverage in place for seasons as short as eight weeks. Gaps in lifeguard coverage arise when lifeguards go off-duty, both at the end of the day and the season. Those gaps can be filled, in part, in several ways.

One strategy to ensure expeditious response of lifeguards to aquatic emergencies that occur after regular lifeguard staffing hours, as well as in post season months (for lifeguard agencies that operate seasonally), has been the organization of special response teams. Two California communities, Los Angeles County and San Diego, have found after hours call volume so high that they keep response teams of lifeguards on full duty 24-hours a day, year-round. In San Diego, this includes a fully staffed 9-1-1 lifeguard dispatch center.

Other communities, unable to justify this level of staffing, have organized community resources, including lifeguards, emergency medical services, dive teams, fire departments, police departments, and allied services to respond in concert when the emergencies arise. Under these systems, an automatic response occurs, with roles of members of the team predesignated and designed to work under the *incident command system* (described in the chapter on *Emergency Planning and Management*). Some members may be off-duty, but on a *callback system,* prepared to respond when summoned, while others may be on regular duty.

Special response teams of this nature require the preparation of emergency operation plans that detail response protocols to ensure cooperation among responders who do not normally work together. In some instances interagency agreements, as well as amendments to local ordinances and state statutes, must be enacted to provide authority for response and to assure that liability and insurance protection is provided for responders.

New Jersey's ANSWER Team: One example of a year-round special response team in an area with seasonal lifeguard protection can be found in central New Jersey. Agreements enacted by adjacent communities (Avon-By-The-Sea, Bradley Beach, Neptune, Ocean Grove) have created the Area Network of Shore Water Emergency Responders (ANSWER). This includes lifeguards as rescue swimmers; a dive team; rescue craft; and EMS, fire and police personnel. Unique dispatching protocols, including the cooperation of the United States Coast Guard's Shark River Lifeboat Station, provide the capability of year-round rescue swimmer response within two minutes. Drills are conducted by the cooperating emergency management offices involving application of incident command system principles and rehearsals of various emergency operation plans.

Some communities address after hours and post-season aquatic emergencies through less structured callback systems, whereby off-duty rescuers are contacted and responded to emergency scenes. A common approach involves issuing pagers or two-way radios to those willing and able to respond as needed. Other agencies maintain telephone numbers of lifeguards residing near the beach. These lifeguards must typically respond in private vehicles and may have little equipment available. It is sometimes difficult to contact them. For seasonal lifeguard agencies, this can be particularly challenging during off-season months, when lifeguards may not reside in the immediate area. Even in cases that lifeguards reside in close proximity, designated personnel may be away from the area and unable to respond when called. Nevertheless, for communities unable to justify the staffing of lifeguards throughout evening hours, a callback system provides some possibility of response of qualified rescuers. The chances of success are greatly improved when persons in a callback mode are provided emergency response vehicles and if times during which response personnel are available is carefully coordinated.

A fourth type of special response team involves communities without available trained lifeguards. In this case, personnel from other public safety services, such as police or firefighters, are trained in aquatic rescue. USLA offers the *Aquatic Rescue Response Team* (ARRT) certification program to help ensure these teams are trained to adequate levels.

WEBBOX

For more information on the Aquatic Rescue Response Team certification program, visit the Certification section of: *www.usla.org*

Agencies which follow the minimum training requirements of this program can help ensure that anyone assigned to effect aquatic rescues has a minimum standard of training and preparedness required of this arduous work. This is especially important in the case of off-hours or post season rescue, which can involve darkness, colder water, and particularly challenging conditions.

The ARRT Certification Program is aimed at members of the agency selected to effect water rescue. For obvious reasons of safety, these are the only members of the agency who should be expected to attempt a rescue of a person or persons in distress in the aquatic environment. This does not however, prevent teams from including support personnel who do not meet the minimum standards, so long as they are not the persons assigned to effect aquatic rescue.

In areas where USLA certified open water lifeguard agencies exist, USLA strongly recommends that any aquatic rescue response team work in concert and under the general direction of that lifeguard agency. Likewise, aquatic rescue response teams are strongly encouraged to tap the resources of a USLA certified lifeguard agency in conducting training, setting policy, and recruiting prospective team members. Since the ARRT program is generally confined to response and rescue, it represents a level of certification more limited in scope than that of the minimum standard for lifeguard agencies.

> The United States Lifesaving Association recommends that all open water lifeguard agencies develop plans to address the need for lifeguard response during all hours of the day and all days of the year to ensure that rescuers qualified at USLA recommended levels can be summoned as needed during these periods.

Maintenance

Beach maintenance is an aspect of preventive lifeguarding. With the exception of routine maintenance of lifeguard facilities and equipment, lifeguards should not be assigned to general maintenance duties, but every lifeguard has a responsibility for monitoring the beach and water for potential hazards. For example, hazardous flotsam must either be removed by the lifeguard or reported immediately to beach maintenance crews for removal. At lake facilities, underwater plant growth should be monitored closely and removed before becoming a hazard.

One purpose of routine beach patrols is to look for beach hazards, including broken glass, abandoned fire pits, and other sharp or hazardous materials. Lifeguard agencies must follow special procedures for protecting the public and themselves when any type of potentially hazardous material is found along a beach area, including medical waste and drums, or containers that may contain toxic waste. In some areas, military explosives may float ashore from time to time. Usually, if explosives float, it is because they are intended to be used as markers in aquatic military exercises. Still, markers are meant to burn and some are quite hazardous.

If hazards cannot be immediately removed from the beach area, lifeguards should keep people away from the area until the hazard can be removed. As a standard practice, beach patrons should be kept at least 500 feet back from any potentially explosive device, further if possible. The local bomb squad or fire department should be summoned for consultation and disposal.

At seasonally protected locations, beach and underwater areas should be closely inspected for hazards prior to each season. Winter storms often cause hazardous submerged objects or other shoreline damage to occur. Dry land environmental hazards include rock outcroppings, cliff areas, and similar topographical features which provide visitors with opportunities to hurt themselves while recreating.

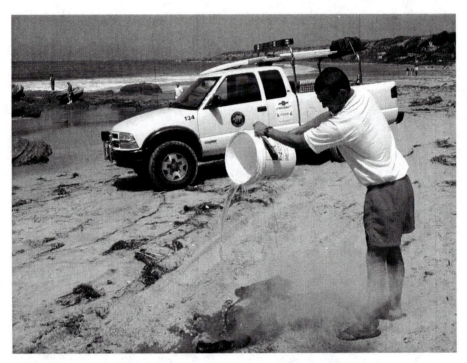

Lifeguard putting out hot coals.
Credit: Ken Kramer

Human made structures and improvements can also inflict injury. These may include bathhouses, piers, floats and docks, parking lots, playgrounds, boardwalks, cycle paths, and so forth. Lifeguards should make it their business to be aware of all the potential hazards in areas under their responsibility, attempting to mitigate them as appropriate.

Facility Design

From conception to construction, beach facilities should be designed carefully with public safety in mind. This is particularly true for any improvements such as roadways, parking areas, walkways, and beach houses. Facility designers and engineers should consider ways to overcome natural hazards, which may include the installation of railings, the removal of water hazards, and even redevelopment of the sandy beach and swimming area.

While most lifeguard agencies are not directly involved in design of public improvements at the beach—except those directly related to lifeguard activities—many lifeguard agencies are actively involved in designing safety into the beach environment. At many flat-water beaches, swim lines are installed to delineate the swimming area and provide emergency flotation support for people caught in deep water. At surf areas, it is more difficult to install safety equipment in the water due to the dynamic conditions of tides and surf. Still, some beaches install swim lines, buoy markers, or flags to delineate swim areas or protected zones. To regulate boat traffic, special "No Boating" buoys may be placed at the perimeters of swim areas to warn boaters away from swimmers. Facility design may also include special safety considerations regarding docks, floats, and any play equipment installed on or near the water, including slides, diving boards or rope swings.

For a discussion of lifeguard towers and related facilities, please refer to the chapter entitled *Lifeguard Facilities*.

Chapter Summary

In this chapter, we have learned that preventive lifeguarding is a primary responsibility of any lifeguard agency and should be considered in the broadest terms. Public education is one preventive strategy. We have learned about using educational materials, recorded information lines, public appearances, mass media, special events, and special programs to reach people before they arrive at the beach. We have learned about the use and enforcement of rules and regulations, including separating incompatible activities. The value of signs and flags has been discussed, including USLA national warning flag guidelines. We have learned about pre-events to accidents and on-site preventive actions that can be taken. Additionally, we have learned about special operation modes, extended shifts, after-hours and post season responses strategies. Finally, we have learned about the importance of beach maintenance and facility design to further minimize the possibility of injury.

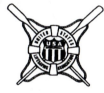

Discussion Points

- Why is it so important to educate people about beach hazards before they arrive at the beach?
- What sort of beach safety educational materials have you seen and how effective did you think they were?
- How might a recorded information line benefit public safety?
- How could the mass media be used to disseminate information on beach safety?
- Why are rules and regulations necessary at the beach?
- What are examples of incompatible activities that might be separated to improve public safety?
- In enforcement of regulations, why is it valuable to provide alternatives?
- What are some of the benefits and limitations of signs and flags?
- What is an example of a pre-event to a drowning?
- What are some on-site preventive actions a lifeguard might take?
- Why might lifeguards need to implement a special operation mode?
- What is the value of staggered shifts to extend hours of lifeguard coverage?
- How might after hours and post season aquatic emergencies be handled?
- What are examples of maintenance and facility design that could be expected to reduce the potential for injury?

Reference

Brewster, B. C., Burgess, G. H., Gallagher, T., Gould, R., Hensler, M., & Wernicki, M.D., P. (2002). United States Lifesaving Association position statement shark bite prevention and response. Huntington Beach, California: United States Lifesaving Association.

Chapter 11
Water Surveillance

In this chapter, you will learn about techniques for effective water surveillance. This includes learning to evaluate beach users to help anticipate who might later need your help and learning to identify signs of distress. Here we provide techniques for effective water observation, which is critical if lifeguards are to rescue those in need in a timely manner. You will learn about establishing areas of responsibility and zones of coverage. You will learn how to maintain vigilance while assigned to surveillance duties; and you will learn about coverage systems.

CHAPTER EXCERPT

In emergency medicine there is often reference to a golden hour—the period of time after a traumatic injury during which effective medical intervention is essential to the saving of life. In open water lifesaving, such a time frame is an unknown luxury. Lifeguards measure the opportunity for successful intervention not in minutes, but in moments.

To prevent injuries or successfully intervene before a drowning occurs, the primary skill a lifeguard must employ is effective observation. Effective observation is not simply a question of vigilance. Accurate assessment and recognition of drowning victims is a skill which requires training, experience, tremendous concentration, and good judgment. Experienced lifeguards can sometimes actually predict which people at their beach will need assistance long before an emergency arises. They do so by using visual clues, many of which will be discussed in this chapter.

Surprisingly, it is not always obvious when a person is in distress or even experiencing panic in the water. This varies depending upon swimming skills, environmental conditions, and the individual. As detailed in the chapter entitled *Drowning*, a nonswimmer who steps off a drop-off into water that is overhead, may display the *instinctive drowning response*, expending all energy trying to stay afloat and possibly appearing, to the untrained eye, like a person playing in the water. (Pia, 1997) A person with good swimming skills caught in a rip current may swim against the current and make some progress, though the swimmer will tire much more quickly than would be the case were there no current. Some people

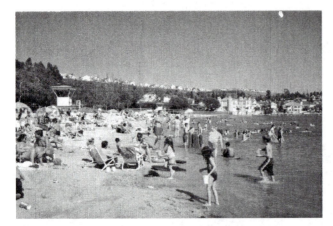

Credit: Lake Mission Viejo Lifeguards

submerge with no prior sign of a struggle whatsoever. (Pia, 1997) For these reasons, lifeguards must be adept at anticipating problems, recognizing when a person is in distress without hearing a yell for help, and understanding the sometimes subtle presentations of people in distress or panic.

In emergency medicine there is often reference to a golden hour—the period of time after a traumatic injury during which effective medical intervention is essential to the saving of life. In open water lifesaving, such a time frame is an unknown luxury. Lifeguards measure the opportunity for successful intervention not in minutes, but in moments.

Recognition and Assessment

In order to provide successful rescue of people in the drowning process, it is important to be able to identify signs that may help to indicate various drowning presentations. Once these signs have been recognized, the situation can be assessed and the lifeguard can respond appropriately.

Dry Land Observation

If possible, observation of beach visitors should begin before water entry. There are a number of clues and statistical facts lifeguards can use to key in on people in their area most likely to experience problems. While these clues can suggest persons who merit particular attention, lifeguards should not exclude any water user from their surveillance.

- *Age*—Very old or very young people should be watched carefully. As explained in the chapter entitled *Drowning,* in the year 2000, drowning was the second leading cause of accidental death for those under 15 years of age and the third leading cause for those 15–35. Infants and toddlers can drown in water no deeper than their arm length due to their inability to easily get to their feet after falling over. Older children may lack the judgment or willingness to recognize their own limitations. Older adults may lack physical strength necessary to fight an unexpected current or to quickly move away from a breaking wave.

- *Body Weight*—People who are overweight may become easily exhausted and are likely to be less able to move quickly to avoid a hazardous condition.

- *Pale or Extremely White Complexion*—If a light skinned person arrives at a sunny beach with no tan whatsoever, it is a reasonable presumption that the person is not a regular beachgoer and therefore may be inexperienced or unfamiliar with

LearnMore

The films *On Drowning* and *The Reasons People Drown,* depicting actual drowning emergencies at a flat water swimming area, are available for purchase at: *www.pia-enterprises.com/*

the open water environment. This is a particularly useful clue in an area frequented by tourists, since they may have a total lack of familiarity with local water conditions.

- *Intoxication*—Those who display a behavior pattern which suggests a probable impairment of normal physical coordination due to alcohol or drugs should be eyed as potential rescue candidates, particularly considering the high degree of drownings which involve alcohol. Slurred speech, an unstable gait, or erratic behavior are some examples of tell-tale behavior.

- *Flotation Devices*—The only truly safe flotation devices are US Coast Guard approved lifejackets which fit the wearer and are properly worn. With that exception, flotation devices such as inflatable rafts, balls, and life rings can be *killers*. While flotation devices are sometimes used by accomplished swimmers for purely recreational purposes, they are also used by weak and nonswimmers. Often nonswimmers use flotation devices to access deep water so that they can stay with friends who can swim; but if the non-swimming user of a flotation device becomes separated from the flotation device, submersion and death can occur very rapidly with little or no observable struggle. One of the most chilling sights to a lifeguard is a flotation device offshore with no one around it.

Parents of small children often give them flotation devices, believing they can pay less attention to their children as a result. It is not unusual to see very small children with inflated rings around their upper arms to assist in swimming, but if such devices deflate unexpectedly or fall off, death by drowning may be the result. Some swimming areas actually ban use of flotation devices due to the danger they present. Since flotation devices can completely prevent a lifeguard from determining whether a person can swim at all, it should be assumed by the lifeguard that a person using a flotation device is a nonswimmer until the lifeguard is certain that the person is competent without the device.

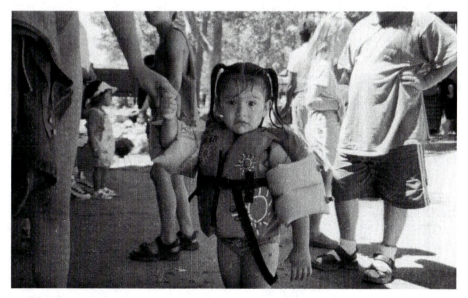

Credit: Dan McCormick

No one should use a flotation device without immediate supervision unless the person has the skill to easily swim to shore from the area where the device is being used.

- *Improper Equipment or Attire*—In most climates, under normal summerlike conditions a swimmer is adequately attired with only a swimsuit. Body surfers will usually equip themselves with swim fins. In cold water, an experienced swimmer could be expected to wear a wetsuit to prevent loss of body heat and exhaustion. Depending on the conditions, absence of such equipment may be a clue of inexperience.

  Any person who enters the water wearing clothes, other than those designed for swimming, should be watched carefully. Clothes offer a negative buoyancy factor and restrict swimming ability. While some people with strong swimming skills may simply lack the funds to purchase swimsuits, the wearing of street clothes while swimming is a likely sign of a lack of water knowledge. On the other hand, it is easy to dismiss from consideration a person who arrives at the beach with an impressive array of equipment under the assumption that the person must have extensive water skills. There is no guarantee however. Particular attention should be paid to those who have unusual difficulty donning their equipment or whose equipment fits poorly. The poorly fitting wetsuit, for example, may be borrowed by a nonswimmer from a friend who is a swimmer.

- *Disability*—People with physical disabilities are increasingly using open water areas for recreation. Some areas furnish ramps for wheelchairs to help wheelchair bound people move across the beach. Other areas furnish wheelchairs specifically designed to move through the sand. Amputees and people with less obvious disabilities also swim. Physically challenged people usually know their limitations and make prudent decisions, just like other beachgoers; but just like other beachgoers, people with disabilities may overestimate their abilities. Given the same hazard (e.g., a rip current) and all other things being equal, a disabled person is likely to have more difficulty than a fully able-bodied person. It is important however, not to presume that a disabled person is an incompetent swimmer. Lifeguards will find that just like able bodied swimmers, there are disabled swimmers who are very strong and some who are very weak. Lifeguards should make their evaluations on a case by case basis.

Swimmer Observation

Once beach visitors are in the water, a number of signs can signal problems. The following are several of these signs.

- *Facing Shore*—The first indication of trouble from people beginning to feel anxiety or experiencing distress is that they normally face shore or continually glance in that direction. This is a very important clue for a lifeguard, particularly at a surf beach where most swimmers will be facing away from shore, watching the waves. Even at a non-surf beach, groups of swimmers may be playing and facing each other, but one may be anxiously looking toward shore. In some cases an offshore platform may substitute for the safety of shore and the swimmer may instead look toward this platform.

- *Low Head*—Competent swimmers remaining in a stationary location hold their heads high. They tread water, breaststroke, or float on their backs. The chin is usually clearly above the water level. Swimmers whose heads hang low in the water demand a focus of attention to determine competency.

- *Low Stroke*—This normally accompanies a low head and can be visualized as a stroke that is very low to the water with the elbows dragging.

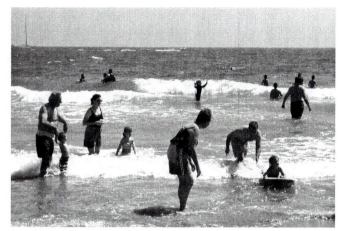

Credit: Ken Kramer

- *Ineffective Kick*—Under normal circumstances, the weak swimmer displays little or no kick. The lack of a break in the surface of the water should cue the lifeguard to a possible problem. In these cases, the body plane changes to a more upright position and little forward progress is made.

- *Waves Breaking Overhead*—Most people who are competent at swimming in the surf dive under waves. When waves wash over a swimmer's head with no apparent attempt by the swimmer to duck under them, it is a strong indicator that this is a rescue candidate.

- *Catching Large Waves Without Body Surfing*—The primary goal of a swimmer in distress is to make it to shore. These people may be willing to pay the price of going over the falls of a large wave to accomplish this goal. Those who allow themselves to be carried by a breaking wave, without making some attempt to body surf or duck under the wave, should be eyed very carefully. Often, weak swimmers who go over the falls on a breaking wave find themselves disoriented and in worse shape than before.

- *Hair in the Face*—The natural instinct of people in control of themselves in the water is to brush the hair out of their eyes. People who make no attempt to do so are usually under stress and concerned about other things—like keeping their heads above water.

- *Glassy, Empty, or Anxious Eyes*—Eyes can be a window to emotion. Experienced lifeguards can read the fatigue and fear in the eyes of a distressed or panicked person. Depending on distance, this may only be detectable with binoculars or not detectable at all.

- *Heads Together*—When other swimmers suddenly converge on a particular swimmer or simply cluster together, it may be an indication that one or more needs assistance. Often people in distress are unable to signal to a lifeguard or don't think to do so. Instead, they call to the people nearest to them for buoyancy or moral support. This request for aid may not be perceptible to the lifeguard, but the actions of other swimmers can suggest that a rescue is needed. When swimmers congregate for any significant length of time, the situation should be investigated with binoculars or in person.

- *Hand Waving*—Waving an arm, particularly in the water, is a natural sign of distress, perhaps because in water it is usually the only way to attract attention other than by yelling. The wave is a particularly important signal in the case of scuba divers who are generally taught in training that they should never wave unless they are in distress. This distress signal is constantly abused by people waving to friends ashore or nearby in the water. Although waving by swimmers in distress is a relatively uncommon occurrence, any person facing shore and waving should be assumed to be signaling for help until it can be ascertained that the person is all right. If it is determined that there is no distress, lifeguards should make an effort to counsel those responsible about the appearance of an emergency that is created by a wave from the water, particularly in the case of scuba divers.

- *Fighting or Being Swept Along by a Current*—Currents are a major source of distress. Lifeguards should know the locations and characteristics of currents that regularly present themselves in the same location. In addition, lifeguards at beaches susceptible to unexpected currents should be constantly on the alert for the appearance of currents and watch current areas with particular scrutiny. The first sign of potential distress in a current is the simple fact that a swimmer is moved laterally or offshore by the current; however, it is impossible to know whether the swimmer will be able to resolve the problem until the swimmer comes to recognize the pull of the current and tries to get out of it. Even waterwise swimmers may initially attempt to fight the current and strong swimmers may succeed in doing so; but once a swimmer begins to fight a current stronger than the swimmer's skills, the drowning process has begun and will only be resolved in one of three ways:

1. The current relaxes.
2. The swimmer swims sideways to the pull of the current and gets out of it.
3. The swimmer is rescued.

When a swimmer concludes that fighting the current will be futile and if the swimmer does not know to swim sideways to the pull of the current, panic will quickly set in. Therefore, as soon as a swimmer nears a dangerous current or becomes caught in it, experienced lifeguards begin preparing for a water rescue.

- *Erratic Activity*—Any activity out of the ordinary should always be given close scrutiny. It may be someone who is showing off or horsing around or perhaps disoriented and out of touch with the reality of the environment. Showoffs intentionally take risks to attract attention and often find themselves in over their heads.

- *Clinging to Fixed Objects*—Swimmers who are fearful or in distress sometimes try to cling to piers, rocks, pilings, buoys, or other apparent objects of security. This is often a good sign that the person is either too frightened or too exhausted to continue swimming and demands close scrutiny. In addition, aquatic life such as barnacles and mussels attached to these objects can cause significant injuries.

Drowning Presentations

There are two particularly obvious signs that a person has gone beyond initial distress and is in imminent danger of drowning, thus needing the most expeditious assistance possible. These are most typically displayed by people with little or no swimming skills.

- *Double Arm Grasping*—Usually the head is tilted back, with the chin up, and both hands and arms are slapping at the water simultaneously and rapidly in an ineffective butterfly type stroke (the instinctive drowning response). This is most typical in flat water when the nonswimmer is suddenly in water that is overhead.
- *Climbing the Ladder*—As the term implies, the action duplicates an upward crawling motion. It is also known as climbing out of the hole. Again, the chin is high with attention focused upwards. Neither action provides any forward mobility. This is typical of people with limited swimming skills.

Effective Water Observation

Firefighters, police, and lifeguards are all expected to respond expeditiously and efficiently once an emergency arises. Firefighters and police most often respond to emergencies based on reports from others who have observed the problem. While lifeguards also respond to such reports, a basic responsibility of lifeguards is to watch over water areas to locate people in distress. In this sense, lifeguards report the emergencies *and* respond to them. In fact, the vast majority of lifeguard emergency responses are self-initiated and therefore effective water observation is a critical skill for lifeguards. Lifeguards must be able to observe, evaluate, identify, and respond to emergency situations quickly and effectively.

Observation Techniques

Because of the suddenness of aquatic emergencies, safe swimming areas should be scanned completely at least every 30 seconds. If this effort is impeded by attendance levels or unusual activity, additional assistance (backup) should be requested by the lifeguard. Good observation techniques include the following basic points:

Visual Scanning

Observation of a swimming area is accomplished through visual scanning. The lifeguard sweeps the area from side to side, checking quickly on each swimmer or group of swimmers. When scanning, lifeguards should move their heads, not just their eyes, because looking directly at an object significantly increases visual acuity. (Fenner, Leahy, Buhk, & Dawes, 1999) If a sign of distress is noted, further assessment of the person in apparent distress should take place. When a distress clue is noted that is less than conclusive, the lifeguard should occasionally scan the rest of the area quickly and return to evaluate the signs of distress further. It is important that the lifeguard not forget to keep watching the remainder of the swimming crowd while making this evaluation. If two or more lifeguards are working together at a station, one lifeguard may alert another guard to a distress sign and study that person or group while the other guard continues scanning. Using two-way communications (e.g., radio or telephone), lifeguards at different locations can contact each other for a second opinion on what is taking place or for a cross-check from another angle.

Scanning is the systematic way of watching your assigned area and your patrons. This coverage should continue at all times that a lifeguard is on duty. Even when a lifeguard is talking to other lifeguards or a member of the public, scanning should continue. Professional open water lifeguards take great pains to avoid ever turning their back to the water, even when they are not specifically assigned to water observation. This is a matter of professional ethics. In some areas it is mandated by agency protocol. Various scanning strategies have been advanced, to ensure a regular and complete scan of the entire area under observation. These may be based on agency protocols. Regardless of what strategy is employed, the goal is to ensure that the entire area is continually scanned. The following are some common scanning strategies used by lifeguards. The practicality of different strategies may depend on crowd and environmental conditions.

- *Patterns*—Sweep the zone from right to left, front to back.
- *Grouping*—Count the swimmers into smaller groups and keep count of each group. Monitor any changes in the numbers in each group.
- *Head Counting*—Count the number of total swimmers.
- *Letters*—Scan your area by using a letter as your pattern.
- *Tracking*—Follow the swimmers submerging to see if they come up or are riding a wave.
- *Hotspots*—Focus particular attention on rip currents, piers, jetties, drop-offs.
- *Pre-Events*—Look for pre-events to accidents (see *Preventive Lifeguarding*).
- *Unusual Activity Areas*—Watch for unusual groupings of swimmers or activities that seem out of place.

Use of Observation Tools

Binoculars are valuable tools for assessing possible distress signs over distance and should be available to all lifeguards assigned to water surveillance. When a potential problem is observed through visual scanning, lifeguards are encouraged to use binoculars to study the situation more closely. The use of binoculars can also let other lifeguards know that a lifeguard has noticed something and has momentarily ceased scanning to focus on a situation. However, since binoculars limit the field of vision in favor of focusing on a small area, they should not be used for continual scanning. Instead, lifeguards should scan with their eyes and use binoculars only when a distress clue warrants further investigation.

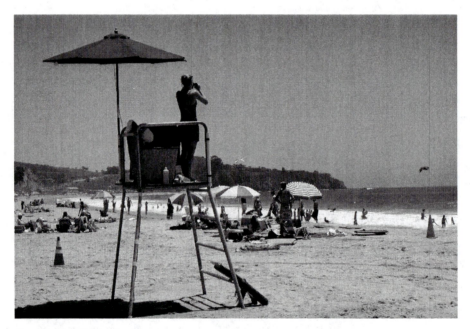

Credit: Ken Kramer

Spotting scopes and high power binoculars mounted on tripods are also used effectively by some agencies, particularly when large beach and water areas must be observed. These scopes sometimes have compass points on them so that coordinates for a boat in distress can be fixed.

Sunglasses are also essential observation tools. Polarized sunglasses are highly recommended because they help eliminate glare, which can obscure large portions of swimming crowds. Sunglasses protect the eyes from blowing sand, wind, and fatigue. This is important to the health of lifeguards, but also to their level of vigilance. Sunglasses used by lifeguards should have frames that protect the eyes, but which do not block peripheral vision.

Overlap

Beaches with multiple lifeguard stations or locations generally divide the entire water area into sections or zones, but it is critical to provide for some type of overlap area between stations to avoid uncovered areas. A standard principle of overlap for a contiguous beach area with several towers is that each lifeguard is made responsible for the water area to the next staffed lifeguard station on either side. In this way, the lifeguards in each tower are equally responsible for the water area between them. One important reason for this overlap is that it is very difficult to clearly define boundaries in the water. It also creates a sense of shared responsibility and doubles the level of protection of swimmers in the area.

Lifeguards should never worry that they might be watching people in another lifeguard's assigned area or ignore distress signs there. Lifeguard administrators should take care to ensure that all lifeguards feel a sense of responsibility for the entire beach area so that egos do not result in a delayed response or lack of response due to fear of embarrassing a fellow lifeguard who may be missing a rescue. A strong sense of group responsibility is essential to effective open water lifeguarding.

Cross-Checking

Glare caused by the sun can cause a serious problem, obscuring large swimming crowds, and essentially blinding lifeguards to a particular water area. Lifeguards must utilize a system of cross-checking to counteract this problem. Whenever a lifeguard assigned to water observation is unable to see a water area for any reason, lifeguards in adjacent locations, should be advised to cross-check. On a beach with several staffed lifeguard towers, this is easily accomplished. In other cases, an alternative method is to post a lifeguard in a vehicle or on foot to cross-check areas with serious glare. At beaches where glare is experienced, standard operating procedures should be developed to address this problem. Cross-checking is also used for purposes of getting a second opinion from another lifeguard as to the need for rescue.

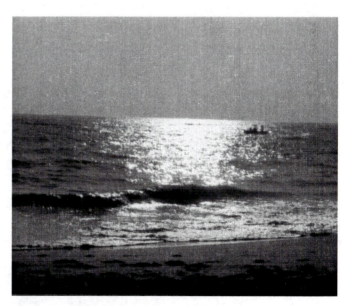

Glare can be a serious problem.
Credit: Paul Drucker

Area of Responsibility

All lifeguard services should define an *area of responsibility* as clearly as possible. The area of responsibility is defined as that area of the water, beach, and related facilities wherein lifeguards are expected to be primary responders. The defined area of responsibility generally includes:

- *Water Areas*—Lifeguards are typically expected to be responsible for all water areas offshore of defined protected beaches, including those above and below the water surface.

- *Offshore Limit*—Some agencies define an offshore limit for lifeguard services, particularly for situations that may involve boating accidents a good distance from shore. If such a limit is defined, lifeguards should be instructed on what other agency or agencies can be summoned if an emergency beyond the offshore limit is observed.

- *Beach Area*—Most lifeguard agencies are responsible for observing beach areas and responding to emergency situations there.

- *Adjacent Facilities*—Many lifeguard agencies, while not actually responsible for observing activities in adjacent facilities, such as parking areas and bathhouses, are subject to calls to emergencies that may occur in those areas.

- *Off-Site Areas*—Off-site areas may include facilities, roadways, business districts, hotels, and residences that are not actually connected to the defined beach facility or park. Some lifeguard agencies are responders to emergencies in these areas due to their relative proximity.

Regardless of the defined area of responsibility, lifeguards must avoid tunnel vision. While lifeguards should concentrate on the assigned area of responsibility, they can provide essential reporting in cases of emergencies or other problems in adjacent areas.

Zones of Coverage

Once the overall area of responsibility has been defined, priority zones should also be defined. This provides lifeguards with a sense of the most important areas upon which they should concentrate. The three major priority zones, in order of importance, are usually as follows:

- *Primary Zone*—The water is a lifeguard's top priority. The primary zone for each lifeguard station is the water area for which the lifeguard is personally responsible. On beaches with several towers, the primary water zone generally extends to the next staffed lifeguard station on either side. This zone auto-

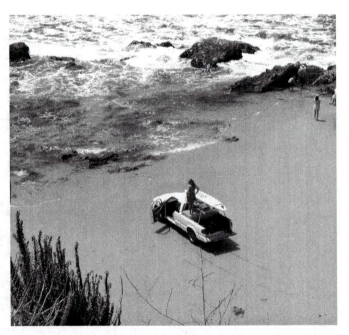

A mobile observation platform.
Credit: Ken Kramer

matically extends when lifeguards in adjacent stations are on a response or the adjacent station is closed.

- *Secondary Zone*—This usually includes adjacent water areas (including primary zones of other lifeguards), the beach, immediately adjacent park areas, the sky, and the water to the horizon. Less frequent scanning of this zone is required, but the lifeguard checks this zone regularly. If the adjacent tower lifeguard is occupied, that part of the secondary zone becomes primary.

- *Tertiary Zone*—Generally the tertiary zone includes all other areas within sight of lifeguards. It could include adjacent streets and parking lots, for example. This zone is scanned least frequently.

Maintaining Vigilance

Lifeguards are, by their very nature, athletes. They must be physically capable of responding quickly and effectively in arduous conditions to save the lives of others. Water surveillance however, is a tedious and sedentary job, with which many athletes struggle. It is both monotonous and stressful. A lifeguard may scan for hours, days, or weeks without observing anything requiring a critical response. Then, a subtle visual clue may indicate a serious, life-threatening emergency. If the lifeguard is not alert, it may be missed and a life lost. Maintaining vigilance is therefore a vital issue for lifeguards.

Many studies of vigilance on the part of people assigned to critical tasks have been conducted over the years. One finding is that vigilance declines over time without regular breaks from surveillance duties. (Fenner et al., 1999) (Applied Anthropology, 2001) Based on available research, USLA encourages limiting continuous assignment of lifeguards to surveillance duties, without a break of at least 15 minutes, to one hour. This break from surveillance duties may include the assignment of other appropriate lifeguard tasks. (Applied Anthropology, 2001) The goal is not to address fatigue, but rather to prevent unintentional declines in vigilance.

Heat has been demonstrated to negatively impact attentiveness. Studies have demonstrated a 30% decline in vigilance in a temperature of 79° and a 45% decline in a temperature of 86°. (Applied Anthropology, 2001) In hot environments, it is therefore advisable to do whatever possible to keep lifeguards assigned to surveillance cool. Air conditioned lifeguard towers are the ideal approach to deal with this problem. Where that is infeasible, ensuring that lifeguards are fully shaded and protected from the sun's rays may help. Additionally, ensuring that lifeguards stay well hydrated can be expected to reduce drops in vigilance associated with heat. (Fenner et al., 1999)

The impact of listening to music or a radio broadcast while involved in water surveillance should be carefully considered. During times of very low beach and water activity, this may have a beneficial effect of relieving boredom. (If lifeguards are permitted to listen to music or radio broadcasts, volume should be kept low and earphones should never be used.) Research suggests however, that as sensory information increases, there may be deterioration in the lifeguard's concentration span and scanning ability. (Fenner et al., 1999) Therefore, particularly during busy periods, music and radios may negatively impact vigilance.

The use of computers, personal digital assistants (PDA), reading materials, and the like are inappropriate for lifeguards assigned to water surveillance. Use of electronic voice communication tools, such as wired telephones, cell-phones, and two-way radios should be restricted to conversations directly related to lifesaving duties. Carrying on personal conversations through these means while assigned to water surveillance poses an unacceptable distraction. When a lifeguard assigned to water observation must interrupt that task to provide medical attention, preventive services, or for other

LearnMore

You can order a video on the Five Minute Scanning Strategy from Aquatic Safety Research Group, LLC 1632 Glenwood Circle, State College, PA 16803.

essential reasons, lifeguards in neighboring towers should be advised, so that they can help maintain continuous surveillance. In some cases, it may be appropriate to send backup during this period.

Most people are at their most alert state mid-morning, with a marked decline in the early afternoon, and a rebound of sorts later in the day. This suggests that lifeguard breaks should be more frequent in early afternoon, but since different people may be affected differently, it has also been suggested that lifeguards be provided an opportunity for input into their break times in accordance with personal experience. (Fenner et al., 1999)

There is little question that fatigue has a negative impact on vigilance. Some sources of fatigue cannot be avoided. This includes the physical exertion involved in rescues and related lifeguard work. Other sources, such as dehydration and exposure to the elements can be limited by ensuring adequate hydration and providing protection to lifeguards. Lifeguards themselves however, must take responsibility for coming to work well-rested, and free of the effects of alcohol or drugs. This includes prescription medication that might be expected to impact vigilance. (Fenner et al., 1999)

Even when lifeguards are given frequent breaks, boredom can negatively impact vigilance. One approach that seasoned lifeguards employ is running imaginary scenarios through their minds. If the man jogging had a cardiac arrest, what would I do? What if that boat turned suddenly toward the surfline? What if one of those three people on the inflatable raft fell off and immediately disappeared? Running these imaginary scenarios has a dual value. It helps the lifeguard remember key skills and helps relieve boredom. The lifeguard must be careful though, not to allow this process to devolve into daydreaming, which would negatively impact vigilance. Running scenarios is an active and intentional mental process.

Another approach to staying alert is the *Five Minute Scanning Strategy* developed by Tom Griffiths (2002). This strategy calls upon lifeguards to change their posture, position, and visual scanning pattern every five minutes. Using a watch with a countdown timer might help regularize this strategy. Even slight movements can help, by stimulating the sympathetic nervous system to keep you alert. Some lifeguards choose to stand during their entire watch to help keep themselves alert.

Staying vigilant is clearly essential to effective surveillance. No matter how effective a lifeguard's scanning techniques may be, if the lifeguard is daydreaming or allowing distractions to interfere the best scanning techniques will be rendered useless. Lifeguards should use the information in this section to develop their own approach to ensuring they remain ever vigilant in watching over those who are counting on their protection.

Coverage Systems

Coverage systems are plans for providing protection to an area of responsibility. The development of a coverage system is a complex task for any emergency service. A fire chief, for example, must consider the size of the community served, the types of fires expected, the size and configuration of buildings and structures that must be protected, concentrations of commercial and residential areas, and other related factors. With that information, fire department managers can determine the staffing level and deployment needed to provide an adequate level of preparedness and response. This is a coverage system.

Like other emergency services, lifeguard agencies must develop coverage systems. Considerations in this process include beach and water attendance, the size of the facility, the area of responsibility, the beach season, water and marine life hazards, the scope of the service, past rescue experience, and so forth. These factors help determine the number of lifeguards, their deployment, and daily scheduling.

Basic Coverage Principles

Basic coverage principles include the following:

- *Area of Responsibility Defined*—The first step to creating a coverage system is a clear understanding of the area of responsibility.
- *Operation Period Defined*—This includes the days of the year lifeguards will be on duty and the times of day coverage will be provided.
- *Protection Provided with No Break in Service*—As with other emergency services, once lifeguard protection begins, using established hours, protection must continue uninterrupted. While some lifeguard services may reduce coverage due to lower than expected crowd conditions, coverage should not be completely eliminated for routine breaks or meal periods. Instead, backup coverage should be provided for this purpose. It is an unacceptable practice for all lifeguards on duty at a beach to leave the beach unprotected for a lunch break. If supervisory personnel determine that coverage should be terminated early due to weather conditions or extraordinarily low attendance, beach patrons should be notified.
- *Working Conditions Are Reasonable and Clearly Understood*—In many areas, working conditions are established through adherence to labor laws and employee contracts. Nonetheless, the paramount concern is that an atmosphere is maintained that ensures safety for both the employee and those being protected.

Example Coverage Systems

As examples of how basic coverage principles are followed, the following are four different lifeguard operations.

Single Site Operation

Whispering Willows State Park is a small day area located on a pond. The area is open from 9 am to 8 pm daily and gates control access to the 60-car parking lot. The beach is approximately 100 yards long and is protected from two lifeguard stands.

Six lifeguards are assigned to work at Whispering Willows, each working a 40-hour week during the summer season, composed of five eight hour days. Two lifeguards have Monday and Tuesday off, two

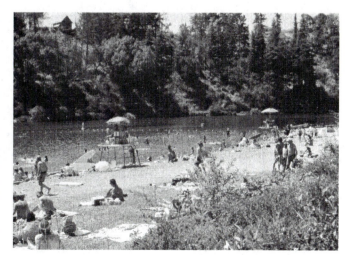

Credit: Lucy Woolshlager

have Wednesday and Thursday off and two have Friday and Saturday off. With this schedule, there are four lifeguards working Monday through Thursday, five on Friday and Saturday, when attendance increases, and all six on Sunday, the busiest day.

The lifeguards cover the beach from 9 am to 8 pm on a rotating schedule. Each day, at least two lifeguards report to work at 9 am and work to 5 pm. Then, at least two report at noon and work to 8 pm. On Friday, Saturday, and Sunday, the additional lifeguards arrive during shifts in between, such as 10 am to 6 pm. Coverage is thereby maintained from 9 am to 8 pm, seven days each week, without a break in service. Backup is available at all times. The lowest level of coverage exists during the early morning and late evening hours when attendance is lowest. The greatest coverage is provided mid-day, when attendance is highest.

Multi-Tower, Independent Operation

Lengthy Beach is a moderate-sized coastal town with a one-mile protected beach. The Lengthy Beach Patrol has established five lifeguard towers along the beach, providing continuous coverage over the one mile beach for the summer season. Fifteen open water lifeguards work 40-hour weeks in addition to supervisory staff, with three lifeguards assigned to each tower on a schedule very similar to that of Whispering Willows. On any given day, two lifeguards will work each tower and provide breaks for each other during the course of the operation day.

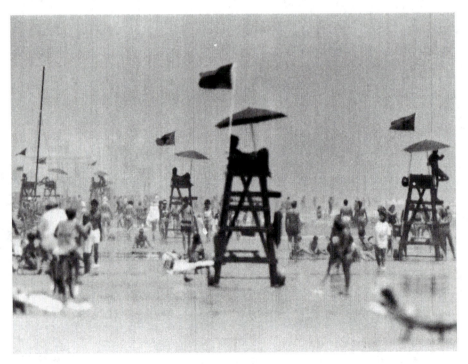

Credit: Mike Hensler

Multi-Tower Operation with Backup

Wide Island County provides lifeguard services over three miles of sandy beach from 12 towers during the summer. Twenty-one seasonal lifeguards are hired for forty hours each week, covering the beach from 9 am to 6 pm. Each tower operates with a single lifeguard. Two lifeguard supervisors work daily from vehicles to provide backup and oversight.

Tower Zero Operation

Surf City, a major population area in a warm climate, operates a lifeguard service year round covering ten miles of beaches. There are several large, fixed observation towers with a wide area of view and numerous smaller, numbered towers spread along the beaches. During the busier season, the operation at Surf City is very similar to Wide Island County. The smaller towers are staffed by seasonally employed lifeguard personnel. The main observation towers are not numbered (thereby the reference to "Tower Zero"). They are used primarily for overall observation and supervision of the area and are staffed by more senior personnel who coordinate responses and backup. The seasonal lifeguard personnel are relieved and backed up by mobile lifeguard units dispatched by lifeguards at the main tower.

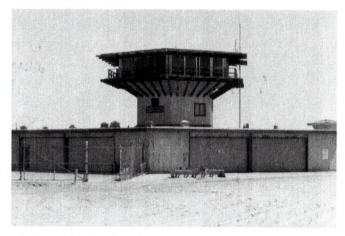

The Tower Zero system requires a main station with a commanding view.

Credit: Rob McGowan

In high season, lifeguards are staffed from dawn to dusk on staggered schedules. The first lifeguards on duty staff only the main observation tower. Those not assigned to water observation prepare equipment and patrol the beach. As mid-day approaches and more lifeguards arrive for their shifts, the smaller, numbered towers are opened, with preference given to those known to have high rescue activity and those furthest from the main tower. During mid-day all towers are staffed. As evening approaches, the smaller towers are closed one by one until all are closed. A lifeguard remains on duty in Tower Zero until the end of scheduled lifeguard protection.

During months of lower attendance, the small towers are not staffed and all observation is provided from the larger, fixed towers. From these towers, a smaller staff of lifeguards can observe the entire beach area using powerful binoculars and communicate with beach visitors over a public address system. They patrol the beach regularly in mobile lifeguard units and when trouble is noticed, mobile lifeguard units are dispatched to the scene.

Chapter Summary

In this chapter, we have learned how to recognize and assess signs that may help indicate drowning presentations. That includes observations before people even enter the water, as well as signs of persons in distress in the water. We have learned methods of effective water observation. We have learned that all lifeguard services should define an area of responsibility and zones of coverage. We have learned about the challenge of maintaining high levels of vigilance and ways to do so. We have learned about coverage systems and have seen some examples of these systems.

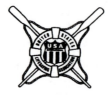

Discussion Points

- Why might it be difficult to know if a person in the water is in distress?
- What are some clues from a beachgoer's behavior on land that they might later need assistance in the water?
- What are some examples that a swimmer is in distress?
- What would double arm grasping or climbing the ladder indicate?
- What are some visual observation techniques that can be used to ensure the entire water area is scanned every 30 seconds?
- What are some common observation tools?
- What are the values of overlap and cross-checking?
- Why should areas of responsibility be defined?
- Why should zones of coverage be defined?
- What are some techniques for maintaining vigilance?
- What are some of the basic coverage principles?

References

Applied Anthropology (2001). Lifeguard vigilance bibliographic study. Paris, France: Applied Anthropology.

Fenner, P., Leahy, S., Buhk, A., Dawes, P. (1999). Prevention of drowning: visual scanning and attention span in lifeguards. *The Journal of Occupational Health and Safety Australia and New Zealand, 15,* 1. New South Wales, Australia: CCH Australia, Ltd.

Pia, F. (1970). *On Drowning.* Larchmont, New York: Water Safety Films, Inc.

Pia, F. (1997). Reflections on element #1 of effective surveillance: water crisis recognition training. In *International Life Saving Federation International Medical-Rescue Conference* proceedings. San Diego, California: International Life Saving Federation, Americas Region.

Chapter 12
Components of a Rescue

In this chapter you will learn the fundamental steps involved in successful accomplishment of an open water rescue. We will break down an open water rescue into the three major components and the steps involved in each component. You will learn what is involved in each component and each step.

CHAPTER EXCERPT

Before a lifeguard enters the water on a rescue, it is important that someone else knows that a rescue is being performed, because the lifeguard will be exposed to a potentially dangerous situation and further assistance may be needed for the rescue.

To the beach visitor, rescues performed by lifeguards may seem dramatic, spontaneous events. Suddenly, a lifeguard springs from the station, runs to the water's edge and plunges in. The lifeguard quickly swims out to a person in distress (a victim) and contact is made. Returning to the beach, the lifeguard assists the victim to dry land and returns to the station, prepared for the next rescue to develop. Those who had riveted their attention on the sudden action go back to their recreational activities. It's all over, for now.

To the experienced lifeguard, most rescues are routine; but while many rescues may seem quite simple, they actually represent a carefully planned response to a specific set of circumstances. The lifeguard first recognizes distress, panic, or drowning signs, which are carefully and quickly assessed. The decision to respond is made. An entire backup network is alerted. Rescue equipment is selected based on the requirements of the rescue. The lifeguard plans an approach to the victim and carries it out. Throughout the approach, the lifeguard maintains constant visual contact with the victim. Upon arrival, the lifeguard calms the victim, signals to shore, and completes the save by bringing the victim to shore. Following these events, the lifeguard evaluates the victim for any complications, completes reports necessary to document the event, and prepares for another response.

The United States Lifesaving Association recognizes three basic components of every open water rescue. Each component includes specific steps. The three components of every rescue are as follows:

1. Recognize and Respond
2. Contact and Control
3. Signal and Save

Specific rescue procedures may differ somewhat from agency to agency; but these three rescue components are valid for all rescue situations, from wading assists to rescues with multiple victims. Each rescue includes all three components. What follows is a detailed description of each component and the subordinate steps involved.

Recognize and Respond

The first component of a rescue—*recognize and respond*—includes four steps:

1:1 Recognition
1:2 Alert
1:3 Equipment Selection
1:4 Entry

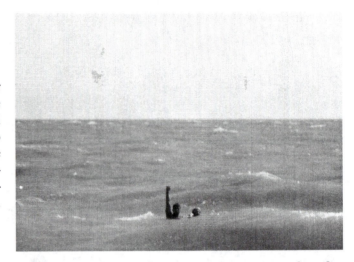

A lifeguard with a victim in a rip current signals for assistance.

Credit: William McNeely, Jr.

Recognition

Before a rescue can take place, there must be *recognition* of distress. Typically a lifeguard determines through observation that a person needs assistance in the water. Perhaps a swimmer has fallen off a floating support in deep water or is being swept into deep water by a current. In some cases, lifeguards are summoned to respond by beach visitors who have noticed something wrong in the water. Although unusual, the lifeguard may actually hear cries for help from the victim. The 9-1-1 telephone system and the marine radio system are also sources of reports of emergencies, particularly for areas outside the direct observation of lifeguards. Occasionally employees of other public safety agencies observe and report the need for a lifeguard response. Regardless of the source of information, the process begins when a lifeguard recognizes the need for a rescue.

Alert

Before a lifeguard enters the water on a rescue, it is important that someone else knows that a rescue is being performed, because the lifeguard will be exposed to a potentially dangerous situation and further assistance may be needed for the rescue. An *alert* to others triggers procedures that will provide backup assistance for the lifeguard. It will also ensure that other lifeguards begin to cover the water area of the lifeguard leaving on the rescue.

Each agency has its own alert procedures based on staffing levels and available communication equipment. A lifeguard may simply alert a station partner before responding to a rescue. At stations where lifeguards work alone, they may use a two-way radio to announce rescues or may trigger an alarm. Some stations are equipped with special telephone systems allowing lifeguards to simply take a telephone off the hook. The off-hook telephone rings into a central switchboard, identifying the station involved. Other alert procedures may include air horns, whistle signals, and similar audible devices. Some agencies use flag systems, but this alert method is least certain in that it relies on other lifeguards who may or may not observe the signal.

The best alert systems allow for two-way communication which enables the responding lifeguard to firmly establish that the alert has been received, to briefly detail circumstances of the response, and to request any special assistance which may appear necessary. The alert for a routine rescue may be very brief, such as, "Tower #1 in on one victim." The lifeguard in Tower #1 states that a rescue of one person is being initiated. For further information on lifeguard communication, please refer to the chapter entitled *Communication Methods*.

The importance of the alert cannot be over-emphasized. Alerts are standard practice in all emergency services, including fire departments, police agencies, and emergency medical services. Without an alert, lifeguards expose themselves to potentially life-threatening situations without anyone else becoming aware. A significant component of drowning statistics is attributable to untrained people who drown while trying to assist others. Although lifeguard training significantly reduces this potential, lifeguards are at risk on every rescue.

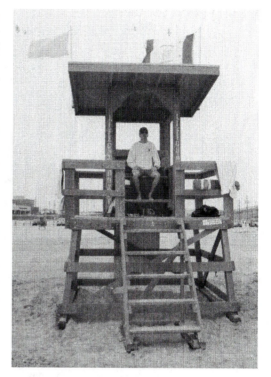

Credit: Peter Davis

Equipment Selection

Once the alert is made, or simultaneous to this notification, the responding lifeguard must make an *equipment selection*. Proper equipment selection requires a thorough familiarity with all rescue equipment maintained by the agency, a proper evaluation of the incident, and the foresight to consider ways that apparent circumstances of the incident may change during the response.

Sometimes the lifeguard who has observed distress develop may actually determine that other personnel should respond based on proximity or the availability of special rescue equipment. For example, a rescue boat may be very near the victim and signaled to effect the rescue. Equipment selection for more advanced equipment is covered later in this text. In our hypothetical rescue, the lifeguard selects a rescue buoy. (For specific information on use of a rescue buoy, please see the chapter entitled *Standard Rescue Equipment.*)

Entry

Once proper rescue equipment has been selected, the lifeguard determines the most efficient path to the victim and effects a water *entry*. It is very important to attempt to maintain visual contact with the victim throughout the rescue. Victims may move with a current or submerge prior to the lifeguard's arrival. In the latter case, lifeguards must be able to fix a *last seen point*.

The water can be very deceiving since there are usually no stationary objects offshore. Once in the water, the lifeguard may be too low to keep a consistent eye on the victim, particularly in waves. For

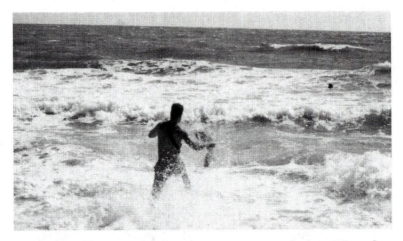

A lifeguard enters the water to rescue a victim. Note the victim's head in the rip current.

Credit: William McNeely, Jr.

this reason, it is sometimes valuable to take a *bearing* from fixed points on land. Buildings, trees, and other stationary objects ashore can be used for this purpose. One of the best methods is to line up two stationary objects ashore that are one in front of the other, such as two trees. By staying a course that keeps the two objects consistently lined up, the lifeguard can maintain a straight line while swimming. This is also known as a *rhumb line*.

The drowning process can progress rapidly through the distress and panic stages to submersion, so speed is important. To increase the speed and efficiency of entries, several points should be considered for swimming rescues:

- *Get There Safely*—As important as speed may be in a water rescue, if the lifeguard is injured en route to the victim, the victim may not survive. Speed is important, but lifeguards must protect themselves at all times.

- *Running Is Faster than Swimming*—Running to the closest point on shore to the victim is usually much faster than swimming a diagonal route to the victim. In planning the entry, lifeguards should usually run down the shoreline to the point closest to the victim before entering the water.

- *Use the Current*—If the victim is caught in a current, the best point for water entry will vary. For example, if the victim is caught on the edge of strong, out-flowing current from a tidal bay, the lifeguard could run to a point adjacent to the victim, jump into the center of the current and be swept past the victim. In this case, as in a river, the lifeguard may need to intentionally enter upstream and swim diagonally toward the victim. At a surf beach, if a victim is caught in a rip current moving perpendicular to the beach, the best entry point will usually be at the rip current feeder. The current then helps carry the lifeguard to the victim. At lower tides, rip current channels are sometimes bordered by sandbars that are waist deep or even shallower. The lifeguard may be able to run out on the sandbar to a point very near the victim before jumping into the rip current channel and swimming to the victim.

- *Run in Shallow Water*—Running in shallow water is faster than swimming. Upon entering the water, the best technique is to kick high out of the water while running to minimize the resistance of the water. This is called high-stepping. At the same time, life-guards should always be conscious of the potential for uneven bottom conditions that can inflict serious joint injuries.

- *Use Surface Dives to Get to Swimming Depth*—On a gradually sloping beach, upon reaching deeper water the lifeguard will be unable to continue the running entry. At this point, however, swimming may not yet be the fastest method of moving forward. Wading to swimming depth is a possibility, but it takes considerable energy and may be quite slow. At surf beaches, incoming waves will further impede forward progress. The lifeguard's goal is to present as little of the body as possible to the oncoming wave. In such cases, when running is no longer effective, but swimming is not yet the fastest method of forward propulsion, a surface dive or surface dives should be used. At a surf beach, the lifeguard dives under incoming waves that are too large to jump over or through. As the lifeguard dives forward, the head and neck must be protected. This can be accomplished by fully extending the hands and arms forward as the dive is initiated.

- *Porpoise*—A more advanced technique involves *porpoising* through shallow water to swimming depth. Porpoising is accomplished by springing forward in a shallow dive with the arms fully extended. If swim fins are used, they are held in each hand. As the forward glide slows, the lifeguard grabs the sand and pulls the feet under the body in a crouching position, then springs forward using the legs in another forward dive. This arcing dive-glide-recover pattern is repeated until swimming depth is reached. Porpoising can be used in both surf and flat water, but is particularly effective in surf.

At beaches with a steep slope, the period spent running or porpoising through the water will be very brief. On the other hand, beaches with long, gradual slopes necessitate extensive running and porpoising through the water. Under either circumstance, *the lifeguard begins swimming when running, wading, or porpoising action are no longer faster than swimming.*

Contact and Control

The second component of a water rescue—*contact and control*—includes the following three steps:

2:1 Approach
2:2 Contact
2:3 Stabilize

Approach

Once swimming depth is reached, the lifeguard approaches the victim as quickly as possible, using swimming strokes that will allow frequent checking on the position of the victim. The crawl stroke is best because it is fastest. Using the heads-up form of water polo players, the approaching lifeguard can usually maintain visual contact with the victim. In some situations, the lifeguard will be unable to see the victim no matter what stroke is used. This may occur when water conditions are rough or when a drowning presentation has progressed to a submersion. In these cases, the bearings that were taken on water entry become critical for fixing the last seen point of the victim.

To further assist, lifeguards ashore must by prepared to provide easily understandable signals to the lifeguard in the water. Upon losing sight of the victim, the responding lifeguard can turn to shore for this assistance. Audible devices, such as public address systems and whistle systems may

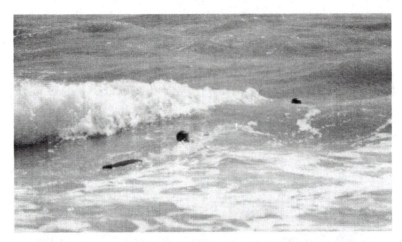

A lifeguard approaches a victim in a rip current. Note that the surf is not breaking in the rip current channel.
Credit: William McNeely, Jr.

be useful, but should not be solely relied upon because the lifeguard in the water may not be able to hear them. Simple shore based arm signals are as follows:

- *Move to Right or Left*—A rescue flotation device (RFD) is extended to the right or left at the end of a fully extended arm by the lifeguard ashore.
- *Go Further Out*—An RFD is held vertically between two upraised arms.
- *Stay There*—Arms are extended horizontally to the sides without holding a rescue buoy.
- *Move Offshore and Wait*—An RFD is held horizontally in both hands overhead. This is generally used when a boat or helicopter is being sent to retrieve the lifeguard and victim.

In addition to these shore based signals, other arm signals intended primarily for use by a lifeguard in the water can also be used by lifeguards ashore. These are covered later in the *Signal and Save* section of this chapter and in Appendix A.

Upon nearing the victim, the lifeguard should begin talking to the victim to provide reassurance and instructions. The lifeguard can watch the victim's eyes and facial expression for signs of fright or panic. It is well worth taking the time needed to calm the victim because a panicked victim can be very dangerous. During final stages of approach, the lifeguard should keep away from a position where the victim can grab the lifeguard.

Usually, the mere presence of another person in the water who seems calm and knowledgeable will have a very positive effect. The presence of the rescue buoy also gives the victim immediate hope. The final few feet of the approach are covered with the rescue buoy extended toward the victim, and the lifeguard using swimming kicks for thrust. The lifeguard assumes a defensive position by pushing the buoy toward the victim.

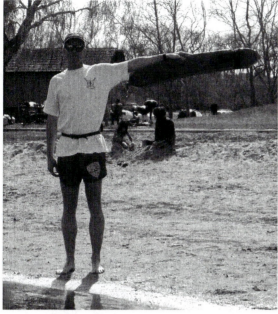

Move right (or left).
Credit: Sandra McCormick

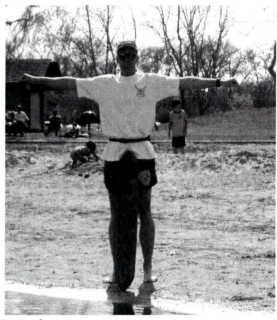

Stay there.
Credit: Sandra McCormick

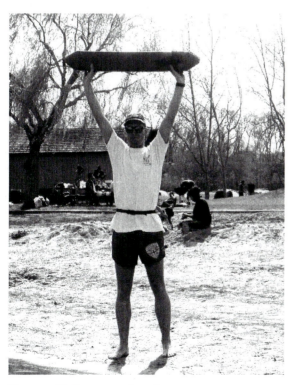

Move offshore and wait.
Credit: Sandra McCormick

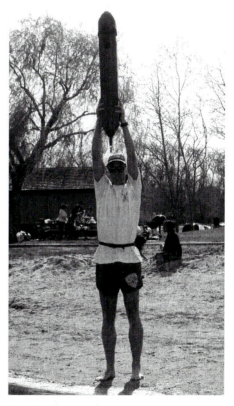

Go further out.
Credit: Sandra McCormick

Contact

Contact of the victim begins when the victim grabs the rescue buoy or is otherwise connected to it. Lifeguards should always avoid direct contact with victims in the water because they can panic, grab the lifeguard and jeopardize the safety of both. For purposes of this description, we will assume a standard rescue scenario in which the victim grabs an extended rescue buoy. The chapter entitled *Standard Rescue Equipment* provides information on more complicated rescues and proper use of an RFD.

If the victim grabs the lifeguard in panic, the lifeguard should immediately stop swimming and submerge. Victims virtually always let go when this maneuver is used. If necessary, the lifeguard can push off from the victim using the feet, then swim away underwater and surface seven to ten feet away from the victim before extending the buoy again.

Stabilize

Once control has been gained in a rescue, the lifeguard can begin to *stabilize* the victim. In most situations, once support in the form of a rescue flotation device has been provided, the panic experienced by the victim will quickly subside. The victim can regain normal breathing, wipe away hair and water from the face, and communicate with the lifeguard. Rational thinking returns, leaving the victim able to understand what is happening and what must be done.

In most rescue situations, lifeguards should take advantage of this reduction of panic before proceeding with the rescue. It is an excellent opportunity to explain to the victim what has happened, to assure the victim that the situation is now under control and to rest before proceeding. Since the immediate crisis has been contained, there is usually no immediate need to proceed with retrieval to shore until extrication is planned and explained to the victim.

Signal and Save

The third and final component of a rescue—*signal and save*—includes four steps:
    3:1 Signal
    3:2 Retrieve
    3:3 Assess
    3:4 Report

Signal

The alert initiated by the responding lifeguard begins a backup procedure that directs the attention of shore-based lifeguards to the rescue and may bring other lifeguards or staff to the beach near the rescue scene. Once control of the situation has been gained and the victim has been stabilized it is important to *signal* to other lifeguards. USLA has adopted four basic signals which all lifeguard agencies should utilize. These simple signals allow for national consistency and effective communication among lifeguards working for different agencies. Each signal, when given by a lifeguard in the water, should be repeated by lifeguards on shore. This lets the lifeguard in the water know that the signal was seen and understood. These signals can also be used by lifeguards ashore to communicate with lifeguards in the water.

USLA Approved Arm Signals

- *Under Control*—Also referred to as "no further assistance needed." The lifeguard touches the fingers together over the head, forming a large circle with the arms. An alternative is to touch the middle of the head with the fingertips of one hand, but this signal is not as visible. Either of these signals simulate the commonly used "OK" hand signal made by creating a circle with the thumb and forefinger. They are used primarily when the lifeguard has determined that the rescue can be accomplished without the help of others and the victim is stable. It is important to note that this does not mean lifeguards ashore can ignore the rescue in progress. The situation can deteriorate and the lifeguard in the water will need to be able to signal the change to someone watching from shore.

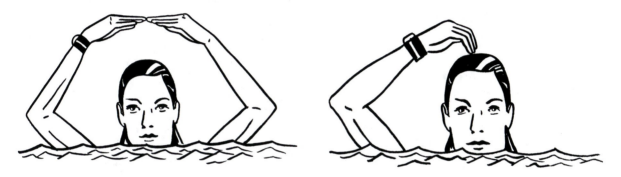

Under Control

- *Assistance Needed*—The lifeguard raises, *but does not wave* one arm. The lifeguard in the water needs further assistance. This could be due to a badly panicked victim, multiple victims, an injury the lifeguard sustained in the response, etc. Backup should be sent immediately.

- *Resuscitation Case*—The lifeguard raises *and waves* one arm. In situations involving non-breathing victims, or those with seriously lowered respirations, backup staff must be advised that some degree of resuscitation will most likely be required once the victim is brought back to the beach. This allows backup staff to prepare resuscitation equipment for use once the victim has been retrieved. It also signals the need for in-water assistance. A single lifeguard in the water is rarely able to effectively manage a non-breathing victim alone. Lifeguards on shore, seeing the lifeguard wave an arm,

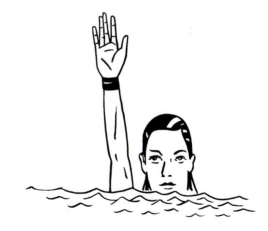

Assistance Needed

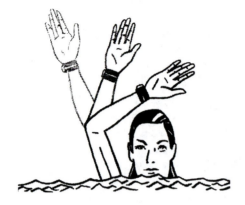

Resuscitation Case

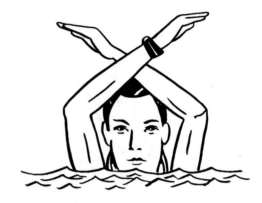

Code X (Missing Swimmer)

may be able to determine that an ambulance will likely be needed and either request an ambulance in advance or place an ambulance on standby. This can greatly lessen ambulance response time.

- *Code X*—The lifeguard raises both arms and forms an X overhead. This is the most serious signal of all. The lifeguard could not reach the victim in time. A swimmer is missing and presumed submerged. The lifeguard in the water believes that search and recovery procedures need to be initiated. This signal allows a lifeguard in the water to advise lifeguards ashore of the need for immediate backup without interrupting an initial search for the submerged victim by having to swim to shore. Lifeguards on shore receiving this signal should immediately take bearings to fix the point of the lifeguard, as well as prepare an appropriate response. For more details, please see the chapter on *Search and Rescue*.

Retrieve

In our example, the victim has not submerged. Once the victim has been stabilized and the signal has been given, the lifeguard will *retrieve* the victim to shore. In calm water conditions, the objective during retrieval is simply to reach water of standing depth. In heavy surf or current conditions, more careful route selection is needed.

If the victim is in a rip current, the lifeguard usually first swims laterally out of the current before swimming ashore. Rescues off rocky shores or near piers and other obstructions may also require lateral swimming before a turn is made toward the beach. Lifeguards should make every attempt to avoid swimming a victim to the beach through sets of very large surf. Lifeguards can either wait for a lull between sets of waves or swim the victim to deeper water for pickup by a lifeguard vessel or rescue helicopter, if available. Another alternative is to swim the victim to an adjacent beach area with less adverse surf conditions. While this may take time and energy, it may also be the safest method.

Once the route is determined, the victim should be informed. In most cases, with lifeguard instruction, the victim will be able to assist by holding firmly onto the rescue buoy and employing a flutter kick or frog kick. By using a backstroke, the lifeguard can maintain constant visual contact with the victim. If a crawl or breaststroke is used, the lifeguard should look back regularly to check on the victim.

Victims should be instructed to continue grasping the rescue buoy until told that they can release it. Upon approaching shore, victims often become more confident or simply embarrassed and let go of the rescue buoy. In rip current rescues and in surf, a victim who releases the rescue buoy prematurely can easily be recirculated back into the rip current.

While swimming to shore at a surf beach, lifeguards must remember to watch for incoming waves. If the victim will be taken in through large breaking waves, the victim should be advised of this and told how to prepare. The lifeguard gets behind the victim and hugs tightly under the armpits with the rescue buoy against the victim's chest. Just before the wave hits, the lifeguard can pinch the victim's nose with the thumb and forefinger and keep the rest of the hand over the victim's mouth to reduce the chances of water being swallowed or aspirated.

In situations where the victim is extremely weak or unconscious, the lifeguard will have to adapt the rescue buoy to provide support for the victim before beginning retrieval. Techniques for proper use of rescue buoys in these cases are detailed in the chapter entitled *Standard Rescue Equipment*.

Remove

Once shallow water is reached, it may be a simple procedure to remove the victim to shore. In most rescues, the victim needs little or no further assistance. Some agencies have established policies that require lifeguards to escort all victims completely out of the water to dry sand, even if the victim appears to need little or no assistance. In some situations, victims will need help leaving the water. Perhaps a weak or tired swimmer is having trouble maintaining balance or wading ashore. Other victims may be unconscious or barely lucid. In these situations, lifeguards will have to carry or assist the victims.

Lifeguards should consider several points important to removing victims from the water. First, lifeguards must have the strength and ability to extricate a victim without assistance. Although there are often other lifeguards, staff, or visitors present to assist with extrication, there may be times when a lifeguard will have to accomplish removal alone. Second, lifeguards should use extrication techniques that will minimize the possibility of personal injury. Victims may be heavy or unable to assist the lifeguard at all. Lifeguards should use techniques that protect the victim from injury during extrication,

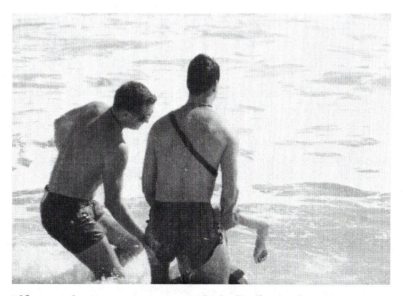

Lifeguards remove a rescued victim from the water.
Credit: William McNeely, Jr.

both from the terrain that must be covered and from the removal technique itself. Two simple removal techniques are offered in this chapter that consider these points.

When victims are able to assist to some degree during the removal process, a *shallow water assist* is recommended. To execute this technique, the lifeguard simply drapes one of the victim's arms around the back of the lifeguard's neck, holding the hand or forearm, and supporting the victim's waist with the other arm. Then the victim is gently directed out of the water to dry sand and assisted in sitting or lying down on the beach. When the victim cannot assist in the removal process, a *longitudinal drag* is recommended. Place the hands under the victim's armpits and attempt to support the head with the forearms. Then drag the victim up the beach. If any spinal injury is suspected, use techniques for stabilizing spinal injuries described in the chapter entitled *Medical Care in the Aquatic Environment*.

Assess

Assess all victims for possible complications after the rescue. This can be done rather informally in routine cases. Does the person have a steady or unsteady gait? Are the eyes clear? Does the person appear alert? Does the person seem fully oriented? In most cases, this will be adequate.

It is a good practice to ask all victims if they are all right upon reaching shore. Can they take a deep breath without pain? Do they think they swallowed or inhaled (aspirated) water? In most cases, it will be obvious if a person is feeling poorly, but lifeguards must remember the tendency of victims to deny problems. Often upon the completion of a rescue everyone on the beach is watching. The victim feels very embarrassed and just wants to leave. Lifeguards should never release victims until reasonably certain they are fine. For details on assessment and treatment of drowning victims, including when they should be sent to the hospital, see the chapter on *Medical Care in the Aquatic Environment*.

Report

The rescue *report* is critical for all lifeguard provider agencies. Rescue reports, including name and address of the victim, should be completed for every rescue performed by lifeguards. The report form should include information such as the name of the lifeguard, the time of day, and the date. Example report forms can be found in *Appendix B*.

USLA defines a water rescue of a swimmer as any case in which a lifeguard physically assists a victim in extrication from the water when the victim lacked the apparent ability to do so alone. For reporting purposes, providing verbal commands or advice to swimmers in the water is considered to be an aspect of preventive lifeguarding, but not a rescue.

Statistics generated through the filing of rescue reports often provide the single most important information in determining needed levels of lifeguard staffing. While stories about rescues are sometimes fascinating, agency administrators need hard facts about the volume of rescue activity when budget-based decisions must be made. This makes the accurate reporting of rescues critical to lifeguards concerned about ensuring that staffing levels meet the need. Some lifeguard supervisors remind their personnel that, "If you don't record it, it didn't happen." While in truth the rescue may have taken place, statistically it didn't happen if a rescue report wasn't filed.

USLA compiles annual statistics on the number of rescues performed at beaches throughout the United States. These statistics have proven essential in helping justify the value of adequate lifeguard staffing levels throughout the country and the need for lifeguard equipment. They are regularly the basis of media reports and research. Each open water lifeguard agency should report the rescues they perform annually, using the USLA national lifesaving statistics form found on USLA's website at:

www.usla.org. Reports should be submitted within a month after the end of each calendar year. Seasonal agencies should report at the close of the season.

Chapter Summary

In this chapter, we have learned about the three components of a rescue and the steps involved in each component. The first component of a rescue is Recognize and Respond, which includes the steps: recognition, alert, equipment selection, and entry. The second component of a rescue is Contact and Control, which includes the steps: approach, contact, and stabilize. The third component is Signal and Save, which includes the steps: signal, retrieve, remove, assess, and report.

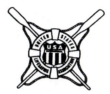

Discussion Points

- Why do you think is it important to know the components of a rescue?
- What are some examples of how distress might first be recognized and by whom?
- What are some ways a lifeguard might alert others before leaving on a rescue?
- Why is it important to alert others before leaving on a rescue?
- Why should a lifeguard usually run as far as possible before swimming to the victim?
- How might current impact a lifeguard's swim to a victim?
- When does the lifeguard entering the water stop running and start swimming?
- What are the signals used by a lifeguard on shore to advise a lifeguard in the water on best actions to take?
- Why should lifeguards avoid direct contact with victims in the water?
- How long should the lifeguard take to stabilize a victim before retrieval?
- What are the four USLA approved arm signals a lifeguard should use to inform those on shore?
- What are some methods for removing a victim from the water?
- Why is it important to assess the victim before releasing the victim?
- Why is it important to complete a report on the rescue?

Chapter 13
Standard Rescue Equipment

In this chapter, you will learn about the basic equipment used by lifeguards throughout the world. You will gain a basic understanding of how this equipment is used effectively. Skills for effective use of rescue equipment require extensive practice and experience. This chapter provides an overview. To effectively utilize the information in this chapter, you will also need to participate in practical training exercises.

CHAPTER EXCERPT

The rescue flotation device (RFD) has become the principal piece of rescue equipment used by professional lifeguards in the United States.

Special training and the use of rescue equipment are essential to professional lifeguard operations. These are the primary factors separating professional lifeguards from amateur lifesavers. The rescue equipment described here is the mainstay of professional open water lifeguard agencies—core equipment which should be available to all open water lifeguards. Under guidelines of USLA, there should be at least one rescue flotation device (RFD) available for each lifeguard on duty, swim fins readily accessible to lifeguards (as appropriate according to local conditions), and spinal stabilization equipment—including spineboard, head and neck immobilization devices, and fastening devices readily accessible at each staffed beach area. Additional equipment required under ULSA guidelines is discussed in the chapters entitled *Search and Recovery* and *Medical Care in the Aquatic Environment*.

Standard rescue equipment is essential for the following reasons:

- *Support of the Victim*—To reverse the drowning process, buoyant support must be provided for the victim. This support must be sufficient to maintain the victim's breathing passages above the water surface.

- *Lifeguard Safety*—A panicked victim, desperate for buoyant support, is a very real threat to an approaching rescuer. The victim may attempt to grab the lifeguard, forcing both underwater and into a mutually life-threatening situation. When buoyant rescue devices are provided to victims they usually have an immediate calming effect as the primary source of fear (submersion) is eliminated. This enhances lifeguard safety.

- *Speed*—Some rescue devices can reduce lifeguard response time, which is a critical factor in drowning prevention.

- *Increased Efficiency*—Many rescue devices provide increased efficiency for the lifeguard by augmenting the lifeguard's swimming skills or by providing support for the victim so that the lifeguard can devote more energy to swimming. For example, rescue flotation devices (RFDs) increase the speed with which victims can be removed from the water and allow the rescue of multiple victims by a single lifeguard.

In the open water setting, most lifeguard rescue equipment consists of devices used during in-water rescues, rather than extension devices such as reaching poles or throwing devices (ring buoys, etc), which are more typically found in the pool environment. This is not to suggest that these devices are of no use in open water. Extension or throwing devices may be useful at open water recreation areas with floats, docks, or piers, since distress may occur at those facilities within easy reaching or throwing distance. Open water lifeguards assigned to flood rescues in swiftwater also use throw bags and similar devices very effectively. At open water areas however, it is a very rare situation that allows for an effective throwing or reaching rescue. Therefore this text will not cover such rescues in detail. Suffice it to say that if a victim can be easily and reliably rescued by throwing a line or extending a pole, this method should be given due consideration. Nevertheless, lifeguards must always be prepared to enter the water to effect a rescue.

Rescue Flotation Devices

The rescue flotation device (RFD) has become the principal piece of rescue equipment used by professional lifeguards in the United States. The two types of rescue flotation devices are the *rescue buoy* and the *rescue tube*. Rescue buoys are also known as rescue cans, torpedo buoys (torps), and Burnside buoys. The latter name stems from designer of the modern rescue buoy. (See the chapter on *Lifesaving History*.) These devices are oblong and molded from lightweight, hard plastic. They have handles molded into the sides and rear, which allow the victim to maintain a firm, comfortable grip during rescue. Rescue buoys are available in different sizes for different conditions. They are very durable and highly visible.

The rescue tube, also known as the Peterson tube after the lifeguard who designed it, is a flexible foam buoy with an embedded strap and a vinyl skin. The embedded strap is connected to the lanyard leading to the lifeguard. In a rescue situation, the tube can be wrapped around the victim and secured. The ends of the tube are typically fastened together with a ring (on one end) and snap-hook (on the other), or by a plastic fastening device. This is particularly useful when taking a victim through breaking surf, wherein the rescuer and victim might otherwise be separated. Rescue tubes are available in several sizes.

The three major components of an RFD are:

- *Float*
- *Lanyard*
- *Harness*

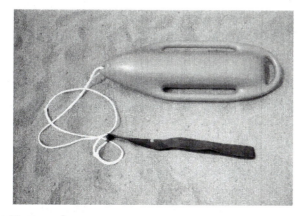

Rescue buoy.

Credit: Dan McCormick

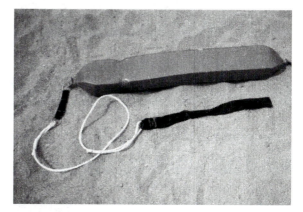

Rescue tube.

Credit: Dan McCormick

The two primary types of RFDs each have distinctive characteristics and many lifeguard agencies select one over another for specific reasons. For example, agencies where multiple victim rescue situations are common may employ large size rescue buoys because of the extra buoyancy they provide. Another approach is to employ both types of RFDs, thus allowing equipment selection appropriate to the rescue.

RFDs should always be available in a number adequate to allow all lifeguards at a beach to use one if a major rescue takes place. In many areas, RFDs are assigned to lifeguards as pieces of personal equipment, for which they are responsible during all duty hours. At other agencies, RFDs are assigned to locations rather than lifeguards. When lifeguards leave these locations, they are always expected to take an RFD along. Some agencies require the use of an RFD on all rescues in addition to other equipment that may be selected.

There are good reasons for such policies:

- *Constant Readiness*—While on duty, lifeguards should be ready at all times to respond appropriately and expeditiously to a person in distress. If a lifeguard is away from the station for some reason, a fundamental piece of rescue equipment should always be at hand for an immediate response.

- *Identification to the Public*—RFDs are very distinctive and recognizable, even more so than uniforms, thus allowing persons in need of assistance to quickly locate lifeguards. The RFD also helps to symbolize the authority of the lifeguard when approaching a beach patron. In a rescue situation, the RFD helps identify a lifeguard during water entry, which may help to clear the way on a crowded beach or help avoid confrontations. When a lifeguard responds to a rescue with an RFD (even a shallow water assist), people will often focus their attention to the water area, which can be helpful in bringing family members to the scene to assist with information or ensure better future supervision. In the water, a victim seeing a lifeguard approach would have no way of knowing the approaching swimmer is a lifeguard without the presence of the RFD.

- *Identification to Fellow Lifeguards*—Like other people at the beach, lifeguards are easily lost in the crowd; but the characteristic shape and color of the RFD allows lifeguards to spot each other much more easily. In the water as well, the presence of an RFD helps other lifeguards quickly locate the lifeguard using it and signals that a rescue is likely in progress. As a signaling device, the RFD helps lifeguards in the water identify lifeguards on the beach and the instructions they are giving. RFDs of different colors can be used to differentiate specially trained or assigned lifeguards, lifeguard supervisors, or junior lifeguards.

- *Multiple Uses*—RFDs can be used in conjunction with other equipment and can be taken along without interfering with other devices. RFDs can be adapted to almost any rescue situation. For example, with a boat tow attached to the rear of a rescue buoy, it can be used to swim a boat away from the surf. They can be modified to carry and store special rescue equipment, such as one-way breathing masks. They can be used for a wide variety of signals on the beach and in the water; and RFDs are even useful as self-defense tools in particularly dangerous public confrontations.

RFD Advantages and Limitations

Each type of RFD has distinct advantages and limitations.

Rescue Buoy Advantages

- *Multiple Victims*—Rescue buoys have particularly high buoyancy, allowing the simultaneous support and rescue of several victims.
- *Victim Avoidance*—A conscious victim can be instructed to use the rescue buoy without any contact with the victim.
- *Durability*—Rescue buoys are generally very durable.

Rescue Buoy Limitations

- *Lack of Victim Security*—Victims can't be attached to a rescue buoy as they can to a rescue tube.
- *Hard Exterior*—Although softer than the original metal design, modern rescue buoys are still hard plastic and can cause minor injuries.

Rescue Tube Advantages

- *Hydrodynamic*—The rescue tube is particularly streamlined, creating very little drag against the lifeguard towing it.
- *Victim Security*—The victim is actually wrapped in the buoy.
- *Rescue Boat Use*—The soft design keeps rescue tubes from bouncing around in a rescue boat.

Rescue Tube Limitations

- *Single Victim Use*—The rescue tube can be used for more than one victim, but is designed for a single victim.
- *Low Buoyancy*—Rescue tubes have a relatively low buoyancy compared to rescue buoys.
- *Requires Physical Contact with Victim*—Wrapping a rescue tube around the victim requires physical contact with a possibly panicked victim.

- *Requires Extra Maneuver*—Unlike the rescue buoy which is simply pushed to the victim, the rescue tube requires that the lifeguard take an extra step of wrapping and fastening.
- *Fending Off*—Rescue tubes cannot be effectively used to fend off a panicked victim.

The snap-hook of a rescue tube can cause lacerations or other injury. This is very unusual, but it is best to secure the tube around the victim to avoid this problem. Rescue tubes are more susceptible to environmental degradation than rescue buoys. They should be stored in an elongated position out of the sun.

Rescues with Rescue Flotation Devices

The basic use of an RFD was described in the chapter entitled, *Components of a Rescue*. The following additional factors must be considered:

- *Water Entry*—RFDs are equipped with a lanyard, which attaches the RFD to the harness, and a harness, which connects the lifeguard to the lanyard. The lanyard and harness can trip the lifeguard during the entry run. Care should be taken to unwrap the RFD and don the harness, while holding the lanyard off the ground. This can be done be holding the lanyard in the same hand being used to hold the RFD. RFDs should be carried into the water until the lifeguard needs to begin porpoising or swimming, since a dragging RFD is dead weight and may collide with beach visitors. At surf areas, lifeguards should expect to feel extra drag after waves pass by, which is caused by the force of the wave against the RFD.
- *Removal from Water*—In many situations, lifeguards can simply drop RFDs as they move to assist or carry victims from the water. In some surf conditions however, an unsecured rescue buoy could be washed with force against the lifeguard or victim, potentially causing injury. If heavy surf conditions are present, lifeguards may want to carry the RFD completely out of the water or have the victim do so.
- *Fouling*—If the lanyard becomes wrapped around an object, the lifeguard can be placed in serious jeopardy. For example, the lanyard could become wrapped in the propeller of a rescue vessel. For this reason, it is essential that the attachment between the lifeguard and lanyard allow for quick release.
- *Lanyard Length*—The length of the lanyard may reflect individual preference of each lifeguard. In general however, the lanyard should be long enough to allow the buoy to clear the kicking feet of the lifeguard while swimming, plus a foot or two. The longer the lanyard, the more likely it is to trip the lifeguard or become fouled, but in large surf conditions, a longer lanyard may better allow lifeguards to more easily submerge under waves. If buoys are shared at an agency, lanyard length should take into account the lifeguard with the longest legs.

Rescues with Rescue Buoys

Most conscious victims will quickly grab and hold tightly to the rescue buoy handles. The lifeguard can then swim toward shore. A weak or unresponsive victim will require assistance. In these situations, the lifeguard should move to the rear of the victim facing the victim's back while keeping the RFD in front of the victim. Then the lifeguard reaches under the victim's arms to grasp a side handle of the rescue

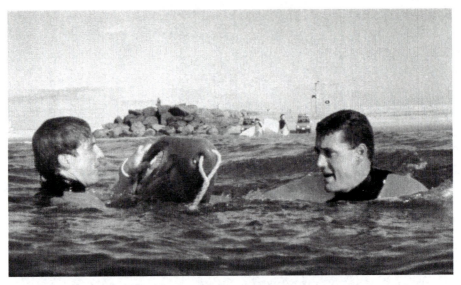

A lifeguard makes contact with a victim.

Credit: Annette Kennedy

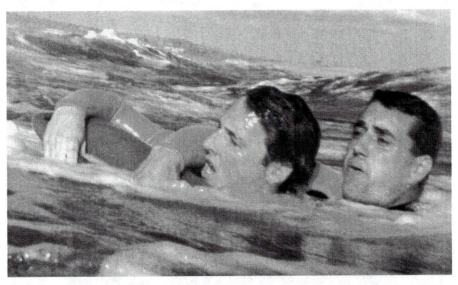

A lifeguard prepares to bring a victim through the surfline.

Credit: Annette Kennedy

buoy. The rescue buoy is pulled close to sandwich the victim between the RFD and the lifeguard. The rescue can now proceed, with forward propulsion achieved by kicking the feet. Swim fins are extremely valuable in these cases. Even with swim fins, it can be difficult to bring a victim ashore in this manner, so additional lifeguard assistance should be considered. This same technique should be used in heavy surf, even when the victim is conscious and alert, to prevent having the victim become separated from the rescue buoy.

Rescues with Rescue Tubes

Perhaps the most valuable feature of the rescue tube is its ability to be wrapped around the victim and secured. It should always be used in this way, not as a device to be held by the victim. In most presentations, the lifeguard should first be concerned with establishing control by providing the support of the tube to the victim and letting the victim stabilize. Then, if possible, the lifeguard can direct the victim to move on the tube to a position where the victim is facing the tube with both arms over it and the tube is nestled under the armpits. The lifeguard can then move to the rear of the victim and bring the ends of the tube together for connection. Note that this requires the lifeguard to come into direct contact with the victim, which should not be done until the lifeguard is certain that the victim will not panic and grab the lifeguard.

If the victim is unconscious or unresponsive, the process of securing the victim in the tube is more difficult. While facing the victim, the lifeguard can pull one arm over the extended tube to armpit level, then carefully work the other arm over the tube to the same position and connect the tube from the rear of the victim. Another technique is to swim to the rear of the victim and provide support with one hand under an armpit while placing the tube in front of the victim's face. From that point, the life-

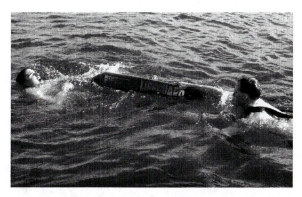

Credit: Sandra McCormick

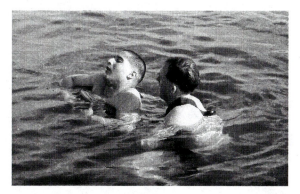

Credit: Sandra McCormick

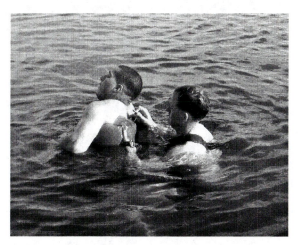

Credit: Sandra McCormick

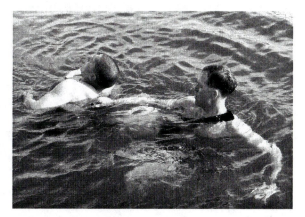

Credit: Sandra McCormick

guard can lift one, then the other arm of the victim over the tube to the armpit level and finally connect the tube at the victim's back.

If a victim must be moved through a heavy surfline, the lifeguard moves to the rear of the victim and holds on to the tube and victim with the lifeguard's face to the victim's back. The lifeguard should check behind frequently, while kicking toward shore, and advise the victim when to expect the force of a wave.

Swim Fins

At many lifeguard agencies, swim fins are issued as part of the lifeguard's basic rescue equipment. The obvious advantage to use of swim fins is the added speed and power that they give to the responding lifeguard. When lifeguards are unable to use arm strokes, due to the need to hold on to victims, swim fins can be essential to making rapid progress. In rocky areas, swim fins provide protection for the feet. They can also be useful during search and recovery procedures requiring diving.

Use and Selection of Swim Fins

The use of swim fins is indicated in rescue situations involving longer approach swims, deep water rescues involving currents, and larger than normal surf. They are also useful when lifeguards need to provide additional support to victims in deep water, such as situations involving resuscitation. Swim fins are not as useful in shallow water rescues or in rescue situations a short distance from shallow water. In these situations, the time necessary to don swim fins can delay response unnecessarily.

Lifeguard agencies are usually very particular in selecting or approving swim fins for lifeguard use. Swim fins must fit the lifeguard precisely, so fins are usually selected and assigned to individual lifeguards. The type and style of swim fins are also important. Shoe-type fins are usually unacceptable because they frequently fall off. Adjustable heel-strap styles are generally less dependable than solid heel-strap styles. Swim fins which float or have neutral buoyancy are very useful because a lifeguard can remove them if necessary, without fear of loss.

Rescues with Swim Fins

When swim fins are used on rescues, the lifeguard dons the RFD harness, then grabs the RFD and lanyard in one hand and both fins in the other, running with them into the water. Upon entering the water, the lifeguard drops the RFD and takes one fin in each hand. At this point the fins can be used as paddles (one in each hand) until the lifeguard is in water approximately chest deep. The lifeguard can also porpoise, holding the heel strap of each fin in each hand. Once swimming becomes the most expeditious manner of making forward progress, the lifeguard stops and

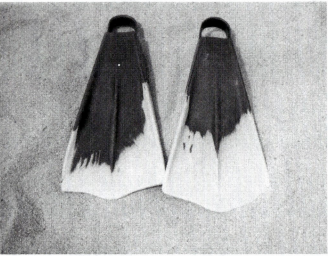

The most common design of lifeguard swim fins.
Credit: Dan McCormick

dons the fins. This can rarely be done with the head above water, therefore, lifeguards who use fins must be adept at donning their fins blind. Experienced lifeguards always keep their fins in the same orientation to each other onshore, so that when they enter the water, they know which side of the fin is up without looking. When the fins have been put on, the lifeguard swims to the victim. Although it takes a few moments to don fins, the increased speed of the lifeguard in swimming to the victim usually offsets this short delay.

Swim fins should not normally be worn while running on shore or in shallow water. An exception to this guideline is a water entry in a rocky area. Swim fins can be put on immediately in this situation, as the fins provide protection for the feet. High strides will cut down the resistance caused by the swim fins.

Upon return to shore, swim fins are usually removed upon reaching shallow water, before the lifeguard begins walking again. Another alternative, if the lifeguard must support the victim, is to walk backwards. In rare instances the lifeguard may need to discard swim fins upon reaching shore in order to support the victim better or to provide resuscitation. Fins that float are particularly useful in such situations, as they can be more easily recovered.

Rescue Boards

Rescue boards (known also as paddleboards and rescue surfboards) are a valuable piece of rescue equipment which evolved from the surfboard. While surfboards and rescue boards have a common ancestor, today's lifeguard rescue boards should not be confused with surfboards. Although these devices may have a similar appearance, rescue boards are primarily designed for rescue, not surfing.

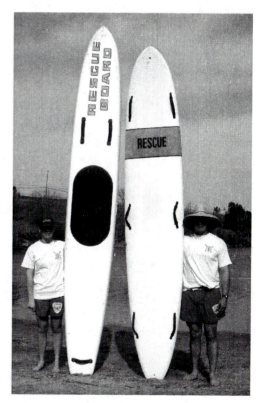

Credit: Sandra McCormick

A rescue board is a buoyant, lightweight craft approximately 10' to 12' long and shaped to move quickly through the water. Most commercially produced rescue boards are manufactured from a shaped, reinforced core of polyurethane foam, which is then covered with a skin of fiberglass, epoxy, or other compound. This skin, like that of most surfboards, can be damaged if struck by or against a hard object. It can also injure those who might be struck by the rescue board. An alternative design involves a deck made of ethylene vinyl acetate (EVA), a material similar to the soles of running shoes. This material is durable, yet less susceptible to damage and less likely to injure those struck by the board.

The rescue board includes a skeg (fin) attached to the bottom of the board at the rear to help maintain stability, acting somewhat like the keel of a ship. Skegs are sometimes quite sharp and can cause serious injuries if they strike a person. A design that helps avoid such injuries is a skeg with a leading and trailing edge made of soft, flexible material.

Rescue boards are often equipped with inlaid handles for use by lifeguards and victims. On hard fiberglass rescue boards, a foam deck pad may be included to improve comfort while knee paddling. Most lifeguard

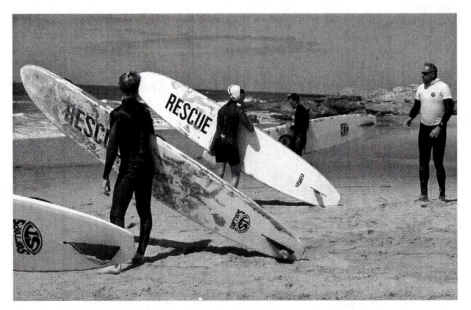

Rescue board training.

Credit: Ken Kramer

agencies prefer commercially manufactured rescue boards to custom-made devices, although some larger agencies order high quality rescue boards to their own specifications. The primary use of a rescue board is water rescue of swimmers. They can also be used in boat rescue, for patrolling, for swim/surf crowd control, and, in a pinch, as a backboard to remove an injured victim from the water or as a platform for CPR, although these latter users should only be employed as a last resort.

Rescue Board Advantages

- *Speed*—When properly used in low to moderate surf, rescue boards can allow lifeguards to cover considerable distances much faster than swimming with fins. In flat water, rescue boards are almost always the fastest method of accessing victims, other than power boats.

- *Buoyancy*—Rescue boards are very buoyant and can support numerous victims. Increased buoyancy can also be useful during situations where resuscitation must be provided in deep water. In rescues involving multiple victims, the rescue board can be used as a raft for several victims to hold while waiting to be ferried to the beach. In calm water, rescue boards can even be used to administer rescue breathing. When rescuing a single victim, the victim is almost completely removed from the water, significantly increasing the victim's sense of security.

- *Lightweight*—Unlike a boat, the low weight of the rescue board allows it to be carried, launched, and operated by one lifeguard and easily transported atop a lifeguard vehicle. On the other hand, a rescue board is heavy and unwieldy compared to a rescue buoy and cannot be easily transported by a lifeguard on foot over a long distance.

- *Viewing Platform*—The deck of the rescue board provides an excellent platform from which the lifeguard can observe the swim area. This makes the rescue board a rudimentary patrol device and a useful tool in surface searches of swim areas.

Rescue Board Limitations

- *Surf Conflicts*—A rescue board is difficult to move through heavy surf. A swimming lifeguard can usually more easily penetrate heavy surf than a lifeguard on a rescue board. Trying to return to shore with a victim in these conditions is quite challenging, particularly with an incapacitated victim. Loss of the rescue board is a considerable danger. If the board is lost, the lifeguard may be left without rescue equipment and lose contact with the victim. Other swimmers may be endangered by an uncontrolled rescue board in surf. Rescue boards with EVA foam skins reduce potential injuries, as do skegs with rubberized edges. Regardless of the type of rescue board though, it is advisable to carefully consider use of a rescue board through large, breaking surf. Due to the chance of being separated from the rescue board, it is a good practice to take an RFD and fins while effecting a rescue with a rescue board, particularly in large surf conditions. In this way, if the rescue board is lost, the lifeguard will retain an ability to effectively complete the rescue.

- *Weight*—Rescue boards may be as heavy as 40 pounds, which can make them difficult to remove from racks or carry to the water, particularly for smaller lifeguards. Some newer rescue board designs reduce this weight to 25 pounds or less. Even so, compared to an RFD, the rescue board is a much heavier piece of rescue equipment.

- *Lack of Maneuverability*—Rescue boards operate best when paddled in a straight line with small corrections in direction made occasionally. A congested swimming area may present the lifeguard with too many obstacles to move around en route to the victim. Similarly, congested swimming areas may provide the lifeguard with difficult obstacles during retrieval.

- *Maintenance*—In comparison to RFDs, rescue boards are expensive to purchase and maintain. Rescue boards with a hard skin can be easily damaged (dinged), which can contribute to periods when the equipment is unusable because of maintenance requirements. Rescue boards in a poor state of repair can cause injury to both lifeguards and victims.

- *Skill Requirements*—Lifeguards must regularly practice rescue board skills to maintain proficiency. Without proper skills and practice, the rescue board can be an awkward piece of equipment that can actually be dangerous to beach visitors.

Rescues with Rescue Boards

Entry

As explained in the chapter on *Components of a Rescue*, running is generally faster than swimming. This is not necessarily the case when using a rescue board, due to its weight and cumbersome nature. Instead, it may be preferable to carry the rescue board directly to the water. Since an experienced lifeguard paddling a rescue board is much faster than a swimming lifeguard, the loss of speed onshore can be offset by a gain in speed in the water.

On most days, a lifeguard can move a rescue board to the water by lifting the board up at the middle and carrying it nose first toward the water at the lifeguard's side. Some rescue boards are equipped with handles or carrying slots to facilitate this. On windy days, the wind may cause the board to sail during this carry and the board may become very difficult to manage. Should this situation present itself, the lifeguard can grasp the forward end of the rescue board and drag the tail (rear) of the board in the sand. Dragging the board is not recommended under normal conditions, since the practice will eventually wear away the board's protective covering. During the launching process, an RFD (if also carried as recommended) can be dragged behind the lifeguard or carried with the board.

In flat water, boards should be launched and mounted at about knee depth. This is important, since attempts to launch a board in shallower water may result in the skeg catching on the bottom, which will stop the board and throw the lifeguard off. On sand beaches the lifeguard can gain good speed by running with the board, with the nose pointed toward the water. When the appropriate depth is reached, the lifeguard grabs the board by each rail (side) at about the center, deck inward and without letting go, throws the board forward. When this motion is followed by the momentum of the lifeguard's weight, the board is propelled at considerable speed for a short distance. When the board hits the water, the lifeguard simultaneously mounts the board, assuming a prone or kneeling position. This is a single, fluid motion, which requires practice. Effective use of the rescue board requires a considerable amount of balance and awareness of the orientation of the board. If the lifeguard is too far forward, the nose

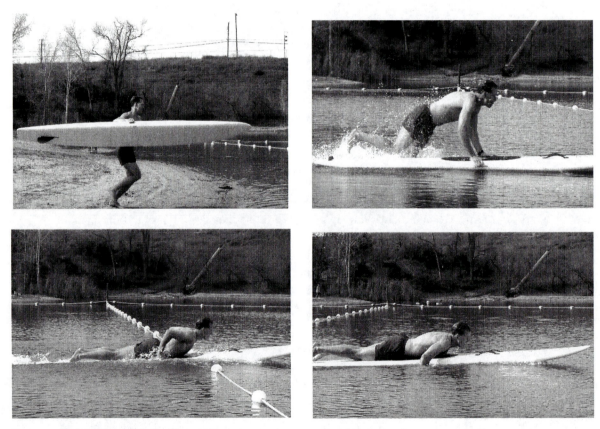

Rescue board launch in flat water.

Credit: Sandra McCormick

dives beneath the surface of the water, slowing or stopping it abruptly. If the lifeguard's center of gravity is too far toward the tail, the board will become unstable.

In surf conditions, one object of launching a rescue board is to initially carry the board over incoming waves. Once the water becomes approximately waist deep, the board can be placed on the water and sledded along the water's surface at the side of the lifeguard. When waves threaten to lift the board above or out of the lifeguard's reach, the lifeguard can swing up onto the deck of the board with the upper body, letting the wave lift both the lifeguard and the board temporarily off the bottom while the lifeguard's legs trail beside the board. When the wave passes, the lifeguard can regain footing and proceed.

Once deep water is reached, the lifeguard must commit to paddling. The board is mounted and a paddling position is assumed. The board must be kept headed directly into the direction of the oncoming wave to keep the waves from throwing the board off to either side. Like surface diving through waves, the aim with a rescue board is to present the smallest possible forward surface to the incoming wave. Generally, this means taking a perpendicular angle to the wave.

The initial goal of using a rescue board in the surf is to get out beyond the breakers. A lifeguard who is swimming can easily duck under breaking waves, but breaking waves landing on a lifeguard on a rescue board sandwich the lifeguard between the force of the breaking wave and the board. In this case, the lifeguard may lose the board or may be thrust into the board by the incoming wave, causing injury. The lifeguard may also be pushed a significant distance shoreward or become separated from the board.

When approaching the incoming foam line of a wave that has already broken, the lifeguard should adjust body weight somewhat toward the tail so that the nose rides up over the foam line. When a wave approaches that will break upon the lifeguard, the lifeguard should try to force the nose of the board down by leaning forward in a push-up position. This helps keep the board from being lifted and carried shoreward by the breaking wave.

Heavy surf conditions may call for an action of rolling the rescue board through the waves (turtling). To employ this maneuver, the lifeguard inhales deeply just before the impact of the oncoming wave and rolls the board over so that the bottom of the board faces toward the sky and the lifeguard hangs underneath. Once the wave has passed, the lifeguard turns the board over and continues paddling.

Approach

Whether paddling from a prone or kneeling position, it is important to maintain a good trim—a position on the board where the board remains flat, or slightly nose high, on the water. In practicing paddling, each lifeguard will find a position on the board that results in the board staying in trim.

The prone position (lying face down on the board) is the easiest to master, since a low center of gravity is maintained for a stable ride. Arms are used in a butterfly stroke motion or a crawl stroke, with the hands and arms dug into the water deeply for efficient movement. In the prone position however, the lifeguard's stroke length is limited and only the arms contribute to forward momentum. This will result in a tired lifeguard over a relatively short distance. Many lifeguards prefer the kneeling position, particularly for distance paddling. It is faster and more efficient, since more of the muscles of the body contribute to the stroke and the stroke is longer, but it requires more skill to paddle in this manner because the lifeguard's weight is concentrated in a single area of the rescue board and balance is more difficult to maintain.

The kneeling position is usually assumed from the prone position. After a few strokes to develop momentum and stability, the lifeguard moves from the prone position to kneeling by holding onto the rails and pulling the knees up to the center of the board, spread somewhat to maintain stability and

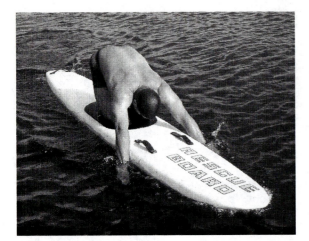

Knee paddling.

Credit: Sandra McCormick

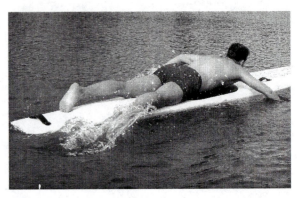

Dragging a foot for direction change.

Credit: Sandra McCormick

trim. The head is kept down to maintain a low center of gravity and the arms dig in deeply to grab water and pull backward. Arms are recovered with hands low and elbows high.

To make small changes in the direction of the board, several techniques can be used. These include dragging a foot, shifting weight, or reaching out and pulling water from the direction of the turn. If the lifeguard wants to turn the board completely around, the lifeguard stops the board by sitting on the deck with legs hung over both sides. The lifeguard then slides back on the board, which picks the nose up. Then, by using an eggbeater kick and/or by paddling with the hands, the board can be twirled to the desired direction.

Approaching a victim with a rescue board should be done in a manner that will place the nose of the board just slightly to one side of the victim. When the lifeguard has drawn nearly beside the victim, the lifeguard slips off the far side of the board so that the board is between the lifeguard and the

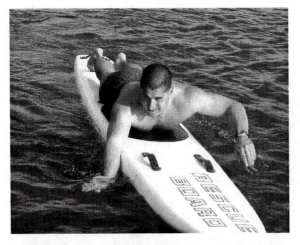

Pulling water from the direction of the turn.

Credit: Sandra McCormick

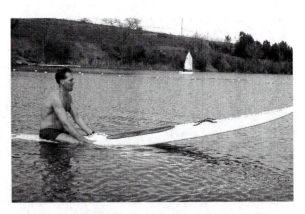

Turning the board completely around.

Credit: Sandra McCormick

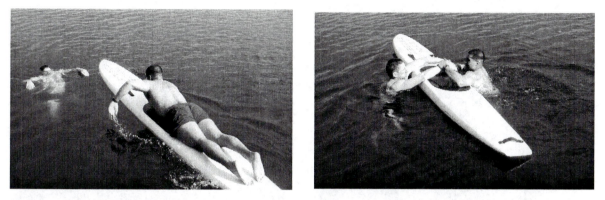

Approach to the side of the victim, then grab the victim from the opposite side.

Credit: Sandra McCormick

victim. Then, if necessary, the lifeguard moves the board to the victim using a swimming kick and the lifeguard reaches over the board to pull the victim to the support offered by the board. This keeps the lifeguard separated from the victim in much the same manner as pushing an RFD to the victim.

Retrieval

Once the victim has been stabilized and the signal has been made, the retrieval process can begin. There is no requirement that victims be loaded onto rescue boards for retrieval. In many situations, lifeguards can simply begin swimming kicks that will move the board and the victim toward shallow water while holding the victim's arms on the board. In other situations, victims may stay in the water and hold onto rescue board handles or the trailing RFD while the lifeguard mounts the board and paddles in.

More skilled lifeguards may choose to bring a strong, conscious victim aboard. One way to do this is to begin by treading water at the nose of the board and stabilizing the board for the victim by holding both sides. The victim is then instructed to mount the board facing the nose. Once the head and shoulders are supported by the board, the lifeguard can assist by pulling the legs onto the deck, if necessary.

If the victim is unconscious or unable to mount the board using the foregoing method, an alternative method of bringing the victim aboard the rescue board involves rolling the board. The lifeguard dismounts the rescue board and turns it over, bottom side up. The middle of the overturned board is positioned between the lifeguard and the victim. The victim's hands are pulled across the board so that the victim's armpits are against the rail opposite the lifeguard. The rescue board is then turned back over flipping it toward the lifeguard. The victim will now be lying across the middle of the rescue board. The final step is to carefully move the victim's body on the board to a lengthwise position.

Once the victim is aboard the rescue board, the lifeguard can assume a position at the tail and push the board to shore by kicking. Alternatively, the lifeguard can carefully mount the board from the tail to assume a position over the victim's hind quarters with the victim's legs on either side. The lifeguard adjusts the board's trim and begins to paddle to shore.

Surf conditions complicate retrievals of victims on rescue boards. At many agencies, lifeguards are instructed not to bring victims through breaking surf on rescue boards. Instead, victims are transferred to rescue boats or to lifeguards with RFDs for retrieval. If a victim must be brought through breaking surf on a rescue board, no attempt should be made to catch or ride waves with victims aboard.

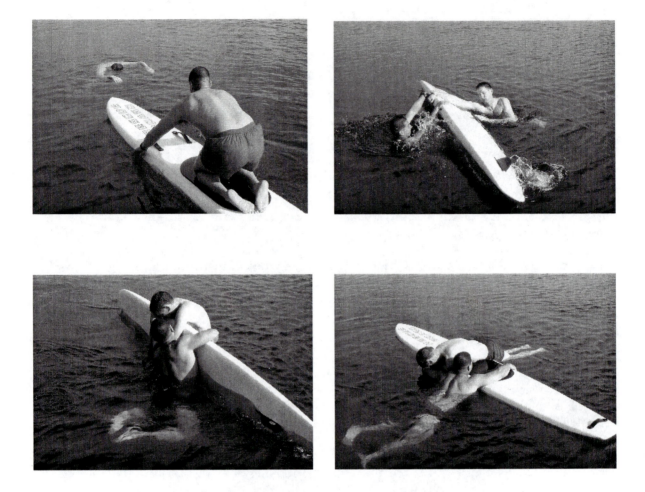

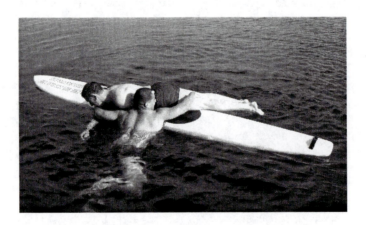

An unconscious victim is brought aboard a rescue board.

Credit: Sandra McCormick

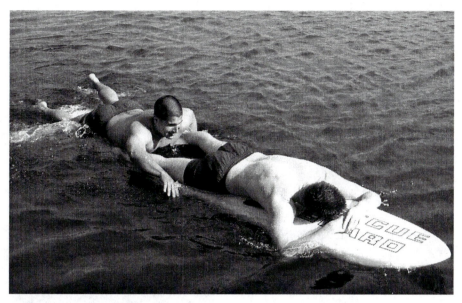

Paddling a victim to shore.
Credit: Sandra McCormick

Lifeguards should keep the board perpendicular to waves and shift weight heavily toward the tail of the rescue board when overtaken by a wave. This may include moving the victim to the rear of the board and sandwiching the victim between the board and lifeguard while holding both rails. The victim should be held tightly, sandwiched between the body of the lifeguard and the rescue board, and advised of what to expect.

Removal from the Water

In most situations, lifeguards must either tend to the removal of the rescue board or removal of the victim. Rescue boards should not be left unattended, especially in moving or turbulent water. Another lifeguard may help with removal of the rescue board while the responding lifeguard deals with the victim.

Maintenance

Care is a must for a rescue board. Fiberglass rescue boards should be kept in a waxed or "non-skid" treated condition. Rescue boards should be inspected daily and any holes or cracks repaired. Any opening in the skin of the board can allow water to seep in and may eventually ruin it. Rescue boards should never be leaned upright against other objects as the wind can sail them into people. They should be stored horizontally or be fully secured if stored vertically.

Spinal Stabilization Devices

Several sources of spinal injury are present at all open water beaches. These include shallow water diving, body surfing, striking a sandbar or other underwater object, wave action, dry land falls, and others. Therefore every lifeguard agency should have spinal stabilization devices available for immediate use. All lifeguards should be fully trained in the necessary techniques. For a discussion of the recognition and treatment of spinal injuries in the aquatic environment, please refer to the chapter entitled, *Medical Care in the Aquatic Environment.*

Spinal Stabilization Device Components

Spinal stabilization devices consist of three parts: spineboard, head and neck immobilization device, and fastening devices to hold the person to the spineboard. Use of spinal stabilization devices may be regulated by local emergency medical service authorities and should be used in a manner consistent with agency protocol and training.

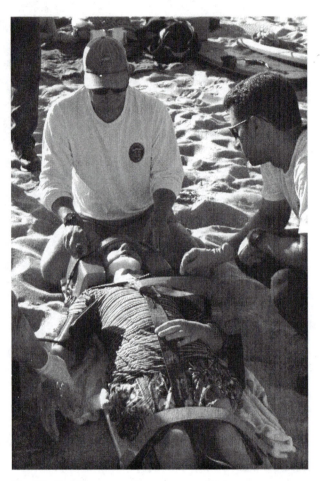

Credit: Ken Kramer

- *Spineboard*—The spineboard is also known as a backboard. A spineboard is a rigid flat surface to which the backside of a person, including head, trunk, legs, and feet can be attached. The most basic version of a spineboard is a flat, rectangular piece of wood of dimensions slightly greater than that of an average male lying supine. Better versions have handles in the sides to improve the grip of rescuers. The most advanced models for aquatic use are made of plastic and metal. These devices float and are slightly contoured. They have handles and specially designed areas for securing straps.

- *Head and Neck Immobilization Devices*—Neck immobilization devices were initially known as cervical collars (C-collars). The original versions were made of foam and lacked reliable support for the neck. Modern versions are quite rigid and significantly limit neck movement. These can be known as hard collars, Philadelphia collars, or by actual brand name. Further stabilization to prevent head movement is provided by head immobilizers. These are placed on either side of the head as the body lies on a spineboard. They may be commercially manufactured or may be improvised material, such as sandbags, rolled towels, etc.

- *Fastening Devices*—Fastening devices are used to secure the trunk, head and legs to the spineboard. These may be pre-designed harnesses, heavy tape, or Velcro straps.

Chapter Summary

In this chapter, we have learned about the standard rescue equipment used by lifeguards. We have learned about rescue flotation devices, including rescue buoys and rescue tubes, their advantages, disadvantages, and how to use them effectively. We have learned about the advantages of swim fins and how they are donned during a rescue response. We have learned about rescue boards, including their advantages and limitations, as well as how they are used effectively. And we have learned about spinal stabilization devices.

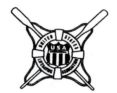

Discussion Points

- Why should there be one RFD for every lifeguard on duty?
- What are some of the values of standard rescue equipment?
- What are some reasons for lifeguards to keep an RFD with them at all times?
- What are the relative benefits of rescue buoys and rescue tubes?
- What is an advantage of a rescue buoy in a multiple victim rescue?
- What is an advantage of a rescue tube in large surf?
- What are some advantages of using swim fins on a rescue?
- What are some advantages of using a rescue board?
- Why might a lifeguard using a rescue board take it directly to the water, instead of running on the beach to a position closer to the victim?
- What are potential problems related to using rescue boards in heavy crowds or large surf?
- What are some reasons that spinal stabilization devices are essential for open water lifesaving work?

Chapter 14

Specialized Rescue Equipment

In this chapter, you will be introduced to some of the specialized rescue equipment employed by lifeguard agencies that can help lifeguards do their jobs more efficiently. Examples include emergency response vehicles, rescue boats, and aircraft. You will learn the advantages of different types of specialized rescue equipment and how each can be used effectively.

CHAPTER EXCERPT

Motorized rescue boats can often move to a rescue location much more quickly than free-swimming lifeguards, or even those in vehicles, and can cover longer distances with minimal lifeguard fatigue. They are particularly valuable at facilitating a rapid response to emergencies which occur well offshore, to remote beach areas, and to vessels in distress.

Emergency Vehicles

One of the most useful pieces of emergency equipment employed by lifeguards is the emergency vehicle. Lifeguard emergency vehicles may be all terrain vehicles (ATVs), pickups, sport utility vehicles (SUV), and the like. Emergency vehicles offer the advantage of increased speed, range, and payload as compared to a lifeguard on foot. Emergency lifeguard vehicles are normally equipped with four wheel drive so that they can be driven on sand and other soft terrain. Full size emergency vehicles (SUV and pickups) are usually equipped with lights and siren for emergency response on the street and on the beach. In addition to rescue flotation devices (RFD), emergency vehicles can carry such equipment as a two-way radio, public address system, extensive medical aid and trauma kit, resuscitator, rescue board, spinal immobilization device, stretcher (litter), automatic external defibrillator (AED), flares, wetsuits, extra fins, face plates, marker buoys for search and recovery, and even cliff

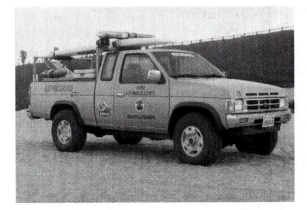

Credit: Rob McGowan

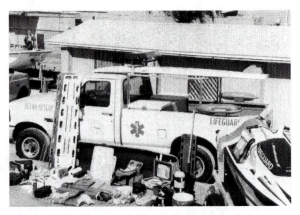

Lifeguard vehicles can carry extensive amount of rescue and medical aid equipment.

Credit: Mike Hensler

rescue gear. Emergency vehicles are of use not only for responding to serious emergencies. They can also function as mobile lifeguard stations, with their mobility allowing a single lifeguard to cover a large area effectively.

Operators of lifeguard emergency vehicles should be thoroughly trained in emergency response driving and in safe use of vehicles on the beach. Some lifeguard agencies have specific training courses for emergency vehicle drivers. This is highly recommended. In developing general training in emergency vehicle operations, local public safety agencies may be a source of information. Driving on the beach however, requires special skills to address the unusual mix of vehicles and beach patrons. Lifeguard agencies with experience in this area should be consulted by those desiring to create such training programs. Of paramount concern in the operation of emergency vehicles is safety. As the size and speed of the rescue vehicle increases, so does the possibility of injury to lifeguards and beach patrons.

Some basics of emergency driving are:

- Prioritize safety over speed
- Drive only as quickly as necessary
- If you don't get there, you're of no help
- If you cause injury in the act of responding to an emergency, you've defeated your purpose
- Follow all laws pertaining to emergency vehicle operation

Even routine driving of emergency vehicles in the beach environment can pose hazards. People are not alert for vehicles on the beach. Although the lifeguard vehicle may be big and brightly colored, people may not expect it or notice it. Small children have a tendency to run in front of lifeguard vehicles toward their parents when a vehicle approaches, particularly in emergency response situations. Parents will sometimes bolt in front of the vehicle to protect their children. Heightened caution is also needed when traveling past pier pilings or other obstructions, such as large rocks. People sometimes seem to jump out from behind these sight obstructions.

When lifeguard vehicles are parked, beach patrons may lie down right beside them, even in front or behind them. Lifeguards should never assume that because they are sitting in an idling vehicle, no one has sat down in the path of the vehicle while it was parked, even for a brief period of time. Before

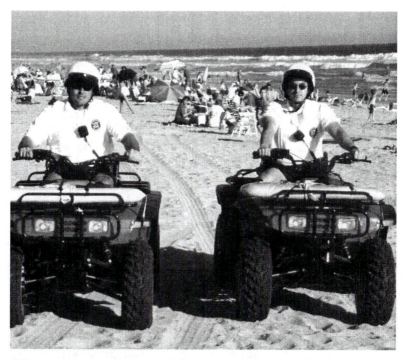

Lifeguards on ATVs patrolling the beach.

Credit: Ken Kramer

leaving from a parked position, the driver should exit the vehicle and visually check in front, behind, and beneath the vehicle. This inspection requires only a few seconds and ensures a safe path.

If the vehicle is to be parked on the beach or in a public area, it's a good idea to delineate the vehicle's parking area. This is ideally done by use of ropes and stanchions. It may also be done by use of traffic cones or flags, but people tend to walk right through these areas. Some lifeguard agencies fence off vehicle accesses ways to discourage pedestrian traffic and indicate areas where vehicles are likely to travel, increasing the likelihood (but not the certainty) that the area remains clear of beach patrons. Cordoning off an area for vehicle parking and access should be done at the start of shift, when beach attendance is low and there is plenty of area to reserve. Signs may also be used. Warning cones may also be placed around a parked vehicle to encourage people to stay back. In any case, the area around vehicles on the beach should then be kept clear of people at all times.

Lifeguard vehicles on routine beach patrol should be driven at an appropriate speed, which is normally very slow. Exceptions include urgent responses, in which case beach patrons should be notified by emergency lights and sirens, as appropriate.

Unlike on the street, where there is little pedestrian traffic, a busy beach is filled with pedestrians and people lying or sitting on the surface upon which the lifeguard is driving. The three most dangerous moves are backing up, right turns, and driving over a berm. During these maneuvers the driver's visibility is impeded. Berms should be ascended or descended at obtuse angles (greater than 90°). Prior to ascending or descending a berm, the best visibility can be attained if the vehicle is positioned with the berm on the driver's side. If the driver cannot see the path ahead, the driver should stop the vehicle and have the passenger check. If alone, stop and exit the vehicle to check the area before continuing. Lifeguards should never drive in any direction if they are unable to visually ensure a safe path.

Rescue Boats

Rescue boats were first used in this country by the original American lifesavers in the 1800s. The variety and sophistication of lifeguard rescue boats have advanced a long way since then. Some agencies still successfully employ variations of traditional manually powered lifesaving craft for purposes of offshore perimeter control and surveillance. As emergency response craft however, the value of these vessels has been eclipsed by motorized rescue boats. They too can be used for offshore perimeter control and surveillance, but are particularly effective for rapid response and more effective coverage of large patrol areas. As explained throughout this text, drownings occur very rapidly. All things being equal, the faster a lifeguard can reach a victim in distress, the less likely that a drowning death will occur. Motorized rescue boats clearly provide a more rapid response and can thus be expected to be more effective in drowning prevention.

In some states, training is mandated for the operation of motorized rescue boats. Regardless of state law, lifeguards operating rescue boats must first be thoroughly trained in their safe operation, particularly considering the potential for injury they pose to both water users and lifeguards.

Rescue Boat Advantages

Size and Stability

Some rescue boats can support the operator and several victims completely out of water. Thus, rescue of a victim and removal from the water can take place almost immediately, effectively fully resolving the victim's distress while still offshore. In a multiple victim rescue, lifeguards in a large rescue boat

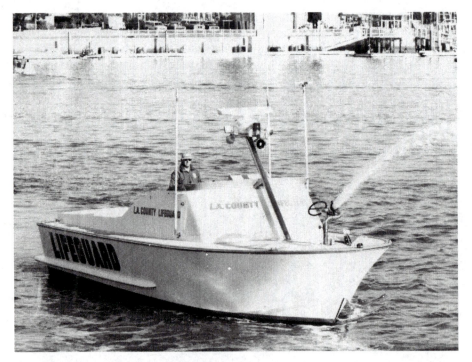

Los Angeles County Baywatch.
Credit: Conrad Liberty

can quickly pluck numerous distressed swimmers from the water, returning them to shore at a later time. This can also assist lifeguards effecting rescues with RFDs. Instead of taking their victims to shore, they can simply swim victims to the waiting rescue boat. In large surf conditions a rescue boat on the outside of the breakers is of particular value.

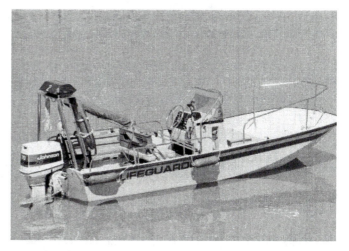

Credit: Leon Skov

Patrol and Observation

Rescue boats are excellent tools for lifeguard patrols. Lifeguards can patrol from rescue boats for long periods with limited fatigue. Depending on the size of the boat, it can be equipped with much or all of the equipment carried in an emergency vehicle, essentially making it into a mobile, offshore lifeguard station.

Rescue boats can provide an observation platform on the outer edge of a swimming area or an offshore recreation area. This provides lifeguards with the ability to monitor these areas and user groups. It allows for early intervention and speedy rescue. Although rescue boats should generally not be used as a substitute for observation by a lifeguard on land, there are many situations where a boat-based lifeguard may be more effective. When glare or large surf conditions interfere with water surveillance by shore-based lifeguards, boat-based lifeguards can be of significant help. If there is considerable offshore activity, a rescue boat can provide additional coverage and surveillance. When evaluating the status of ocean users for possible distress, the boat based lifeguard can usually speak directly with the victim, instead of trying to evaluate status from a distance, as must the shore-based lifeguard.

Speed

Motorized rescue boats can often move to a rescue location much more quickly than free-swimming lifeguards, or even those in vehicles, and can cover longer distances with minimal lifeguard fatigue. They are particularly valuable at facilitating a rapid response to emergencies which occur well offshore, to remote beach areas, and to vessels in distress. In areas with difficult accessibility to land entry, such as cliffs, or lack of beach or street access, rescue boats can quickly and effectively transport lifeguards to distressed swimmers, avoiding potentially dangerous terrain. Some types of motorized vessels can move through large surf with ease and can be reliably operated inside breaking surf. For lifeguard agencies serving large geographic areas, motorized rescue boats can respond to emergencies many miles away faster than vehicles impeded by traffic problems ashore; and upon arrival, the vessel is already offshore, where the problem is likely to be. Manually powered vessels are much slower in comparison and more apt to be deterred by surf conditions, but they may be faster than swimming lifeguards under some circumstances.

Versatility

Some agencies use boats to effectively mark the limits of the swim area and staff that boundary with lifeguard boat operators. Rescue boats can also be used for general crowd control when water users need to be separated or swim area boundaries exist. During special events such as open water swimming competitions, lifeguards in rescue vessels can easily monitor the status of swimmers on the course. Rescue boats are also useful in advising water users of shark sightings or other potential marine hazards, while ensuring the safety of the lifeguard. Rescue boats allow for emergency medical treatment to begin while still in the water. This can greatly improve patient outcome in some cases.

Boat Rescue, Enforcement, and Firefighting

For some lifeguard agencies, a major responsibility of the rescue boat fleet is response and assistance to boaters in distress. The popularity of personal watercraft, kayaks, and kite surfing has added to the volume of these incidents. Rescue boats can be equipped for marine firefighting and lifeguards from several American lifeguard agencies are primary responders to boat, marina, and pier fires. Boats are extremely valuable in enforcement of boating regulations. One of the most frustrating experiences for a lifeguard is watching an errant boater buzzing a swimming crowd. This is extremely dangerous, but the shore-based lifeguard can do little about it. A lifeguard in a rescue boat can quickly resolve such a problem. Moreover, lifeguards from some agencies use rescue boats for general law enforcement, including boating safety enforcement and enforcement of environmental laws.

Rescue Boat Limitations

Size

Rescue boats can be large and heavy. Unless berthed at a dock or pier, launching a boat can be a strenuous process that may take more than one lifeguard. Because of their size and weight, boats can be dangerous in heavy surf and must be handled expertly in negotiating a surfline during a rescue. The boat can become a hazard to swimmers should it be overcome by surf.

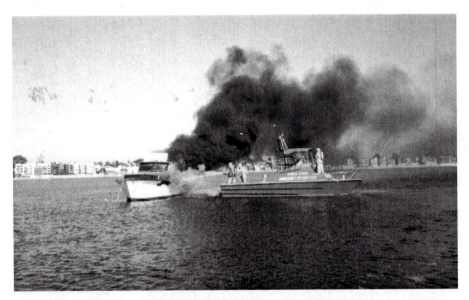

San Diego lifeguards battle a boat fire. Note that lifeguards are wearing full firefighting gear.

Credit: San Diego Lifeguard Service

Crowded Beaches

Heavy water attendance can cause problems in effecting rescues from boats because of the size of the boat and the area necessary to maneuver. Crowds can also make launching and recovering a boat difficult and hazardous. Like motor vehicles on the beach, rescue boats must often be maneuvered very close to people and must therefore be operated with tremendous caution.

Wind and Waves

Because of their high profile in the water, rescue boats are subject to the forces of wind and waves. Although these challenges can usually be overcome with good operating skills, weather conditions can complicate a boat rescue to the point that other rescue equipment may sometimes be a better option. Heavy weather rescue boat operations require special operating skills and should not be undertaken without extensive training.

Expense

Boats can be expensive to purchase and operate depending on their size and how they are equipped. Training requirements are proportional to the complexity of the vessel.

Personnel Requirements

Boats require operators. This may be obvious, but under most circumstances a rescue boat operator cannot leave the boat to effect a rescue. This is different from a lifeguard in a rescue vehicle, for example, who can park the vehicle and leave it to rescue a victim. On the other hand, in many cases, the rescue boat can be brought directly alongside the struggling victim, unlike a vehicle. A properly equipped rescue vessel includes throwable flotation devices in case victims cannot be immediately brought aboard.

Types of Rescue Boats

A wide variety of boats are employed by lifeguards in carrying out their responsibilities. The following are the types most commonly employed by lifeguards at American beaches. Some agencies have boats of several types, employing different boats for different purposes. Lifeguards from these agencies can select the best tool for the job, depending on the circumstances of the rescue. Other agencies focus on a single boat design for purposes of economy and to help reduce training time.

Personal Watercraft

The invention of the Jet Ski™ changed boating dramatically, with many new people becoming involved. The original Jet Ski™ (a manufacturer's trade name), required the operator to stand while riding. Subsequent designs by a variety of manufacturers allow the operator to sit astride the craft. These small jet powered craft have become generically known as *personal watercraft*. PWC are typically less than 13 feet in length and have a basic V hull configuration. They are steered through use of a jet of water which is directed toward the stern by a motorized pump and usually directionally controlled by handlebars. This lends to a limitation of the craft, which is that they cannot be steered unless water is coming from the jet. In emergencies, operators sometimes suddenly back the throttle down to idle, leaving themselves unable to control forward direction.

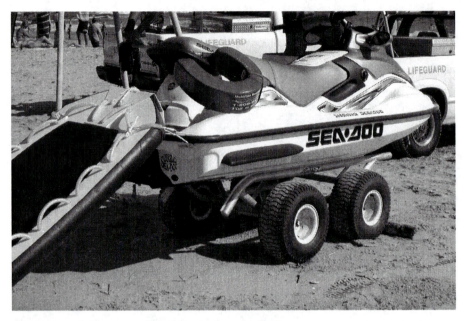

A personal watercraft with a rescue sled.

Credit: Ken Kramer

PWC are very effectively used by many American lifeguard agencies. They are highly maneuverable, have a relatively low maintenance cost, are often unaffected by being capsized (or rolled), and are sometimes available from the manufacturers on a loan basis, thus greatly reducing cost. Appropriate training is essential prior to operation and rescue procedures, although learning to master the PWC generally requires less up-front training than other motorized rescue boats. A single lifeguard without a crewmember can operate a PWC. While these craft typically weigh 500—800 pounds, they can be beach launched with assistance of a properly designed dolly. PWC are valuable in breaking surf and can also be very effective in open water swells and even in high wind conditions.

The high speed of PWC makes it essential that the operator vigilantly monitor the surrounding area for swimmers and other craft. They can be operated near large swimming crowds by skilled lifeguards, but their hard hulls are unforgiving if a swimmer is struck. It is also important for the operator to take care not to become launched into the air over a wave. Personal watercraft leave the operator exposed and often wet. They are therefore not well-suited to cold environments.

Like other boats, PWC have mandatory equipment requirements according to federal law. These requirements include a personal flotation device (PFD) for each person on board, fire extinguisher, sound producing device, and backfire flame arrester. State regulations may require the wearing of PFDs and may prohibit nighttime operation. Additional personal protection equipment recommended by USLA includes helmet, visor, gloves, goggles, wetsuit, and footwear. Many PWC have kill switches to ensure that if the operator becomes separated from the PWC, the motor turns off. These are usually activated when a lanyard, attached to the operator, pulls the switch. It is important to always attach this lanyard to the operator prior to operation, as well as to don appropriate personal protective equipment.

Most PWC are designed to hold only an operator and one or two passengers. Thus, rescue capacity is limited. Furthermore, it can be difficult and dangerous to attempt to pull a victim out of the water and aboard a personal watercraft, since they ride high in the water and are unstable when not underway (which can lead to rollover). To address this issue, rescue sleds are employed, which are towed behind PWC and greatly enhance rescue capabilities. The sled allows for a second lifeguard to ride prone or kneeling on the rescue sled. This lifeguard is responsible for the rescue and emergency medical treatment of victims brought aboard the craft, while the PWC operator is responsible for safe operations. Rescues sleds allow for quick and efficient multiple victim rescues and transport of more than one person at a time. The use of a PWC without an appropriate rescue sled is not recommended.

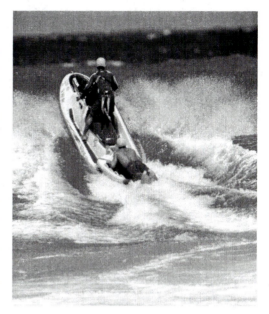

Desirable characteristics in rescue sleds are lightweight, yet rigid construction, multiple handles along the perimeter of the sled, and a top surface that provides enough friction to keep the crewmember from sliding, but not so much so as to tear wetsuit material or cause abrasions to the lifeguard or victim. It is also advantageous to have reinforced handles that do not protrude through the bottom of the sled. The size and shape of sleds vary by manufacturer. Rescue sleds should have a template that matches, or is narrower than the trough, or wake, created by the PWC when underway. The sled

Credit: Mike Waggoner

should ride on top of the PWC transom to avoid pearling (submersion of the nose of the sled).

The attachment system is an important element in the way the rescue sled integrates with the PWC and its ability to maneuver. If only a single point connection is used (similar to the trailer hitch on a car), the sled can pivot in a wide arc, causing problems of maneuverability and safety. On the other hand, a rigidly attached sled that does not articulate during turns impedes the ability to turn the PWC and decreases the overall turning radius. To avoid this, a three point attachment system is used. The center tow point allows the sled to pivot, but the two side points prevent over articulation to either side.

Inflatable Rescue Boats (IRBs)

Inflatable rescue boats (IRBs), also known as inshore rescue boats, were first employed by the lifesavers of Australia and New Zealand. These boats are typically 12 to 14 feet in length and utilize a small outboard of 25 to 35 horsepower for propulsion. Most often they are staffed by an operator and a crewmember, who sit on opposite gunwales while holding handles. The relatively low weight of these craft (about 300 pounds) allows them to be moved and launched fairly easily. To keep the vessels light, fuel cans are replaced with fuel bladders made of a synthetic material. A propeller guard is commonly attached to the outboard for safety. This is highly recommended.

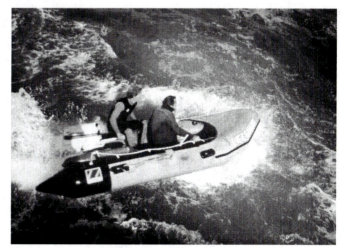

Credit: B. Chris Brewster

IRBs are versatile boats. Used by trained operators, they can successfully handle very large surf conditions and be operated in the surfline for extended periods of time. These boats are relatively fast, because they draw little water as they float across the surface, but not as fast as a PWC. They can be launched from a beach or returned to the beach with relative ease. As a result, a nearby harbor is not needed and response is immediate. In a pinch, an IRB can hold several victims. In a mass rescue situation, the IRB can be used as a raft to which many victims can cling until brought to the beach individually by swimming lifeguards. IRBs can be successfully employed in very close proximity to large swimming crowds with limited danger presented.

IRBs have detractions. They are small open boats wherein the operator and crew can be subjected to heavy bouncing over waves and wet conditions. IRBs are not reliable in high wind conditions because of the instability created by the air filled hulls. A well trained operator can turn an IRB in a very tight circle, but when used to tow other vessels, IRBs are very difficult to steer due to lack of a deep keel. IRBs can be inexpensively maintained, but require regular maintenance. When caught in the wrong orientation by a breaking wave, IRBs can flip. Even in this circumstance however, they are generally less hazardous than other types of rescue boats because of their soft sides. Properly employed restart procedures can result in complete salvage of an outboard that has been fully doused.

Rigid Hull Vessels

Some lifeguard agencies operate large, motorized rigid hull vessels, equipped for full service response to swimming rescues, boat rescues (including fires and towing services), and other emergencies. These vessels can be equipped with a full compliment of rescue and emergency gear such as two-way radios, firefighting equipment, positioning equipment, medical gear, scuba gear, depth finders, and public address equipment. In some agencies, these vessels combine traditional lifeguard duties with those of harbor patrol, general law enforcement, and special rescue missions.

Rigid hull vessels are particularly useful for offshore rescues or for long distance rescues to remote beach areas. They can carry numerous victims from the head of a rip current. They can also accommodate a victim on a stretcher or allow for full CPR. Some lifeguard agencies actually utilize rigid hull rescue boats inside the surf in a manner similar to an IRB; however, this is uncommon and requires unique skills. Large, rigid hull rescue boats offer the greatest degree of protection for operator and crew. Depending on

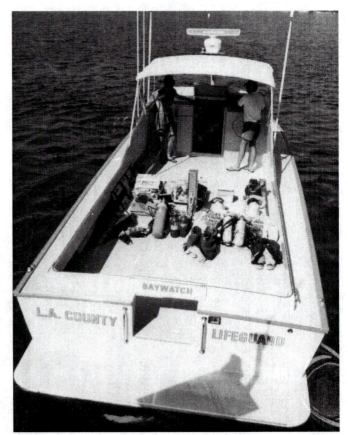

Credit: Conrad Liberty

their size, most larger rigid hull vessels are either difficult to beach launch or cannot be beach launched at all. A nearby harbor is usually needed, along with docks and storage facilities.

Rowed Boats

At most major beach areas in the United States where rescue boats are employed, manually powered (rowed) rescue boats have been replaced or augmented by motorized rescue boats. In a few areas, such as New Jersey and the Great Lakes, rowed rescue boats remain in use. These boats are most typically known as lifeboats, surfboats, dories, or rowboats. Usually they are rowed by one or two lifeguards.

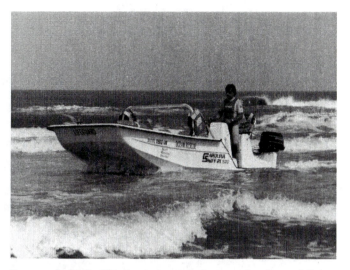

Some rigid hull rescue vessels are designed for work inside the surfline.

Credit: Mike Hensler

Manually powered boats include hollow draft surf rescue dories. These are designed to cut through the surf, while retaining adequate stability to be used as an effective observation platform. Rescue dories feature a square stern that facilitates foot placement for the rear crewmember, who can propel the boat from a forward facing standing position. The square stern also allows boarding of the victim over the transom. On the surf beaches of the Great Lakes and at many other inland lakes, a wide variety of wood, fiberglass, and aluminum boats are employed.

Rowed vessels are dependable in that they do not rely on motors, which can fail. They are clean, in that they involve no emission of used or unused fuel. Compared to powered vessels however, rowed vessels are very slow and easily delayed or even stopped by surf conditions. In almost every case, a swimming lifeguard responding from the beach will reach a distressed victim far more quickly than a vessel which is launched and rowed to the victim. On the other hand, when deployed outside the swimming crowd, the lifeguard aboard a rowed rescue boat can quickly observe and rescue a distressed victim.

Kayaks

The least expensive type of rescue boat is the kayak. While less versatile than a motorized rescue boat, kayaks are light, maneuverable, inexpensive, and in some ways superior to a paddleboard for observation. Open top kayaks used in lifeguarding are plastic, highly maneuverable craft that can carry a personal flotation device (PFD), rescue buoy, and limited medical gear. Rather than sitting inside, the operator sits on top of the craft. Kayaks are easily carried to the water's edge by a single lifeguard.

Kayaks provide a relatively dry platform for patrol and observation. Lifeguards in kayaks can sit in an erect position, easily observed by swimmers. These craft can be useful for rapid approach, control, and stabilization of a victim or multiple victims. Retrieval though, is more difficult. With minimal skills, lifeguards can propel kayaks quickly through light and moderate surf. Kayaks are particularly useful in choppy light surf conditions that make the use of rescue boards or dories difficult.

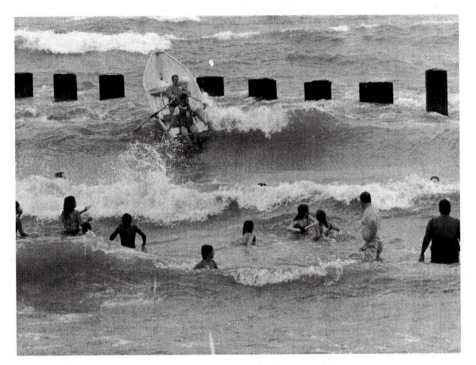

Credit: Al Shorey

Use of Rescue Boats

The following is an overview of the techniques commonly used to operate lifeguard rescue boats. Actual operation of rescue boats, particularly motorized rescue boats in the surf environment, requires extensive training under the supervision of a skilled and experienced operator.

Alert

The most common source of alert to the need for a rescue boat response is observation by a shore-based lifeguard. A rescue boat may be sent because the victim is a significant distance from shore, because there are multiple victims, or because a patrolling rescue boat is close to the rescue. There are a variety of other reasons to utilize a rescue boat, but these are the most common.

Boat operators may also observe distress while on patrol. Lifeguards in a rescue boat are at a lower level than lifeguards in an observation tower and lack the ability for broad observation of the entire swim area, but they are also much closer to the swimming crowd and can make more direct evaluations of those who appear to be in distress. At some agencies, lifeguards in rescue boats are expected to patrol unguarded beaches that, due to remoteness and low attendance, lack on-site lifeguard supervision. In these cases they may be the only source of supervision, albeit sporadic. Lifeguards in rescue boats may be alerted to vessels in distress by observation of a flare, waving flags, whistles, or by a marine radio broadcast. The marine VHF radio band is publicly available to all mariners and many boaters carry them. By monitoring the calling and distress frequency (channel 16), lifeguard rescue boat operators and crew can keep abreast of emergency calls initiated by boaters. Boaters are also increasingly likely to carry cell phones, which may be used to call 9-1-1. Rescue boat operators may be notified by radio of such calls.

When lifeguards ashore spot a problem that calls for a rescue boat response, they must have a method to immediately alert the rescue boat crew. Likewise, when lifeguards in a rescue vessel observe people in distress requiring their assistance, they need a reliable method to advise lifeguards ashore of the incident so that proper backup can be sent. Effective use of rescue boats requires two-way radio communication capabilities, both to shore and to other rescue boats. This can be problematic for small rescue boats which lack a waterproof location for even a hand held radio, but there are several sources of waterproof containers that effectively resolve this problem.

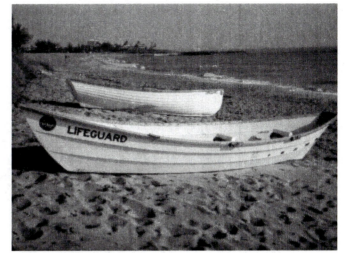

Credit: Paul Drucker

When radio communications break down or in cases that radio communications are not available, it is important to have a backup method. This may include an air horn, flag, etc., but it must be emphasized that such methods are unreliable and limited in value, in that lifeguards ashore cannot provide details on the nature of the rescue, while lifeguards in the rescue vessel cannot provide information on victim status or other observations.

Entry

When a drowning presentation is detected by lifeguards patrolling in a boat, they can move directly from alert to contact and control of the victim. Beach-based boats however, will have to go through an entry. At flat water beaches, boats can be positioned at the water's edge with the bow of the boat in the water, ready for response. At surf beaches, boats will usually be positioned on the beach close to the waterline, but above the uprush. If significant tidal changes are present, the boat will need to be moved regularly to keep it close to the shoreline. Some agencies utilize rollers placed under the hull of the boat or small trailers to facilitate launching. It is important to minimize any hazard to the public that might be presented while rescue boats are positioned on the beach. As an example, if a trailer is used to launch the rescue boat, agencies may wish to mark the trailer tongue with a bright noticeable object, such as a road cone. An unwary individual playing Frisbee or chasing a ball is more likely to notice the marker than a low lying metal trailer tongue.

Boats should be prepared for instant use, with all equipment aboard and accessible. Proper preparation and maintenance is required to ensure that when an emergency occurs, the boat is fully serviceable. A motorized rescue boat, for example, will be of little use, and perhaps seriously impede an expeditious rescue response, if the motor won't start. For this reason, lifeguards should never completely rely on a boat response to a rescue. A lifeguard ashore should always be prepared to effect the rescue if the boat response encounters problems. At some agencies it is a standard practice to respond a lifeguard from shore in all cases, even when a boat is responding from nearby. The shore based lifeguard can always return to shore if the boat based lifeguards complete the rescue first. This practice can also be useful if the rescue boat is needed to respond to another more critical rescue. The shore based lifeguard can assume control of the victim, freeing the rescue boat to respond where needed.

Safe entry protocols require that the launch area first be cleared of water users. Flat water entry is straightforward—lifeguards simply push off from shore and respond; but surf entry can be very challenging, particular as surf size increases. It is important to select an area with few or no swimmers around. There is always the possibility of losing control of the boat in the surf and having the boat pushed to shore by incoming waves, striking swimmers. It is also difficult to see over waves to determine whether a swimmer is ahead, and if the operator is focusing on getting through breaking waves, attention can be distracted.

The primary rule of operating a rescue vessel inside the surfline is that the boat should be kept perpendicular to incoming waves and foam lines of broken waves. This presents the least resistance to the power of the waves and allows the design of the vessel to efficiently deflect wave energy. Skilled operators of powered craft can learn to take broken waves at almost parallel angles while the vessel is moving forward at significant speed, but this requires advanced training.

When a manually powered rescue boat is employed by a single lifeguard in the surf environment, the lifeguard will push from the stern into the water with the bow perpendicular to incoming waves. The boat is pushed to a comfortable rowing depth, usually waist deep water. The lifeguard then vaults over the stern, enters the vessel, and begins rowing. Likewise, a personal watercraft operated by a single operator is pushed to a depth needed to operate, started, and the operator jumps aboard.

Beach based vessels which utilize two lifeguards are IRBs, and sometimes PWCs and dories. Entry with these craft with a crew of two persons is quite similar. At first, both lifeguards push the boat toward an adequate depth for rowing, for the IRB outboard to be dropped from the cocked position without striking bottom, or so that the PWC jet will not to draw sand and other debris into the jet drive pump. Once this depth is reached, one lifeguard boards the vessel while the other keeps the bow perpendicular to oncoming waves. The goal is to prepare to exert forward momentum adequate to make way against the waves before the second lifeguard boards the vessel. The PWC operator boards the craft, ensures that the safety lanyard (kill switch) is attached to the operator, then starts the motor. Once the operator gives the command, the second lifeguard boards the rescue sled. The IRB operator starts the engine, while the first lifeguard in the dory simply assumes a rowing position. Once the lifeguard in either vessel determines that forward progress can be made which will allow the boat to make headway without further assistance from the lifeguard in the water, this lifeguard is advised to climb aboard.

The position of the operator of an IRB is usually sitting on the *port* (left facing forward) pontoon near the stern. The crewmember sits on the *starboard* (right facing forward) pontoon toward the bow. These positions help keep the vessel balanced.

In a dory, the rowing position can be a standing one, facing forward (known as "boating") or a sitting one facing toward the stern. The latter position requires less skill and allows for more efficient rowing, but it is more difficult to maintain visual observation over the victim in this position. Directions from beach based lifeguards may be needed.

An essential role of the lifeguard in command of a rescue boat is to avoid taking a direct hit from a breaking wave. This can injure the crew; it can swamp an IRB, killing the engine; it can significantly impede the progress of a manually powered rescue boat or carry it all the way to shore in the foam line; and it can knock the operator and crew member of a PWC off the craft or rescue sled. In any case, the rescue boat response is slowed or curtailed and persons inshore of the boat can be threatened by the unpiloted incoming boat.

In larger surf, boat operators time their approach to traverse the surfline carefully, often hanging inshore of the breakers until the boat can be moved quickly forward between breaking waves. The inside of the surf break is a difficult area in which to maneuver because the water is moving shoreward so quickly and the water is heavily aerated, providing low buoyancy; but a breaking wave is most dan-

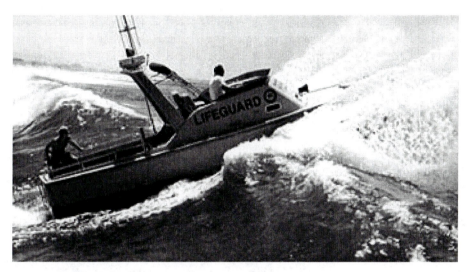

Rescue boat moving outside the break

Credit: Huntington State Beach

gerous and to be avoided. In large surf, operators of IRBs and PWC may move the craft back and forth inside the breakers, waiting for the right moment to make it through.

When a two person rescue boat is clearly about to be caught by a breaking wave which will break directly on top of it, the lifeguard in command of the vessel advises the crewperson. In an IRB, the crewperson braces by grabbing the bow line and lying face down between the bow pontoons, head first. This maneuver adds weight to the bow to reduce the chance of the boat riding up the wave and being flipped. On a PWC, the best action on the part of the operator is to flatten to the seat. The lifeguard riding on the rescue sled presses tightly to the sled while holding tightly with one hand on a side handle and the other on an opposite forward handle. The crewmember's head position is down and away from the stern of the PWC to avoid impact. The operator of a motorized craft may decide to try to punch through the wave in a last minute burst of speed. This may allow the boat to avoid much of the power of the wave which would otherwise break directly on the vessel. In any case, a direct perpendicular orientation to the wave is critical or the boat will likely broach and be pushed ashore.

Great care must be taken if the rescue boat rides up the steep face of a wave about to break and when the bow plunges downward on the other side. Powered vessels are very susceptible to being launched over an incoming wave and becoming airborne. Lifeguards can be seriously injured or even ejected from the boat. Personal watercraft are particularly prone to this problem due to their high power and speed, but any boat can become airborne given the right circumstances. The goal in all cases is to get to the other side of the wave without being caught in the break, but to try to stay in contact with the water at all times. This is done by using no more forward power than is needed to get past the wave and by rapidly decelerating as soon as it is clear that the boat will reach the other side. With all rescue craft, when operating in breaking waves it is critical that operators plan their route to ensure that bathers and swimmers are not placed in peril should the craft be disabled or lose power.

Contact and Control

Safely approaching a victim with a rescue boat, particularly in rough conditions, requires great skill and extensive practice. The obvious goal is to rescue the victim expeditiously without further injury. If an oar, propeller, or boat hull strikes the victim, injury is likely. In rescue boats with two persons aboard, if a safe approach will be difficult or the victim's condition is poor, one lifeguard can simply enter the water with an RFD to assist the victim, then swim the victim to the waiting rescue boat.

In flat water or gentle swells outside the surfline, a manually propelled rescue boat is rowed within ten to twenty feet of the victim, then a fast rowing pivot is performed to present the stern to the victim. Stern presentations are preferred for rowed rescue boats because the transom is the most stable area of the vessel. The lifeguard then backs toward the victim. If there is only one lifeguard aboard, the lifeguard ships the oars and moves to the stern to assist the victim aboard. If there are two, the sternmost lifeguard provides this assistance.

In these same conditions, an IRB is simply brought alongside the victim and the victim is brought in over a pontoon with the assistance of the crewmember (preferably over the mid to forward portion of the port pontoon). The transom is not used because of the hazard presented by the outboard. On a personal watercraft with a lone operator, the victim is helped aboard with a one arm assist from the operator who must take care not to allow too much weight to shift to one side. If a rescue sled is towed, the boat is positioned so that the victim can be grabbed by the lifeguard on the sled and held there in a prone position, usually under the arms of the lifeguard, who grabs the outer handles of the sled.

The most difficult area to effect a boat-based rescue is inside breaking surf. Generally, only the IRB and personal watercraft are suitable for rescues in this zone because they are best able to maintain position inside breaking surf without being overcome. In either case, the ideal is to bring the vessel alongside the victim maintaining a constant bow out (toward the breaking surf) position. The victim is then brought abroad as previously explained. It is particularly important to effect this action very quickly when inside the surfline for obvious reasons.

Highly skilled IRB and PWC operators utilize a maneuver in critical rescues between breaking waves which can rapidly extricate a victim. This involves approaching the victim at moderate speed and turning sharply around the victim in a counter-clockwise direction. In the case of the IRB, this brings the port pontoon down to water level. The crewmember leans over from the starboard side and grabs the outstretched arms or armpits of the victim. The victim is then rolled into the boat. For the PWC, the operator maneuvers the craft to locate the rescue sled in a position that the crewmember can grab and roll the victim onto the rescue sled as the operator accelerates away from the breaking wave. Due to the hazard involved, this technique is appropriate only for highly skilled operators in critical situations.

Larger rescue vessels generally approach the surfline from the outside and back down into the waves, keeping the bow out. A crewmember then jumps into the water and brings the victim out to the rescue boat. Great caution is needed in operating large rescue boats near the surf because of the danger involved in having a large hard hull vessel overcome and pushed into the beach toward swimmers.

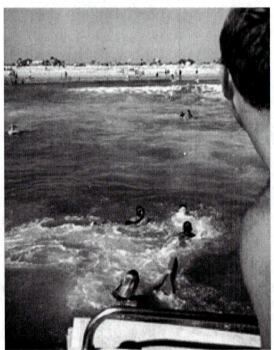

Deckhand assisting a multiple person rescue.

Credit: Huntington State Beach

Retrieval

Once the victim has been brought aboard the rescue vessel, expeditious retrieval to shore is not normally necessary. Exceptions include cases where the victim needs medical attention or where the rescue vessel is immediately needed for response to other emergencies. Usually however, lifeguards can take the time to carefully consider the return route to shore.

For flat water, the rescue boat is simply returned to shore. Manually powered boats are best beached stern toward the beach to allow the victim to exit over the transom. Powered vessels must usually be beached bow first.

Returning to shore in significant surf conditions requires careful planning and timing. The lifeguard in charge should first select the best area for this return. Considerations include avoiding areas where swimmers are present, selecting areas with less severe surf breaks (if available), and bringing the vessel to a safe shore area (devoid of rocks, debris, etc.).

Powered vessels that can be beached can normally outrun incoming surf. The operator waits to gauge the incoming sets of waves, then simply drives straight to shore between breaking waves. As an IRB approaches shallow water, the operator kills the engine and raises it to the cocked position. This is very important because striking even a sandy bottom can damage the engine and transom. PWCs can be accelerated over breaking waves and the operator stops the jet prior to running the craft up onto the beach. It is important to ensure the beach area is clear as the craft can travel a considerable distance up the beach depending on the speed of exit.

Rowed boats usually cannot outrun the surf. When returning to shore in surf conditions that threaten to overwhelm the boat, the stern lifeguard can ship oars and drop over the transom to stabilize the boat by holding onto the transom with the hands and extending the body to act as a sea anchor and rudder. Some agencies prefer that dories are pivoted so that the bow is toward the waves and the boat is rowed backwards toward shore for a more stable ride. This depends on the design of the craft. Either of these maneuvers may be impractical depending on surf size. If there is a significant hazard in retrieval of the victim to the beach, an alternative is to simply swim the lifeguard to shore with a crewmember from the rescue boat or a lifeguard from shore.

Aircraft

Few lifeguard agencies have aircraft available for regular use; however, many agencies have rescue, medical, and law enforcement aircraft they can call upon when needed. Fixed wing aircraft can be useful for covering wide areas in the case of a search, but are of little value in transporting a lifeguard to a rescue or evacuating a victim. Of all the forms of transportation available to lifeguard services, the helicopter is the fastest, most agile, and most versatile.

Helicopters can transport lifeguards over long distances expeditiously, then drop them to victims. Properly equipped helicopters can lift victims and lifeguards from the water and some can even land on the water. This is particularly valuable in very large surf conditions where the victim is taken outside the surfline or in rescues of persons aboard offshore boats. Larger helicopters can be configured to carry PWC to an offshore location where they can be deployed by being pushed out the door.

Helicopters are ideal in searches for persons lost at sea because of their high vantage point and mobility. When necessary, they can be used to transport medical supplies to offshore locations or drop pumps to sinking vessels. Helicopters can provide night lighting for water and cliff rescues. They can also be extremely valuable in flood rescues, when victims are trapped by moving or rising water. Some lifeguard services develop a working agreement with a helicopter provider that results in having a helicopter on standby for large surf conditions, heavy crowds, or inclement weather.

Victim Extrication Using Aircraft

There are two primary methods of extricating victims from the aquatic environment using helicopters—hoist and static line. The hoist is typically available on larger helicopters specially equipped for rescue, notably those of the US Coast Guard. Using a powered reel, a cable is lowered to the victim from a hovering helicopter, the victim is secured and the helicopter continues to hover as the victim is reeled up. The victim is then swung inside to safety.

The static line method is used by smaller helicopters which lack powered hoists. This involves a line hung from the helicopter to which the victim is attached. The victim is elevated from danger as the helicopter gains altitude. This technique is somewhat more difficult because the victim must hang from the static line as the helicopter pilot flies the victim to safety and the victim must then be gently set down.

The US Coast Guard generally uses a yoke system to attach the rescue line to the victim. This is simply a circle of material similar to fire hose. The yoke (also known as a horse collar) is placed over the victim's head and under the armpits with the hoist line on the victim's front side. As the victim is hoisted, the circle closes and the victim holds the sides. This method is very rapid.

Static line rescue systems typically employ a pouch made of netting attached to the end of the line. The net is lowered into the water and the victim climbs inside. Once the victim is inside, the heli-

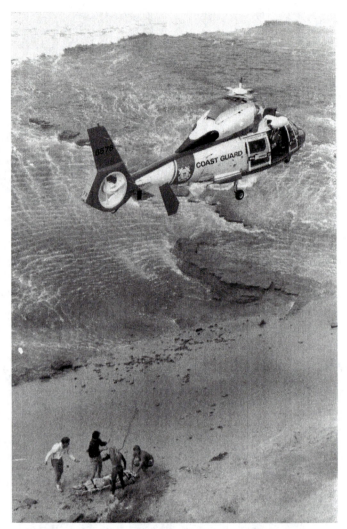

Lifeguards and a Coast Guard helicopter crew prepare to extricate a victim by hoisting the stretcher from a beach area bordered by high cliffs.

copter pilot lifts off. An injured victim in a stretcher can be evacuated using either the hoist or static system so long as a proper harness is used that will keep the stretcher level and the victim is properly strapped inside.

A third extrication method, often used in flood rescue, is to have a helicopter actually touch down one skid or even land, allowing the victim to climb inside. The one skid method is extremely challenging for a helicopter pilot in that flight must be maintained simultaneously to touching a stationary object. The simple addition of weight to one side of a helicopter from a victim boarding can cause the aircraft to yaw, creating the potential for a loss of airworthiness.

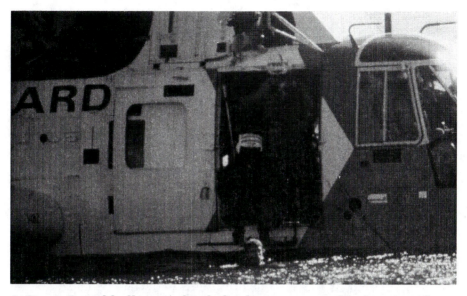

A Coast Guard helicopter lands in the ocean outside large surf to pick up a victim from a swimming lifeguard.

Helicopters build up static electricity which is discharged upon touching the ground. In order to create a partial discharge without hazard when a metal cable is lowered to the lifeguard or victim, the cable should first be allowed to touch the boat deck, water, or ground. Once this contact is made, there is no further concern for this discharge, as the winch cable will continually act as a ground.

It is vital that a cable or line attached to a helicopter never be secured to a rescue vessel, unless it is a small rescue vessel being hoisted. Helicopters must have the freedom to move according to changing wind currents and cannot in any way be secured to substantial surface craft.

When removing a victim from a boat, helicopter pilots often prefer to head into the wind and maintain minimum airspeed for stability. This requires that the boat be headed in the same direction at the same speed.

Landing on a Beach

If a helicopter must be landed on a beach, lifeguards must create and maintain a secure landing zone (LZ) of adequate size. As a general rule, an LZ which is 100 feet in diameter should be considered a minimum. Helicopter pilots also appreciate the existence of a wind indicator in the immediate area, but outside the LZ. This can simply be a flag atop a lifeguard station, for example, or a smoke bomb. Another option is to draw a large arrow in the sand pointing toward the prevailing wind direction.

The rotor wash of a landing or departing helicopter creates a small windstorm which can carry sand for hundreds of feet. It can also blow beach items like umbrellas and tents, which can injure beachgoers. When a helicopter is expected to land on a beach, beach patrons should be advised to collapse umbrellas and secure light items.

A helicopter landing on a beach always draws a crowd, but poses a danger. Adequate crowd control measures should be implemented prior to landing. It is a good practice to summon local police well in advance of landing a helicopter on a crowded beach so that they can assist in securing the LZ. Lifeguards should remember that they are not immune from the problems of rotor wash. Most experienced lifeguards take shelter behind emergency vehicles or other stationary objects to protect themselves during landing and take-off—the times of most intense rotor wash.

While helicopters are extremely valuable for lifeguard rescue, extensive training is needed before lifeguards can properly employ them. Lifeguards must be conversant with protocols needed in approaching a helicopter on the ground, because the blades can be lethal. When working in close quarters with a helicopter, it is important to keep eye contact with the pilot if at all possible and to be prepared to back off quickly if necessary. Helicopters hovering over water can create a tremendous amount of water disturbance and noise which can be very disorienting and curtail verbal communication.

These concerns notwithstanding, with proper skill and training of the personnel involved, helicopters are an invaluable tool for lifeguards. It is strongly recommended that lifeguard agencies with the local availability of helicopters create appropriate liaisons, develop contingency plans, and conduct regular training exercises.

Boat Tow

The boat tow is one of the simplest and least expensive pieces of rescue equipment a lifeguard will use. It can make the difference in successfully rescuing boats worth tens of thousands of dollars and the persons aboard. A boat tow is a length of line approximately six feet long, with a loop spliced in one end and a large snap hook on the other end. When a boat is observed to be in distress, perhaps disabled and drifting toward rocks or surf, the lifeguard runs the boat tow through the rear handle of a rescue buoy and pulls the snap end through the loop end of the line. The snap end of the line is then pulled tight. There is now a six foot piece of line securely fastened to the rear handle of the rescue buoy, with a snap hook on the far end. The lifeguard swims to the boat and clips the hook into the bow eye of the boat. The lifeguard then swims the boat away from danger. This process is surprisingly effective for vessels up to 30' long and larger. Swim fins are highly desirable when using a boat tow. Little progress will be made without them.

The lifeguard using a boat tow must always be prepared to jettison the rescue buoy if the vessel is caught by surf while the tow is underway. The lifeguard must also maintain a position so that the lifeguard is not caught between an incoming wave and the boat. The goal in using a boat tow is to tow the vessel from immediate danger. Obviously a swimming lifeguard cannot keep a boat away from danger indefinitely. Once this is accomplished, if there is an anchor aboard it is used. If a rescue boat is available, it is dispatched to take over the tow.

Landline

The typical landline device is a length of line (usually 200 or more yards), with a snap hook on the lead end and a spliced loop or snap hook on the tail end. It is kept coiled on a reel or laid in an easily transported, open container. Some agencies keep their landlines in inexpensive plastic laundry baskets.

The landline provides an added level of security and safety for both the open water rescuer and victim by establishing a link with assistance on shore. The rescuer dons the harness of the landline or attaches the end of the line to an RFD and swims to the victim. Once control and stabilization are attained, assistants ashore can rapidly retrieve both the rescuer and victim(s) by pulling in the line. Therefore, while the rescuer must swim the line to the victim, once the victim is reached no further swimming is necessary.

While use of the landline is in decline as it is supplanted by lifeguards with swim fins, motorized rescue boats, and other lifesaving tools, it remains in use along parts of the New Jersey shore and on some beaches of New York, New England, and the Great Lakes. Availability of landlines is required by regulation in a few states. In some cases, public safety agencies whose employees may not meet standards recommended by USLA, such as fire department and rescue squads, use landlines, primarily to reduce safety risks to rescuers. Standard protocols in these cases involve rescuers wearing personal flotation devices, swim fins, and, depending on water temperature, wetsuits. (USLA does not recommend that any person engage in in-water rescue unless trained in accordance with either the USLA *Lifeguard Agency Certification Program* or *Aquatic Rescue Response Team* certification program.)

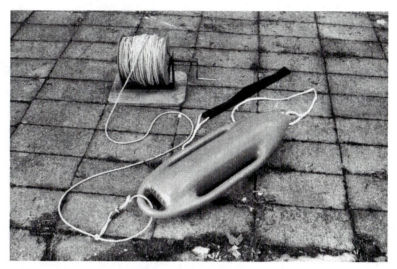

Rescue buoy attached to a landline on a reel.
Credit: Dave Foxwell

Landline Applications

The open water lifeguard agencies which use landlines indicate that while they are not generally the rescue tool of first choice, they are sometimes effectively employed in the following applications:

- Surf conditions which prohibit use of rescue boards or rescue boats
- Multiple victim rescues
- Situations where the victim (and rescuer) might otherwise be thrust upon rocks or reefs by currents or surf
- Lateral current situations as in swiftwater rescues
- Landlines also can be adapted to boat rescues, crowd control and many other situations where a length of line can be useful

Landline Limitations

- Landlines contribute drag on the swimming rescuer and therefore slow approach to the victim(s)
- Landlines require more than one lifeguard to perform a rescue thereby removing them from other duties
- Landlines require significant training and coordination for effective use
- Landline rescues are limited by the length of the line
- Problems can be encountered with crowds, piers, or other obstructions to the clean play of the line

Landline Rescue Techniques

Landline rescues are similar to RFD rescues with the exception of the retrieval phase. There are two primary landline evolutions based on either two or more than two lifeguards. Landlines are most effectively used with a rescue buoy.

Two Lifeguards

The first or responding lifeguard dons the rescue buoy harness and attaches the landline to the rear handle of the rescue buoy using the snap hook on the landline. (The rescue buoy may be prepositioned with this attachment.) The responding lifeguard then enters the water and approaches the victim as the line plays out. The second or assisting lifeguard monitors the line and tends to any tangles that may occur. The responding lifeguard contacts and controls the victim, sandwiching the victim between the lifeguard and rescue buoy, then signals the assisting lifeguard, who pulls them to shore. When shallow water is gained, the responding lifeguard signals for cessation of the pull and removes the victim from the water.

Three or More Lifeguards

The first responding lifeguard dons an RFD and proceeds with a free swimming entry, approaching, contacting, and stabilizing the victim. The sec-

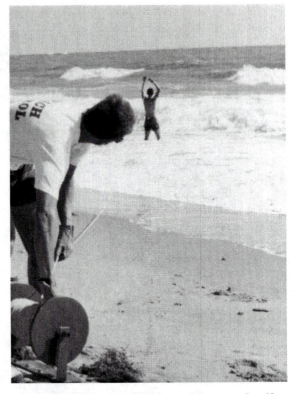

A second lifeguard helps play out the line as the rescuer swims to the victim.
Credit: William McNeely, Jr.

ond lifeguard dons a landline harness or fastens a rescue buoy to the landline snap hook, and swims the landline out to the responding lifeguard and victim. The line is then fastened to the responding lifeguard's RFD. The third lifeguard, onshore, monitors the landline, tends to any tangles that may occur, and pulls victim and responding lifeguard toward shore when signaled.

Additional responding lifeguards assist by keeping the line free of obstructions and interfering spectators while being played out and in assisting on landline retrieval. They may also expedite the playing out of the landline by holding it above their heads through the surf to minimize drag. If there is a possibility of the initial landline not being long enough to reach the victim, a second landline should be placed in preparation for use.

Additional Landline Considerations

- It is important to move the landline to the entry point before commencing the rescue. The entry point may be on the beach directly perpendicular to the victim or at a point along the beach off which onshore currents may carry the victim.
- An alternate method to select an entry point when a rip has carried a victim at an angle to the shore is to place the landline on the shore perpendicular to the point where the

responding lifeguard anticipates the victim will be when contact is made, then run to the base of the rip, enter the water, and use the speed and force of the rip to help overtake the victim. This technique is known as the pendulum.

- If use of the landline results in unmanageable tangles or exceeds the length of line available, the landline should be immediately discarded and a free swimming rescue should be performed.

- Landlines are pulled in facing the victim either hand-over-hand or by grabbing the landline and walking backwards away from the water.

- When retrieving the landline, assisting lifeguards must closely monitor the lifeguard and victim for signals to cease pulling and for swells and waves overtaking the lifeguard and victim. Speed of retrieval is less important then steady pulling. One exception to steady pulling is that the landline retrieval must be slowed or stopped while the swell or wave passes the lifeguard and victim to prevent them from being temporarily submerged. No hand signals are involved. The technique and timing of this retrieval pause should be practiced in drills.

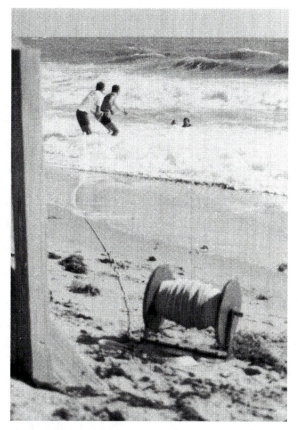

Two lifeguards retrieve a rescuer and victim on the end of a landline.

Credit: William McNeely, Jr.

- After landline rescue the equipment must be carefully recoiled and prepared for immediate use.

- If a second landline rescue is initiated for multiple victims, assisting lifeguards must be certain to know which lifeguard and victim they are supporting to avoid confusion upon retrieval.

Chapter Summary

In this chapter, we have learned about some of the specialized rescue equipment used by lifeguards. We have learned about lifeguard emergency vehicles, which can move lifeguards and equipment rapidly over land, but which require careful operation. We have learned about rescue boats of a wide variety, which can enhance lifeguard surveillance, patrol, and response to aquatic emergencies. We have learned about the value of aircraft, particularly helicopters. We have learned about boat tows. And we have learned about landlines.

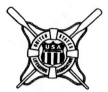

Discussion Points

- What are some potential advantages of lifeguard emergency vehicles?
- What sort of equipment could be carried in a lifeguard emergency vehicle?
- What are some considerations while involved in an emergency response using a lifeguard emergency vehicle?
- What are some ways to avoid injury to beach patrons while using emergency vehicles?
- What are some advantages and limitations of rescue boats?
- What characteristics differentiate a personal watercraft (PWC) from other rescue boats?
- What are some advantages of inflatable rescue boats (IRB)?
- Why must most hard-hull rescue boats stay outside the surfline?
- What are some safety considerations in use of a helicopter?
- Why should a lifeguard using a boat tow be prepared at all times to disconnect from the RFD harness?
- If a landline is used and three lifeguards are available, what is the role of each lifeguard?

Chapter 15
Special Rescues and Defenses

In this chapter you will learn about special types of rescue situations, including defenses from panicked victims. The majority of rescues are routine, requiring basic rescue skills covered earlier in this manual. Yet not all rescues are of a routine nature. Here we will learn about rescues in rip currents, multiple victim rescues, rescues without equipment, rescues of panicked victims who grab the lifeguard, surfer rescues, diver rescues, rescues of persons attempting suicide, rescues in fog or darkness, rock and jetty rescues, pier rescues, boat rescues, rescues involving automobiles in the water, rescues of aircraft crash victims, rescues of shark bite victims, flood rescues, ice rescues, and cliff rescues. With the exception of rip current rescues at surf beaches, special rescues are less frequent than other rescues and often much more challenging. Thorough training and preparation are essential to ensuring that special rescues are successful.

CHAPTER EXCERPT

Effective use of lifesaving equipment increases the efficiency of rescue, while providing additional safety for the lifeguard. All lifeguards should be provided with the necessary equipment to effect rescues.

Regardless of the complexity of a rescue, the three points of a rescue are always followed. As a reminder, these are:

1. Recognize and Respond
2. Contact and Control
3. Signal and Save

Rip Current Rescue

The United States Lifesaving Association estimates that rip currents are the primary source of distress in over 80% of swimmer rescues at surf beaches. Rip currents can pull people into deep water very quickly, creating an immediate hazard to those with moderate or poor swimming ability. Non-swimmers will rapidly submerge after being swept into deep water by a rip current. Even strong swimmers can tire and panic in a very short period of time as they swim against a rip current.

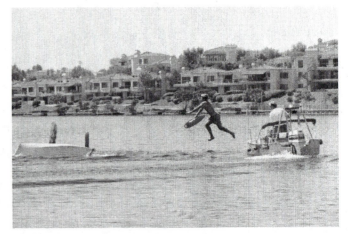

A lifeguard leaps to rescue a submerging swimmer beside a capsized boat.
Credit: Leon Skov

Regardless of the equipment used for rip current rescues, two basic techniques can be employed to the lifeguard's advantage in these situations:

- *Use the Rip Current to Expedite Approach*—The rip current pulls victims away from shore; but most victims fight the current in an effort to swim directly to shore. A lifeguard who enters the current and swims with it can usually more rapidly approach the victim.

- *Avoid the Rip Current to Expedite Retrieval*—Once contact and control are accomplished, the lifeguard should normally plan the retrieval outside the rip current. This may not always be necessary, but there is little point in fighting a strong rip current when it can be easily avoided. To do so, the lifeguard swims parallel to shore until well away from the current, then swims directly to shore. Another option is to swim diagonally toward shore, but since some rip currents pull diagonally away from shore, care must be taken to avoid swimming directly into the force of the current.

Rip currents usually dig a channel in a sandy bottom, leaving water depth in the rip current deeper than that to either side. Therefore, simply moving to the side of the current channel will often help to more quickly locate shallow water. This lessens the distance the lifeguard must swim with the victim. In strong or lengthy rip currents, swim fins are essential and the skill required to quickly don swim fins is critical. In cases of multiple victims or rip currents pulling far offshore, it may be best to swim victims with the current to an offshore rescue boat, if available. In such cases, the power of the rip current can be used both in the approach and in retrieval to the offshore location.

Multiple Victim Rescue

Lifeguards are sometimes faced with two or more victims in a distress or panic presentation. These multiple victim rescues (also known as mass rescues) present unique challenges.

Multiple victim rescues commonly occur when:

- A panicked person grabs on to another for support, but the other person is incapable of providing support or rescue.
- A current suddenly sweeps several people into deep water.

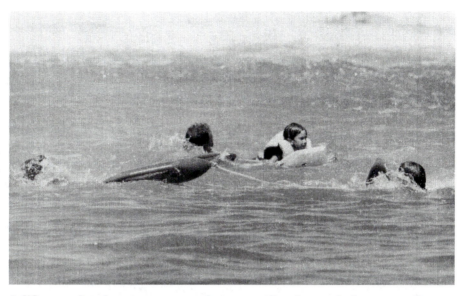

A lifeguard using two rescue buoys pulls three victims to safety.
Credit: Mike Hensler

- A boat capsizes or sinks forcing victims into the water.
- An unexpected wave washes several unwary bystanders into the water.
- A would-be rescuer becomes a victim in a failed attempt at rescue.

The two keys to successful rescue of multiple victims are *flotation* and *backup*. Adequate flotation is essential to allow lifeguards to gain control of a rescue. Panic is usually greatly diminished once victims have something to hold which keeps their heads above the water. This also diminishes the immediacy of the need for assistance. The victims may still be caught in a current and being pulled away from shore, causing significant alarm, but the immediate fear of submersion is eliminated.

If available, a lifeguard selecting equipment for what appears to be a mass rescue should take more than one RFD. At beaches where multiple victim rescues occur with regularity, large rescue buoys should be standard equipment, since they can provide flotation to more victims. A rescue board can be extremely valuable for a multiple victim rescue. Although it can be difficult to rescue several persons using a rescue board in a surf environment, the speed and superior flotation provided by the rescue board can be extremely valuable until backup lifeguards arrive. Lifeguards using a rescue board should also tow an RFD in the event the rescue board is lost, ensuring that the victim(s) will still have a means of flotation. The rescue board is particularly valuable at a calm water beach where the lifeguard can quickly access the victims, then slowly move toward shore with all of them holding on. In any case, providing adequate flotation greatly reduces fear of drowning.

Backup is critical on mass rescues. Information provided in the initial alert by the lifeguard who first spots the emergency unfolding is very important. If this lifeguard advises of the need for backup, it can be dispatched expeditiously, simultaneous to the first lifeguard entering the water. If no backup is immediately available and the lifeguard is unable to adequately control the situation, others nearby with flotation devices can be solicited for help. Several victims can hold onto a surfboard or bodyboard, for example, until additional lifeguards arrive to bring them ashore. Caution should be exercised though, when requesting help from untrained citizens. Lifeguards should closely monitor the situation taking control of the most critical victims.

A rescue boat is an excellent tool for a mass rescue. If it is large enough, the victims can be brought aboard. If not, the boat can simply be used as a raft for flotation until the victims can be ferried ashore by swimming lifeguards.

As a general rule, a lifeguard should not swim past one victim to reach another. If the lifeguard is approaching a victim and sees another further out, the lifeguard may chose to tow the first victim to the second or leave the RFD with the first victim and swim to the second without equipment, physically supporting that victim until backup arrives. Similarly, when using a rescue board, the lifeguard

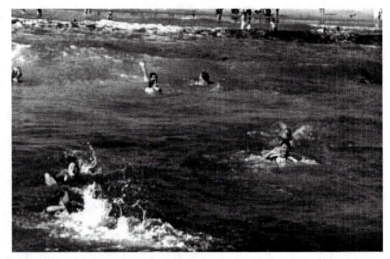

Multiple victim rescue.
Credit: Huntington State Beach

may leave the RFD with the first victim, then paddle to the second with the benefit of being able to provide flotation. In cases where several victims are some distance apart, the lifeguard should try to select the person in the most immediate distress and assist that victim first, then move to the next most distressed person, and so forth. Swim fins are particularly valuable when a lifeguard must support a victim without an RFD.

Rescues Without Equipment

Effective use of lifesaving equipment increases the efficiency of rescue, while providing additional safety for the lifeguard. All lifeguards should be provided with the necessary equipment to effect rescues. Nevertheless, lifeguards must be prepared to effect rescues without equipment if none is unavailable. This may occur in a multiple victim rescue if the RFD must be given up to support one victim, while another is aided elsewhere. Another possibility is that rescue equipment may be lost or damaged on a rescue. While off-duty, the lifeguard may be at an unguarded beach when a drowning presentation is recognized. These are just a few examples.

- *Alert*—Particularly in the case of an off-duty rescue attempt, it is critical to ensure that someone, somewhere knows that a rescuer is in the water on a rescue. Call for help. Draw someone's attention. Direct bystanders to call 9-1-1.

- *Equipment Selection*—Look around. Can something nearby be adapted to use as rescue equipment? Are there ring buoys mounted nearby? Does anything nearby float that can be pushed out to the victim? Are others using flotation devices that can be used? Can some object be extended to the victim to prevent direct contact with a person in panic? A shirt? Rope? How about a surfboard? Many items may be used to improvise rescue equipment.

- *Approach and Contact*—Sometimes victims in distress can make it to shore with encouragement. If so, avoid contact, calm them, and try to talk them in. A rescuer forced to approach a victim without equipment should approach from the rear. This can be difficult or impossible because the victim's tendency is to turn to watch the rescuer, if able. Swim wide and circle around the victim or surface dive in front of the victim and swim under and past the victim to surface behind. If this is not the best option, approach the victim from behind and move swiftly to control the situation. If the victim is clothed, try grabbing their collar and tow using sidestroke. If this is not feasible, one of the following three tows may be effective:

- *Cross-Chest Tow*—Throw one arm over the victim's shoulder and across the chest until your hand is in contact with the victim's side just below the victim's armpit. Immediately secure the victim between the arm and hip (right arm to right hip or left to left). The victim's shoulder should be secured in the rescuer's armpit. Concentrate on keeping the victim's face out of water. While this control method supports the victim and maintains an airway, it may not place the victim in a position that produces a feeling of security, with the face and head out of the water. Struggling may continue as the victim attempts to lean forward out of the water.

- *Modified Cross-Chest Tow*—Quickly place an arm under the victim's arms and across the lower chest (or upper abdomen) of the victim to secure the victim between the arm and hip (right arm to right hip or left to left). The victim's buttocks should be supported on the rescuer's hip. This position usually provides the support that allows the victim to sit forward and remove the head from the water. Panic usually subsides more quickly; but this position may result in the lifeguard remaining nearly or fully submerged, due to the added weight being supported out of the water. This position should be used when there is a short retrieval distance to standing depth, since the lifeguard will not be able to maintain this tow for long.

- *Armpit Tow*—The rescuer takes a position on the back facing the victim's back. The hands grasp the victim under the armpits with the thumbs up and the arms slightly bent at the elbow. The rescuer kicks in using a breaststroke kick. An alternative is to grasp with only one hand, moving to shore with a kick and single stroke. The major advantage of this retrieval method is that the victim is kept high in the water. The major disadvantage is very limited control. It is not appropriate for a surf retrieval.

- *Stabilize*—Attempt to reduce the victim's panic while providing support by using a breaststroke or sidestroke kick. Additional support and momentum can be gained by sculling or pulling the water with the free arm. If the victim struggles, the free arm can be moved to lock onto the supporting arm, pulling the victim more tightly to the supporting hip. If this is unsuccessful, move the free arm to the victim's back and quickly push the victim away. Swim away, reconsider the approach and try again to gain control.

- *Retrieve*—Once control is gained, turn and make progress toward shore a stroke appropriate to the type of tow.

- *Assess*—Treat or resuscitate the victim if necessary. Monitor breathing for signs of complications. Be prepared to assist responding personnel in completing necessary reports.

Defenses

A lifeguard responds to several people in distress who have been suddenly swept into deep water by a current. The lifeguard enters the water and approaches the group, studying people to determine those most in need of assistance. Pulling the RFD in to approach a victim, the lifeguard feels a hand on the back, quickly followed by a vise-like grip around the head, applied by a panicked swimmer who couldn't wait for assistance. For the moment, the rescuer has become a victim.

Lifeguards must be constantly aware of the dangers presented by people experiencing panic in deep water. Distressed swimmers often move toward responding lifeguards and may desperately grab the lifeguard for support. In unusual situations, some victims may even choose the support of the lifeguard over the support of an extended RFD and will make a quick grab for the lifeguard during approach and control. Preventing these situations is the best strategy.

- Do not turn your back on unsupported or unstable victims.
- Do not move through a group of unsupported or unstable victims.
- Do not place yourself in a position in which a panicked person can jump onto you.

Defensive Techniques

Behavior of panicked victims is quite uniform. The victim sees that the lifeguard is buoyant and tries to climb to safety. The victim will grab at any exposed part of the lifeguard and quickly pull into a hugging position at the highest point of support; usually the head. The lifeguard is submerged, either due to the victim trying to climb to safety or simply the added weight of the grasping victim. People experiencing the panic of a drowning presentation can demonstrate extraordinary strength. Children can incapacitate adults. Anticipation of victim movement and quick, decisive actions can often prevent the establishment of a firm head-hold. The following are some strategies to employ.

- *Go Limp and Submerge—This is the best and most effective defense.* Use it before the others. Since the victim grabs the lifeguard in an attempt to climb up for air, if the lifeguard no longer provides buoyancy, the victim will almost always immediately release. Swim away from the victim underwater and reconsider the best approach.
- *Turn Toward the Attack*—Bring the lead arm up in a sweeping, blocking movement.
- *Assume a Tuck Position*—Drop the head lower to the shoulders, draw the knee or knees up and present feet and arms toward the attack. Present as small a target as possible toward the victim. Lean back, away from the attack.
- *Block and Push*—If the victim is close enough, the lifeguard should not hesitate to block an attack by placing a foot on the victim's chest, pushing away and swimming in the other direction. The lifeguard should continue to face the attack while swimming to safety.
- *Ditch the RFD*—In some situations, panicking swimmers may use the RFD lanyard to pull themselves toward the lifeguard instead of toward the floating buoy. Disengage from the RFD and swim away.

In a front head-hold, the victim is facing the lifeguard with arms around the lifeguard's head or neck. If submersion does not result in release of the hold, place the hands on the hips of the victim and push away while tucking in the chin. If needed the rescuer once underwater can bring the rescuer's hands up to victim's elbows and push hard up and away from rescuer. Once the release is accomplished, swim back and away from the victim.

In a rear head-hold, the victim is behind the lifeguard with arms around the lifeguard's head or neck. The lifeguard should grab a breath of air and submerge, turn the head and tucking the chin to one side. When ready, the lifeguard drops the shoulder to the side where the head is turned and turns quickly to face the victim. Leverage can then be applied to the hips as previously described to break the hold and escape from the victim. If needed the rescuer once underwater can bring the rescuer's hands up to victim's elbows and push hard up and away from rescuer. Once the release is accomplished, swim away from the victim.

Surfer and Bodyboarder Rescues

Most surfers and bodyboarders have better than average water skills. They also have with them an excellent flotation device. In the surf environment, most use leashes so that they don't lose their board. Do not assume however, that a surfer or bodyboarder will not need rescue just because they have flotation. Not all users of these devices are skilled. Leashes can break and sometimes injuries occur when a fiberglass surfboard or the skeg strikes a person.

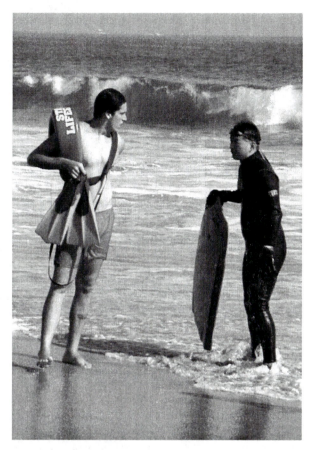

Credit: Ken Kramer

Signs surfer or bodyboarder distress include:

- *Bodyboarders Arm Paddling*—Bodyboards are designed to be propelled by kicking and most users employ swim fins. The use of arm strokes indicates weak ability and possibly distress or panic.

- *Surfers Trying to Kick*—Unlike bodyboards, surfboards are designed to be propelled by paddling, not kicking. A surfer who attempts to use a kick may be showing signs of distress or panic. This usually indicates a novice.

- *Surfboard Positioned Sideways*—A surfer who tries to use a swim kick to move forward may find this very difficult because the surfboard keeps the feet above the water. Some will turn the board sideways, so that their feet are in the water, but their body is out of the water. This is a sign of a novice surfer with very limited ability.

- *Imbalanced Surfboard*—Surfers who are not well balanced on their board with either the nose of the board plowing through the water or the nose elevated well above the surface indicates limited ability.

- *Weak Paddling or Kicking*—Surfers making little progress while paddling and bodyboarders with a weak or flailing kick are likely novice and may be in distress.

- *Falling Off*—Surfers and bodyboarders who continually fall off the board are likely novice.

- *Losing or Abandoning the Board*—Surfers and bodyboarders who lose the board or abandon it may not only be novice, they may be poor swimmers in immediate need of rescue. The use of leashes greatly lessens the possibility of drowning and should therefore be encouraged.

- *Caught by a Rip Current*—Experienced surfers and bodyboarders may use a rip current to quickly make their way offshore, just as a lifeguard might; but most avoid these areas once they reach the surfline. Waves usually don't break well in a rip current due to depth of the rip current channel and conflicting water movement. A surfer or bodyboarder who lingers in a rip current is probably a novice and will quickly tire.

When surfers or bodyboarders need rescue, the three components of a rescue are employed. In many cases, the board can be used to help stabilize and control the victim prior to retrieval. Caution should be used however, in entering the surfline with a victim who has a surfboard. The board can cause serious injury or be lost to the waves, injuring swimmers toward shore. One alternative is to allow the board to be pushed to shore by the waves in an area where swimmers will not be endangered, then to swim the victim in with an RFD. Another is to use a rescue boat.

Occasionally surfers and bodyboarders become trapped outside the surfline at rocky beaches. This occurs because the victim is able to paddle out through the surf away from shore, but is fearful of being injured on the rocks upon return to shore. The responding lifeguard may also conclude that a safe retrieval is unlikely, particularly in large surf. In these cases, it is usually best to summon a rescue boat or helicopter for assistance outside the surfline.

While rare, surfers using leashes can become entangled in pier pilings, or fish, crab, or lobster trap lines. This has caused drowning deaths in several cases. These situations are extremely hazardous, especially in large surf conditions, making the job of responding lifeguards difficult. Agencies with these conditions should train for them and keep equipment on hand to help expeditiously resolve the situation. A blunt tipped knife or even trauma shears are effective tools for cutting surfboard leashes and buoy lines. Preventive actions, when possible, are recommended. The California Fish and Game Code (section 9002) was amended at the request of surf lifeguards to allow them to lawfully remove a trap, buoy, or line located in or near breaking surf or adjacent to a public beach if they believe that the trap poses a public safety hazard.

In rescues of wave riders, spinal injury should be considered a possibility. Sometimes the victim will go over the falls—that is, be caught by the breaking wave and dumped in its force. If the victim strikes bottom or is torqued in heavy surf, spinal injury can result.

Diver Rescue

In many beach areas, people skin dive (diving with mask, fins, and snorkel) and scuba dive (using compressed air tanks). Lifeguards are encouraged to become scuba certified. This training provides insight into the sport and helps greatly in understanding scuba rescue techniques, as well as the pathophysiology of diving injuries. For a full discussion of diving injuries, refer to the chapter entitled, *Scuba Related Illness and Treatment*.

Skin diver rescues are no different than those of swimmers, with exception of the fact that a typical source of panic is having the mask fill with water. Often, simply removing the mask resolves the problem. Since skin divers do not breathe compressed air, they are not susceptible to related problems. Rescues of scuba divers are more involved.

All scuba divers should be trained and certified prior to diving on their own. Several national organizations certify instructors, who certify scuba divers. Reputable dive shops will not provide compressed air refills to persons without a training certification card. In addition to a mask, snorkel, swim fins, and often a wetsuit, scuba divers use a tank of compressed air (not pure oxygen) and a regulator.

The regulator reduces the pressure of compressed air in the tank to a lesser pressure which can be breathed without damaging the lungs.

Scuba divers also use weights and a *buoyancy compensator* (BC). Weights counteract the natural surface buoyancy of a fully equipped diver so that the diver can submerge more easily. They may be carried around the waist on a weight belt, or by some another means. Since scuba divers become progressively less buoyant as they descend, the buoyancy compensator, which is most often an inflatable vest, is gradually inflated by the diver using compressed air from the tank. Divers attempt to maintain neutral buoyancy or to be slightly positively or negatively buoyant to aid in ascending or descending. This requires adjustment of the amount of air in the buoyancy compensator when moving from one depth to another. The recognized depth limit for recreational diving using compressed air is 130 feet. Recreational divers should not descend below this depth.

Divers can experience distress for all of the reasons that swimmers experience distress, but the vast majority of diver deaths are directly attributable to diver error. Equipment failure is rare. The most prevalent factors contributing to diver deaths are insufficient air, entrapment, and rapid ascent. Insufficient air and rapid ascent are closely related in that running low or out of air typically causes the diver to ascend rapidly. Other contributing causes include panic and alcohol or drug use. Physical conditioning is a significant factor in diver deaths and cardiovascular disease is a particular contributing factor.

Running out of air is demonstrative of very poor judgment and is a factor completely under the control of the diver (except in the rare case of equipment malfunction). Divers are strongly encouraged to use the buddy system, diving in pairs, so that if one diver has trouble the other can assist. About 50% of diving fatalities are sustained by solo divers and divers who have become separated from their buddy. For this reason, a lone diver may be viewed as a high risk taker. When two divers embark from shore and one surfaces alone, lifeguards should be very concerned. This means the buddy is now diving alone and may be in distress.

Divers may be entrapped due to entanglement in weeds (particularly kelp) or fishing line or inside a confined space, such as a submerged wreck or cave. Divers are encouraged to carry knives to cut themselves free of entanglement. Divers over 40 and those who are obese should maintain strong physical

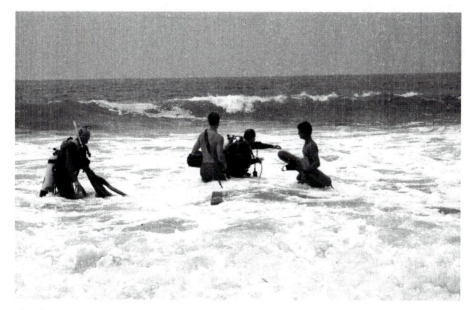

Credit: Ken Kramer

conditioning for scuba diving. Diving gear is heavy on the surface and use of it can strain the cardio-vascular system. An obese diver should be viewed as a high risk candidate for rescue.

Lifeguards with experience in diver rescue know that preventive lifeguarding involves first sizing up divers before they enter the water. In conversation, lifeguards can learn whether the diver is certified and the level of experience. They can be sure the weight belts are fastened with quick release buckles and note the location of the buckle. They can look for ill-fitting equipment, which may indicate that it is borrowed and the diver is novice. If divers are drinking alcohol before a dive, they should be cautioned not to dive. Good judgment is critical while diving and alcohol impairs judgment. It is a good practice to warn divers of any unusually rough or hazardous conditions. Responsible divers will simply avoid diving on a day that conditions are poor.

Divers use hand and arm signals to indicate when they are doing all right. The most commonly used is the OK hand signal, made by forming a circle with the thumb and forefinger. Another is the overhead OK signal, which is similar to the USLA approved arm signal for lifeguards. The diver touches one hand to the top of the head, forming a circle with the arm. Divers also use hand and arm signals to indicate distress. A wave is a sign of diver distress; but it is not the only evidence of diver distress.

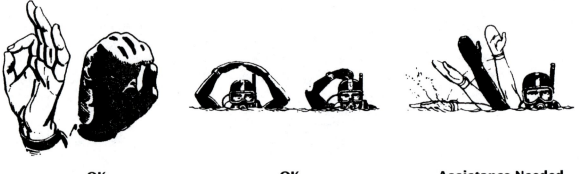

OK   **OK**   **Assistance Needed**

Signs of distress of a diver may include:

- Waving toward shore
- Blowing a whistle
- Surfacing alone with no sign of the buddy
- Surfacing and remaining motionless
- Breaking the surface very suddenly or even explosively
- Hurriedly ripping off a mask or other equipment
- Swimming toward shore, but making no progress

Diver rescues follow the three components of all rescues: recognize and respond; contact and control; signal and save. The initial alert to other rescuers prior to entering the water is particularly important in the case of scuba divers. In these rescues there is a heightened potential for physiological complications contributing to the distress and diver rescues are generally more difficult than those of free swimming persons.

When approaching a diver in apparent distress, the lifeguard should ask about the nature of the problem if it is not obvious. Divers have their own source of buoyancy, though they may become panicked and unable to use it. Other sources of distress are a physiological problem related to diving, a current, or separation from the buddy. The presence of the lifeguard usually significantly reduces fear.

Caution should be used in the approach. Divers often have spears or spearguns with them, which can be lethal. If the diver has a spear or speargun, it should be handled very carefully and always kept pointed away. If necessary to safely complete the rescue, it should be jettisoned.

If the diver is having a buoyancy problem, there are two immediate options. The simplest is to pull the quick release buckle on the weight belt, jettisoning it. This of course results in loss of equipment and should be avoided unless clearly necessary for rescue. The other option is to inflate the buoyancy compensator. The RFD may provide sufficient buoyancy, but if a diver is negatively weighted, inflating the BC or releasing the weight belt is sometimes necessary and can significantly increase comfort of the diver. The buoyancy compensator is usually inflated via breathing into a mouthpiece or by triggering an automatic inflator valve attached to the BC. Some BCs have a CO_2 cartridge which can be triggered to immediately, fully inflate the BC. These techniques should be practiced by lifeguards working in areas frequented by divers.

Once buoyancy has been stabilized, any obstruction should be removed from the diver's face and an airway ensured. A relaxed diver may prefer to leave the mask on and even continue breathing from the tank. For a panicked diver, it may be necessary to remove the mask and snorkel or regulator from the mouth.

If a diver advises that a dive buddy is missing, the diver should be asked if this is normal or if the diver is concerned. Some divers routinely split up upon diving and separation in and of itself is not unusual for them.

A swimming lifeguard with buoy and fins is ill-equipped to perform an underwater search for a missing diver who may be in very deep water or some distance away. Usually such searches require trained dive teams. Nonetheless, the first responding lifeguard can make a few quick surface dives to perform a cursory search and look for bubbles on the surface.

If a diver is observed beneath the surface who is tangled in something, a surface dive should be performed in an attempt to assist. A knife in the possession of either the diver or lifeguard can be very helpful in such cases. If an apparently lifeless diver is observed beneath the surface, the lifeguard should dive down, release the victim's weight belt, and swim to the surface with the victim. The BC should not be inflated unless this is necessary to bring the diver to the surface, since rapid inflation of the BC of a submerged diver can cause the diver to rocket to the surface. Upon reaching the surface, the lifeguard should signal for assistance and begin rescue breathing.

Retrieval of a conscious, distressed diver is essentially the same as for any victim, but complicated by the heavy equipment and relative lack of mobility of the diver. Surf rescues of divers can be hazardous because the tank and regulator can strike the lifeguard, causing serious injury including loss of consciousness. Appropriate caution should be utilized and, if necessary, the equipment can be removed.

Rescued divers should be carefully evaluated for physiological complications related to breathing compressed air. Sometimes these problems are instantaneous, other times they become evident after the dive. Such complications can be immediately life-threatening and should be taken very seriously. Often lifeguards learn of such problems when an afflicted diver walks up to the lifeguard for medical advice. For information on recognition and treatment of diving illness, see the chapter entitled, *Scuba Related Illness and Treatment.*

Lifeguards in rescue boats should be made aware of divers submerged in the patrol area so that they can be avoided. Divers sometimes use a flotation device to mark their location and to warn boaters. The most common is an inner tube with a diver flag. The flag is either red with a diagonal white stripe or the alpha flag, which is a white and blue flag with blue dovetails.

Fugitive Retrieval

Lifeguards at some agencies have police powers, at others they do not. Regardless, occasionally suspects of crimes attempt to elude arrest by escaping into the water and lifeguards are called upon to retrieve them. Often suspects in such cases are actually very poor swimmers and simply desperate to get away. In these cases, superior water skills usually place lifeguards at a distinct advantage. There are several important considerations in these cases:

- *Maintain Personal Safety*—The primary concern of the lifeguard in these cases should be personal safety. Avoid any confrontation likely to result in injury.
- *Take Your Time*—While police officers often become very concerned in these cases and desirous of immediate action, rapid intervention is not called for unless the suspect is in imminent danger of drowning. Many times, it is best to simply watch the fugitive from nearby and wait. In fact, the more time passes, the more fatigued the suspect becomes, reducing the likelihood of effective resistance. Eventually, the fugitive may actually request assistance. Be prepared though, for immediate rescue as necessary.
- *Wait for Police Backup*—Usually, a suspect has been chased into the water by police and they are nearby. If qualified law enforcement personnel are not at the scene, summon them and wait for their arrival. The situation is better managed by leaving the suspect in the water than by bringing the suspect to shore without someone to take control of them.
- *Is a Weapon Involved?*—Lifeguards should determine if a weapon is involved before any approach. A handgun may be usable even after being submerged and a knife is a hazard regardless.

If it is decided to approach the victim, it is highly recommended to use at least two lifeguards, as one may be able to approach from the fugitive's rear. Upon approach, lifeguards should first try to talk the fugitive into surrender. A reminder to the fugitive that there is no escape may be successful. Often, the simple fact that people are approaching in the water causes the suspect to give up, realizing the hopelessness of the situation. Lifeguards should always try to avoid direct contact with victims. This is particularly true for fugitives.

If this is unsuccessful, lifeguards should work to a position that requires the fugitive to turn away from one lifeguard. The lifeguard who is able to work behind the fugitive, then immediately throws an arm over the shoulder and across the chest. The wrist of that arm is grabbed by the other hand for additional control.

If the fugitive is a poor swimmer, the control of the lifeguard is likely to cause a cessation of resistance. If not, the lifeguard should try to kick in toward shore while maintaining a grasp of the fugitive. If control is lost, kick away. As in the case of a panicked victim, the best escape if the fugitive grabs the lifeguard is to submerge and wait until the fugitive releases to surface for air.

Suicide Attempts

It is not uncommon for people to try to take their own lives in or near the water environment. People may jump from piers, cliffs, or bridges. They may swim directly out into large water bodies. They may even attach themselves to weights. While many of these suicide attempts will occur at more remote areas or at times when lifeguards are not present, lifeguards may be called to respond.

The most difficult aspect of a suicide presentation is the fact that those attempting suicide presumably don't want to be rescued. They may swim away from approaching lifeguards and refuse to grasp extended RFDs. In these situations, it may be necessary to take physical control using techniques described for fugitive retrieval. Another option is stay nearby, but to wait for the person to tire. This will ultimately help to reduce resistance. Stay near enough however, so that if the person intentionally submerges, immediate retrieval from below the surface is possible.

It is recommended that two or more lifeguards participate in approaching a person attempting suicide, as responders can expect resistance from initial contact through and perhaps beyond removal from the water. Response to a suspected suicide attempt should automatically trigger a call for police assistance, since a weapon may be involved and police will eventually be needed to transport the person to a treatment facility.

Responses to suicide attempts involving jumpers attached to weights can be particularly difficult for lifeguards as these presentations are often very sudden and involve immediate submersion presentations. Search procedures should be initiated upon arrival at the scene and may require tools necessary to free victims from attached weights.

A consideration in suicide attempts is that they may occur in response to having contracted a life-threatening communicable disease which appears incurable. Lifeguards should use universal precaution appropriate for such cases if communicable disease seems to be a contributing factor. For more information on universal precaution, see the chapter entitled, *Lifeguard Health and Safety*.

Fog and Night Rescue

Fog and darkness have a similar effect of drastically reducing visibility. They also reduce beach activity, so the volume of rescues declines as well. Nonetheless, rescues that do occur in these conditions are typically more difficult for a variety of reasons. Lifeguards need to be prepared for rescues in fog and darkness.

People sometimes travel to the beach from areas where no fog is present, only to find the beach shrouded in fog. Fog may also appear quickly and unexpectedly. In either case, lifeguards may be placed in a position where protection of swimmers must continue when the primary means of victim recognition—visual scanning—is greatly diminished or eliminated.

Some lifeguard agencies simply elect to close the beach to swimming as a safety precaution in fog conditions or at night. In other areas, foggy conditions will activate special fog patrol procedures. When approaching fog is noticed, warnings should be issued to beach visitors. Public address systems can be used to make these warnings and announcements or other audible signals can be made at regular intervals once fog covers the beach, to provide a directional beacon for people still in deep water.

Since visual observation is no longer effective, fog patrols should be commenced to place lifeguards closer to the water's edge in vehicles or on foot. While on patrol, lifeguards should be constantly alert for cries of help or the sound of boat engines from boats mistakenly operated close to shore. Fog patrols are best made in teams of two lifeguards. If a rescue is indicated, one lifeguard can enter the water as the other lifeguard remains ashore to call for backup assistance and to sound an audible device (such as a vehicle horn or siren) at regular intervals. This device serves to help the responding lifeguard determine the direction of shore and helps backup find the location of the response. In surf conditions, shore direction can generally be determined by swell direction and the sound of crashing waves, but lateral position along the beach is more difficult to ascertain.

Lifeguards who become lost in the water in foggy conditions or in the dark should stop and listen for waves, voices, lifeguard fog alarms, vehicle traffic, or other noises that may indicate the direction of shore. In most coastal areas, when wind is present during fog, it is likely to be blowing toward land. Calling for help can also be effective. The lifeguard who starts swimming toward shore should stop frequently to recheck the current position using the clues previously mentioned. Underwater flashlights or waterproof strobes can be attached to RFDs for better identification of lifeguards in the water.

Fog can be particularly dangerous for boats suddenly caught in a fog bank without electronic positioning equipment. Lifeguards should be prepared for this possibility and continue regular patrols in an effort to locate wrecked vessels.

Rock and Jetty Rescue

When compared to smooth, sandy beaches, rescues from rocky shores can be quite difficult and dangerous for lifeguards, especially in surf conditions where incoming waves can throw a lifeguard into the rocks. Rocks often have shellfish attached to them, such as barnacles and mussels. These can cause serious lacerations. Urchins may be present in tidepools. Rocks can be very slippery, particularly when seaweed is attached, and it is easy to fall during response and retrieval.

While rescue procedures at rocky areas involve the three basic components of all rescues (recognize and respond, contact and control, signal and save), special considerations are in order.

The following is a partial list:

- *Protect Your Feet*—Water entry over rocky areas can sometimes be made easier by donning swim fins for foot protection prior to entering the water. Another option is amphibious footwear. The benefits of foot protection should be carefully weighed against maneuverability.

- *Wear a Wetsuit*—Use of a wetsuit can greatly diminish the potential for injury from striking or being abraded by rocks.

- *Use Care During Entry Dives*—Shallow diving entries can be made from ledges, docks, and outcroppings, but should be made with great care to avoid head injury. Keep hands extended above the head and plan the shallowest dive possible. In surf conditions, dives should normally timed for entry into the high point of a wave rather than the trough between waves. Wait for the upsurge of the arriving wave and jump into it.

- *Swim Away Quickly*—Begin swimming as soon as possible upon entry into the water, even in knee to waist-deep water. Continue to keep the hands in front to feel for and fend off rocks.

- *Beware of Underwater Obstructions*—Avoid ducking under incoming waves unless water depth is known.

- *Expect Unexpected Waves*—At rocky beaches with surf, the surf can break suddenly and unex-

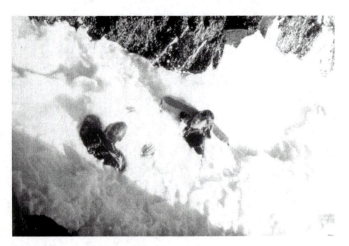

Rescue among rocks.
Credit: Laguna Beach Lifeguards

pectedly due to underwater rocks that lessen depth. Unlike a more even sand bottom, rocks can cause very unpredictable surf breaks.

- *Retrieve to a Safe Area*—Once the victim has been approached and controlled, retrieval should be made away from rocky shores if at all possible, especially in surf conditions. This is an excellent indication for rescue boat backup. Another option is a long retrieval swim to the relative safety of a neighboring sandy beach. The time and effort involved may greatly reduce the potential for injury.

- *Protect Yourself*—A primary rule for lifeguards involved in rescues near rocks is to protect themselves first. The lifeguard will be of no assistance if injured and a serious injury to the lifeguard will greatly delay assistance to the victim.

- *Protect the Victim*—If it is absolutely necessary to make a retrieval to a rocky shore in surf conditions, stay close to the victim rather than towing the victim behind on the RFD. If using a rescue buoy, position it in front of the victim, reach under the arms of the victim (from the victim's back) to grasp the handles, and use the RFD to fend off rocks during retrieval as needed.

- *Know the Area*—The greatest aid to lifeguard response at rocky areas is experience and knowledge of the area. Those who work at a beach with rock areas should get to know those areas well by studying them regularly in all weather and tide conditions. Underwater rock formations should be of particular interest.

Pier Rescue

At many surf beaches across the United States, piers on reinforced pilings extend out past the surfline. Unlike piers at flat water beaches, surf piers are usually constructed at a considerable height over the water to protect the pier deck and any structures upon it from the highest anticipated surf. Most of the time, they are therefore well above the sea surface. Piers provide fishing opportunities, scenic promenades, and special activity or amusement areas for beach visitors.

Surf piers can pose challenges for lifeguards. Pier pilings can create or magnify rip currents. They are unyielding to those pushed into them. Pier pilings are a collection point for fishing lines and plant life, presenting the possibility of entanglement to surfers and swimmers. People sometimes fall or jump from piers. Piers can even become attractive if not dangerous challenges for imprudent surfers, boardsailors, and boaters who may try to operate around the pilings.

To save time on a rescue response near a pier, lifeguards may choose to jump from the pier rather than approaching from the water. Special training and regular practice is required for this entry method. To safely accomplish a pier entry, the lifeguard must know the water depths at every point around the pier. These water depths can be influenced by tides, surf, and sand movement. There may also be flotsam in the water that can cause serious injury. Normally, the best option is to enter outside the surf break. The water will be deepest if the lifeguard times the jump to enter the water on an incoming swell.

Entries from piers should be made feet first. The proper entry method is to hold the RFD in one hand and swim fins in the other. Jump well clear of the pier, preferably on the side that is shoreward of incoming waves. The RFD is raised over the head vertically with one hand and the swim fins with the other. The legs are crossed to protect the groin. Eyes are focused on the horizon to avoid eye injury upon water contact. As the feet hit the water, the lifeguard should let go of the rescue buoy. This helps to avoid shoulder injury as the buoyancy of the RFD might otherwise pull on the arm during submersion. Swim fins that float are of great value in pier entries.

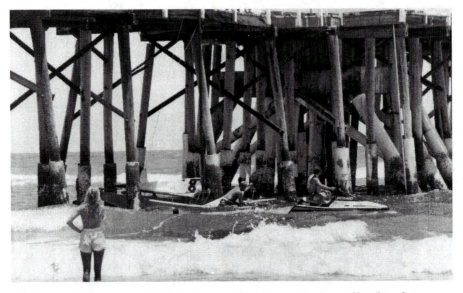

A lifeguard on a personal watercraft attempts to pull a hapless boater out of pier pilings.

Credit: Mike Hensler

Lifeguards should pay particular attention to prevent having the RFD lanyard become wrapped around a pier piling. This is especially important in large surf conditions. Injury can result when the force of a wave pushes a trailing RFD around a piling. If the RFD becomes tethered to the piling the force of the wave can shock load the line, injuring the lifeguard. To avoid this situation, the RFD should be held in front of the lifeguard when maneuvering through pilings with any excess line in hand.

Panicked victims are sometimes inclined to grasp pier pilings and to try to climb them. Shellfish on the pilings can cause painful wounds, as can water movement, which grates the victim's skin against the rough surface of the piling. Still, it is sometimes difficult to convince victims to release the piling in favor of the support of the RFD. In some situations, it will be necessary to forcibly remove the victim from the piling. Once this has been accomplished, the lifeguard should move the victim a safe distance away from the pier as rapidly as possible, and then to shore or a rescue boat. In the event of entanglement, a knife may be required to free the victim. Careful maneuvering when near pier pilings is crucial, with the RFD placed in a position to be used as a fender. The lifeguard must take care at all time to protect from incoming waves that may drive both lifeguard and victim into the pilings.

Boat Rescue

Distressed boats can present lifeguards with several rescue situations, ranging from stalled craft needing assistance to serious boat collisions. Sailcraft, including boardsailors, can also get into serious trouble, often due to inexperienced operators. How a lifeguard agency responds to boat rescues may depend on the equipment available to lifeguard staff.

In larger agencies, lifeguard rescue vessels can be used for a wide range of boat rescues, including towing and firefighting. At smaller agencies, lifeguards may have to respond to serious boat accidents as first responders, relying on other agencies or individuals to provide the equipment necessary for the

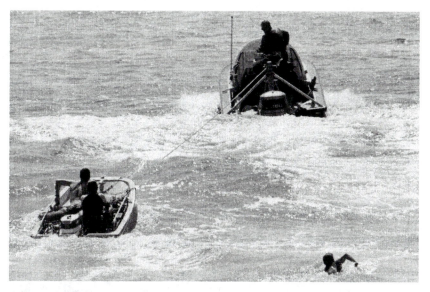

A lifeguard pulls a swamped vessel out of the surfline as his crewmember, who swam the tow line in, lies prone in the bow of the swamped vessel beside the owner.

Credit: Annette Kennedy

safe recovery of boats and their passengers. Whatever the response policies of a lifeguard agency, there are several points for lifeguards to consider in making boat rescues:

- *Recognition*—Distress clues for boaters can be obvious or subtle. A collision, capsizing, fire, or explosion indicate a need for immediate assistance. Other presentations may be less clear. Boardsailors who appear to be in control of a craft may actually be stranded offshore, unable to return against the wind. Small capsized sailcraft may be in distress, or involved in training exercises. The following are some specific indications of possible distress:
  - People working on a boat engine
  - People on board waving anxiously toward shore
  - A boat positioned broadside to the wind or waves
  - Boats with no one on board or on deck
  - Boats continually circling
  - Sailcraft continually *in irons* or with the sail ruffling but catching no wind
  - Repeated falling from a sailboard, especially when no progress is made toward shore
  - Any boat approaching a surfline or swim area with obvious lack of control
- *Alert*—In determining if a response is necessary, lifeguards should remember the established area of responsibility. Boat problems outside of it should be immediately reported to the proper agencies for their response, but if lifeguards can provide immediate lifesaving assistance, agency policy usually calls for a lifeguard response

regardless. If a lifeguard response is appropriate, the alert should contain enough information to inform backup staff of the situation and required equipment.

- *Equipment Selection*—Rescue boats, rescue buoys, and swim fins are good equipment choices for response to boat rescues. If a swimming approach will be used, a boat tow should be fastened to the rescue buoy. If there is any indication of spilled fuel in the water, face masks should be taken for eye protection.

- *Approach*—Great care should be taken in approaching any craft still under power. When approaching a boat drifting toward the surf, avoid an approach from the shoreward side of the vessel. A disabled vessel may overturn at any moment, pushed by the wind and waves. Instead, approach from the seaward side. During approach, if there are people in the water, identify those most in need of assistance and aid them first. Ensure, through conversation with the skipper and passengers, that all passengers are accounted for. If you will need to board the boat, explain to the skipper your intentions. If lifeguards will be in the water around the boat, advise the skipper to turn the engine off and keep it off. For sailing vessels, direct the crew to drop the sails. Carefully evaluate the potential for fire. For example, a slick may indicate leaking fuel. If the boat is in a safe condition and a safe position, encourage people to stay with the boat for support and direct them to don PFDs while awaiting backup assistance.

- *Signal*—Once initial control has been gained and the situation is assessed, signal ashore to indicate if backup response is necessary. In serious boat accidents, lifeguards should continue to stabilize victims while awaiting backup assistance. In flat water conditions or well offshore from breaking surf, anchors may be dropped. When backup assistance arrives, injured passengers can be immobilized if necessary and extricated to stable vessels for retrieval.

- *Flat Water Retrieval*—In the case of minor problems involving disabled boats or inexperienced operators, the lifeguard can offer to retrieve the boat and passengers. Small, capsized sailboats can often be righted. Swamped or capsized small craft can usually be towed ashore with passengers aboard or holding on. Boardsailors can drop their sail across the board and be towed ashore while riding the board. To assist by towing, uncoil the boat tow and have the boat operators attach it to the bow of the craft to be towed. The lifeguard can then swim, paddle, or row while towing the rescued vessel and passengers.

- *Surf Retrieval*—Disabled vessels approaching the surf present a dangerous situation for passengers, lifeguards, and beach visitors. Should the vessel enter the surfline and be catapulted through it, serious injury and damage can occur. To prevent this, lifeguards will often have to assist by keeping the craft out of the surfline, while awaiting backup assistance in the form of a rescue vessel. Depending on surf conditions, towing a vessel up to about thirty feet in length can usually be accomplished by a single lifeguard equipped with a boat tow and swim fins. Upon approaching a boat (from the seaward side), the lifeguard should gain permission to give assistance and request that all lifesaving equipment be donned by the passengers or at least placed on deck. Request that running engines (if providing no propulsion) be stopped and that sails be dropped. If anchors are being used but are not effective in stopping progress toward the surfline, they should be pulled up. Toss the free end of the boat tow to a person aboard with instructions to secure it to the bow eye. The lifeguard can now swim the boat away from the surfline to calmer water to await rescue vessel assistance. If towing cannot prevent a disabled boat from entering the surfline or if the boat swamps, passengers should be directed to jump off to the seaward side. The lifeguard must be prepared to jettison the RFD, which, if attached to the tow line, may pull the lifeguard with the boat through the surfline. Rescue efforts in the water are now focused on people who have abandoned the craft, while efforts on shore focus on clearing the water and minimizing damage to the boat.

Automobile Accidents in Water

Many roads parallel or terminate at the beach. The occupants of motor vehicles can accidentally or intentionally find themselves in the water, presenting lifeguards with a sudden submersion. These cases can be complicated by victim entrapment and possible injuries associated with the vehicle accident. Lifeguard response to vehicle submersion accidents often involves a coordinated effort with local police and rescue agencies. There are several objectives in automobile rescue.

- Determine the exact location of the submerged vehicle.
- Determine the number and location of vehicle occupants.
- Respond necessary equipment and personnel to the scene.
- Plan and execute measures to extricate accident victims for resuscitation and treatment.
- Protect emergency responders from harm.

These types of accidents are relatively rare, so lifeguards are typically seen as the experts expected to handle the situation. Once a submerged vehicle accident has occurred, emergency plans are activated and all responding agencies are notified. These agencies may include police, fire and rescue agencies, and special responders such as tow trucks (extrication of victims may require extrication of the vehicle first). If the lifeguard agency is first on the scene, free-diving lifeguards usually attempt to determine the location of the vehicle and make first attempts at locating and extricating victims. One clue to finding a submerged vehicle is rising bubbles. The ideal tool for rapid dives in these cases is the *bailout bottle*, a small scuba tank that can be strapped on the waist and used by lifeguards certified in scuba for a hasty search. Along with a mask and swim fins, an immediate underwater search can then be initiated. The alternative is free diving lifeguards.

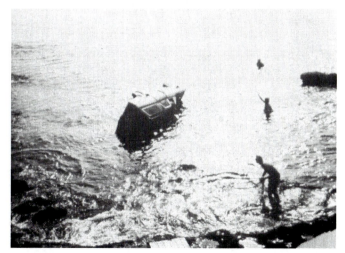

When the vehicle is located, a marker buoy should be fastened to it. An RFD is an excellent alternative if the lanyard is long enough. While initial dives take place, fully equipped lifeguard dive teams should respond and prepare to enter the water. Other responding lifeguards and allied personnel (police, firefighters, etc.) should inspect the scene for victims who may have escaped the vehicle prior to immersion or to interview witnesses in an attempt to determine how many people were in the vehicle.

Because of damage sustained on impact and pressure variances associated with a submerged vehicle, access to victims can be extremely difficult. The best access to a submerged vehicle is normally through the side windows. Side windows are usually made of tempered glass, which is highly resistant to breakage, but which shatters into small, relatively harmless fragments when the glass is pierced. A tool designed for this purpose is the spring-loaded hole punch, but any sharp object, such as an awl, may be effective.

Lifeguards should not assume that all victims are in the vehicle. Some may have been thrown clear during the accident. Checks of the surrounding water, especially pilings or other structures close to the accident scene are important, particularly at night. Lifeguards should also assess prevailing currents to devise a search pattern.

The greatest hazard in rescue of persons in submerged vehicles is laceration from exposed metal and jagged glass. Personal protective equipment such as a wetsuit and gloves should be worn to lessen the chance of injury. There is also potential for entrapment, so lifeguards should use great caution in entering a submerged vehicle. RFD harnesses should be removed. Petroleum products are often present in the water which can be toxic, particularly to the eyes. Use a mask and take care not to swallow the water. If there is a current, try to approach from up-current, since the petroleum will flow down-current.

The value of pre-planning such responses is high, since they are very unusual, but present an extreme emergency involving potentially trapped and possibly seriously injured victims. The possibility of a person trapped and in imminent danger of death always creates a very high degree of concern on the part of lifeguards and bystanders. It is important to stay cool and to remember to operate as safely as possible, as quickly as possible.

Aircraft Accidents in Water

Aircraft commonly cruise over beaches and adjacent waters. In many areas, aircraft traffic is fairly heavy during peak season, with planes towing advertising banners, people sight-seeing from the air, and media or law enforcement helicopters occasionally hovering overhead. Near-shore crashes occur on occasion. Lifeguard response to aircraft accidents should be handled in a manner similar to that of automobile accidents in the water. The aluminum used in aircraft is particularly likely to have jagged edges, so great caution is appropriate.

Some lifeguard agencies are positioned near airports. Over the years, many airliner crashes with multiple casualties have occurred in the water. These cases are particularly challenging due to the number of victims involved. Rescue boats are extremely valuable in these cases. Lifeguard agencies near major airports should have contingency plans worked out with airport authorities and local safety responders. Airports are required to have such plans in place and may be a source of funding for rescue equipment.

Flood Rescue

Flood and particularly swiftwater rescue is extremely dangerous. Unlike surf, which allows for lulls between sets of waves, swiftwater is relentless. A person trapped against a stationary object by swiftwater can easily drown and even the strongest swimming skills will be useless. This section is intended as a brief introduction to flood rescue. Any person who will be assigned to flood rescue response should receive thorough, specialized training and equipment.

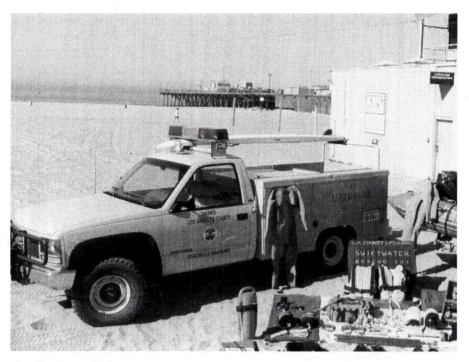

Credit: Conrad Liberty

One of the most dangerous hazards is the low head dam, which can be natural or human made. A low head dam is an obstruction across the path of a river which increases the upstream water level, but allows the river to flow over the top. In these cases, the water flowing over the dam can form a continual cyclical current back toward the dam itself. It thus becomes a self perpetuating, drowning machine. A person caught in this cyclical current, even with a personal flotation device, can be trapped and repeatedly recirculated under the water, unable to break free.

Another, similarly hazardous phenomenon in swiftwater is a strainer. This involves debris in the water, like logs or rocks, which the water can easily move through, but to which any large object will be pressed and held by the current. If trapped underwater in a strainer, it can be impossible to extricate oneself. Even trained rescue teams may have great difficulty removing someone from a strainer.

Lifeguards who lack special training in flood rescue should make every effort to avoid attempting a rescue that requires use of a boat or actual entry into the swiftwater environment. Instead, consider methods which allow lifeguards to stay onshore. One simple, but effective method for shore based rescue is known as the *pendulum technique*. As the victim is swept along by swift moving floodwaters, the rescuer ashore uses a bag of line known as a *throw bag* to manually throw a line to the victim. The rescuer holds one end of the line while the weight of the line in the loosely open ended bag causes it to uncoil toward the victim. Before throwing, several coils of line should be pulled out of the bag out at the rescuer's end to adjust to the force of the load from the weight of the victim and pull of the current. In order to minimize range error, the bag should be thrown directly over the victim so the line drops over the victim's head.

When possible, the rescuer should choose a site, both along the waters edge and in the water, that is free of obstructions such as rocks and trees. The optimal site provides the rescuer freedom of movement downstream. This will assist the rescuer in bringing the victim ashore by lessening the risk of being overloaded by the weight of the victim. It will also allow the rescuer to control the exact landing point of the victim along the water's edge. The bag is best thrown in an underhanded fashion. This is easier to learn and has better accuracy results. Overhand throws may be necessary to clear obstacles. Only one bag should be thrown at a time. Other rescuers should be positioned downstream for other attempts, should the first be unsuccessful. Before the bag is thrown, the rescuer should get the attention of the victim by yelling "rope" or whistling. When the bag is thrown, the rescuer braces and when the victim grabs the line, the force of the current combined with the pull of the line causes the victim to swing to shore (pendulum) on the rescuer's side of the river. If a victim is expected to be swept under an overhang, such as a bridge, netting may be lowered or rescue tubes snapped in the closed position may be dangled to allow the victim an easy purchase.

Other considerations, particularly for victims stranded on objects midstream is use of a fire department ladder truck, with the ladder extended, or a helicopter. In any case, always wear a highly buoyant personal flotation device, a helmet, gloves, and footwear when working around floodwater. Since floodwater is usually contaminated by sewage and other toxins, rescuers should be inoculated against likely maladies, such as hepatitis.

Shark Bite Rescue

In 2002, as a result of several high-profile shark bite incidents during the prior year, the United States Lifesaving Association developed a position statement on shark bite prevention and response. (Brewster, Burgess, Gallagher, Gould, Hensler, & Wernicki, 2002) This section is taken from that position statement. The most current version of USLA position statements can be found on the USLA website at: *www.usla.org*.

Data on sharks suggests that their behavior must always be regarded as *unpredictable*. The United States Lifesaving Association is unaware of any proven techniques whereby an unprotected swimming rescuer can successfully or safely intervene when a shark bites another swimmer. However, rescuers are rarely victims of shark attacks. In fact, of 438 unprovoked shark bite incidents investigated by the International Shark Attack File that involved attempted rescue by another person, only 14 (3.2%) resulted in the rescuer being injured. Of those 14, only two (0.5%) involved injury to a beach-based rescuer who responded to assist. One of these two cases was fatal. Since most shark bites occur quickly and can cause serious, sometimes life-threatening lacerations, there is great value in the availability of trained personnel to rescue the injured swimmer, provide emergency medical care, and arrange rapid transport, after a shark bite has occurred.

The best protective equipment for a lifeguard attempting a rescue of a shark bite victim is an enclosed rescue boat with high gunwales. A personal watercraft may be an alternative, but most personal watercraft provide less protection to the lifeguard and may not be adequate to safely evacuate a seriously injured victim. While a rescue board or kayak may elevate the lifeguard from the water, some sharks have bitten surfers and kayakers, apparently after mistaking them for seals or sea lions. In areas where shark bites have occurred with higher than normal frequency, lifeguards should consider stationing a rescue boat in the vicinity that can allow a rapid, safe response to such incidents.

If a lifeguard observes a shark bite in progress, the lifeguard should immediately notify other lifeguards and determine the most appropriate course of action. This should follow the agency's overall emergency response plans and any specific plans that may exist for shark bites. USLA cannot issue a blanket recommendation that that a lifeguard without protective equipment attempt to intervene during a shark bite incident, due to the potential danger. International Shark Attack File statistics however, suggest that danger to the lifeguard in an attempt to intervene is extremely limited. Moreover, in the vast majority of cases, the shark will effect a bite, then leave the victim alone, well before the lifeguard could possibly intervene. Once injury has been inflicted to the victim, heavy bleeding is likely, so rescue from the water and immediate medical aid may be essential to victim survival.

If a rescue boat is not available and if, as is most typically the case, the shark bite appears to be a typical single hit and run incident, and if the lifeguard considers it safe and within agency guidelines to enter the water, the lifeguard should perform a rescue and treat the wounds of the victim. Once the victim has been evacuated to shore or to a rescue boat, appropriate emergency medical assistance should be provided, in accordance with the lifeguard's training. In addition to normal emergency medical priorities, particular attention should be paid to stopping bleeding and treating for shock.

Ice Rescue

The work of lifeguards normally takes place in warm water; but drowning occurs in cold water too. One of the most dangerous types of rescue is of persons who have fallen through the ice. A study of ice related deaths in Canada by the Lifesaving Society (1998) found that 52% of the people who died in attempted rescues were public safety professionals. While few lifeguards are directly assigned to ice rescue response units, as aquatic rescue professionals lifeguards are expected to have an above average understanding of aquatic rescue wherever they may find themselves. This section is intended to provide a brief overview of the principles of ice rescue. Those who will be assigned to ice rescue teams will require more thorough information and training.

The majority of accidental ice related deaths occur as a result of recreational activities. These include activities such as ice skating and ice fishing, but may also include simply walking on the ice. Consistent with the trends of drowning deaths, younger people are the most likely victims of ice related deaths and more than 80% of the victims are male. More than a third of fatal ice related incidents involve multiple victims. The Lifesaving Society of Canada found that, "The two kinds of conditions most often involved were thin or soft ice, and open holes." (Lifesaving Society, 1998)

For nonswimmers, falling through the ice can be similar to stepping off a drop-off into deep water. Unless able to hold on to the ice or a floating object, the nonswimmer may quickly die by drowning. For swimmers who fall through the ice and are able to keep themselves afloat, two primary challenges are presented. One is the effects of cold water, including cold shock and hypothermia. Eventually, the victim is no longer able to stay on the surface, submerges, and dies by drowning. The other is the tremendous difficulty in getting out of the water and back onto the ice. Cold limbs and a slippery surface with nothing to grip make self-rescue very difficult.

Lifeguards in areas of the U.S. where waters freeze over in winter should include information about ice safety in their drowning prevention education programs. It is easy to overlook this serious problem when considering the traditional role of a lifeguard, but all lifeguards should be concerned with drowning prevention and any information that can prevent drowning is of value to everyone.

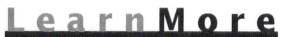

LearnMore

The Lifesaving Society of Canada has published *Ice: The Winter Killer, A Resource Manual About Ice, Ice Safety and Ice Rescue*. Find it on the Web at: *www.lifesaving.org/store.*

Ice Accident Prevention

- *Keep Kids Away*—Curious children and teenagers are likely victims of ice related accidents. Each year before ice forms on local waters they should be reminded of the dangers, and then reminded again when waters begin to freeze over.
- *Stay Off Unless You're Sure*—Don't venture onto ice unless you can be sure it is safe. For walking, it should be at least four inches thick and fully hardened. Even so, there are no guarantees.
- *Never Go Alone*—If you are going onto the ice, go with a friend, but stay separated. If one person falls through, the other can call for help and may be able to assist.
- *Wear a Thermal Protection Buoyant Suit*—These suits maximize the amount of time you can survive in cold water and keep you on the surface.
- *Wear a PFD*—If you don't have a thermal protection buoyant suit, wear a PFD. This will keep you afloat if you fall through and lengthen survival time.
- *Carry an Ice Staff*—An ice staff can be used to check the ice ahead for integrity.
- *Carry Ice Picks*—Ice picks can be used to pull yourself out of the water and on to the ice. They can be made inexpensively with two four inch sections of a broom handle or dowel, a strong nail driven into the end of each dowel and sharpened on the exposed end, and a string to hang the picks around your neck (drill a hole through the ends of the dowels for the string).
- *Carry Rope*—With rope, you may be able to help yourself or others.
- *Carry a Phone*—Have a means of summoning help in an emergency.
- *Stay Low and Spread Out*—If you sense instability in the ice, retreat quickly. If you can't, then spread out your weight by lying on the ice and moving slowly to safety by crawling or rolling.

Self-Rescue from Ice Accidents

- *Stay Calm*—Heat loss is a serious problem. Do what you can to avoid over-exertion.
- *Cry for Help*—Don't hesitate to request help if someone is within earshot. It's best to have help on the way in case you can't extricate yourself.
- *Maintain Warmth*—Keep your clothes on, keep yourself as high out of the water as possible by placing your arms on the ice, avoid swimming any more than necessary to stay afloat, and keep your legs together.
- *Don't Let Your Rescuers Become Victims*—Advise them to stay back in a safe area and to attempt to reach you with a pole, rope, or similar device.
- *Use Sharp Objects*—If you have no ice picks, use keys or any other objects you may have on your person to gain a grip on the ice as you try to extricate yourself.
- *Kick Out*—Face the direction from which you came, extend arms onto the ice with whatever sharp objects you have, and kick hard to get yourself up on the ice. Keep trying if it doesn't work the first time. Once on the ice, don't stand up! Spread your weight out and roll or slide slowly to safe ice.
- *Get Warm and Dry*—Once out of the water, hypothermia is a very serious concern.

Rescue of Others

- *Protect Yourself*—Ice rescuers become victims very quickly. This can result not only in mortal danger to the rescuer, but may also seal the fate of the original victim. Act thoughtfully and deliberately. According to the Lifesaving Society of Canada (1998), "… even with considerable training and good equipment, it is sometimes not possible to save someone. Do not die trying to save one person when you can live to save 20."

- *Use Personal Safety Equipment*—If available, use a thermal protection buoyant suit and a PFD.

- *Leash Yourself*—Tie a stout line around yourself and have others hold it so that you can be pulled to safety if needed. They can pull both you and the victim to safety in a reaching rescue.

- *Low Risk Procedures*—If you can talk the victim to shore by advising of self-rescue techniques or if you can throw a line to the victim or reach the victim with an extended pole or ladder, try this first. Of particular value is a throw-bag or a rope with a PFD or RFD attached.

- *High Risk Procedures*—Venturing on the ice to rescue another person is a very high risk decision. If you feel you must do so, use great caution. Make sure an alert has been sounded and backup requested. Don all available personal protective gear, including a leash held by others in a safe position. If available, push a boat, such as an IRB or flat bottom aluminum boat ahead of you and toward the victim. The boat should also be tethered to a safety line. Maintain a position at all times that cause you to fall into the boat if you break through the ice. If no boat is available, consider any other floatable object, such as a personal watercraft rescue sled, bodyboard, or similar device. If no floating device is available, find something you can use to extend your reach, even a tree branch, rope yourself in with assistants onshore, and crawl slowly toward the victim, flat on the ice, with the extension forward.

- *Treat Hypothermia*—After rescue, hypothermia is a serious problem. Replace wet clothes with dry ones or blankets, find a warm place, and get advanced medical help.

Cliff Rescue

Some lifeguard agencies have jurisdiction over areas that include high rock outcroppings or cliff areas adjacent to protected beaches. These areas may experience special rescue presentations involving people who fall or jump from these heights into the water. Cliff rescues can be complicated by difficult extrication routes and the possibility that the victims may be injured as the result of a fall or jump.

Many agencies will plan rescue approaches and retrievals for these presentations from the water, rather than from the cliff. In these cases, responses are made from adjacent beach areas using rescue boards or boats. Some agencies with nearby cliff areas employ special floating stretchers, which allow entrapped water to drain rapidly while holding the victim firmly inside. These devices are particularly useful when victims have been injured or are suffering from shock. Once victims have been controlled and stabilized, they are extricated to deeper water for retrieval to a waiting vessel or to adjacent beaches.

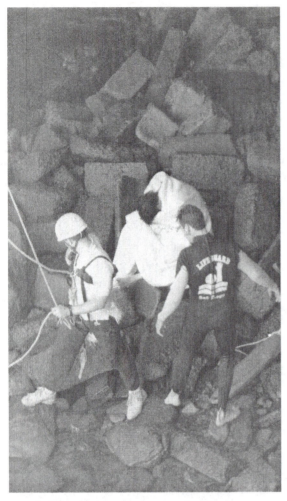

Two lifeguards come to the aid of a victim trapped at the bottom of a cliff. One lifeguard swam to the victim, the other rappelled down the cliff.

Credit: Paul Hansen

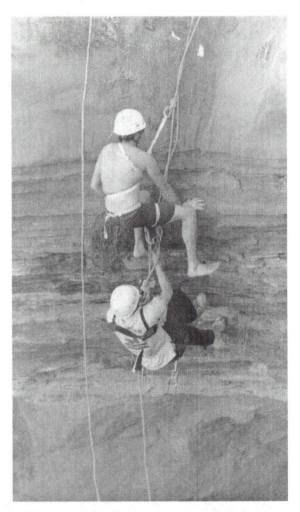

A lifeguard (below) assists a victim as they are hoisted by lifeguards at the top of the cliff.

Credit: Paul Hansen

Some lifeguard agencies are also responsible for rescuing victims trapped on cliffs or who fall from cliffs or rock outcroppings onto dry land. These agencies are outfitted with special extrication tools, equipment, and vehicles for these rescues. The San Diego Lifeguard Service, for example, handles 30 or more rescues each year on cliffs up to 300 feet in height, perhaps more than any other public safety agency in the US. This lifeguard service maintains a special rescue vehicle with a crane and mechanical cable to aid in cliff rescue. Coastal cliff rescue is similar to alpine rescue. It requires extensive training which will not be covered in detail in this manual.

Chapter Summary

In this chapter, we have learned about many special rescue situations that develop due to environmental conditions and the activities of people. We have learned how to successfully rescue victims from a rip current. Since rescues sometimes involve multiple victims, we have learned how to rescue more than one person at a time. We have learned techniques for situations in which rescues must be made without rescue equipment and what to do in case a panicked victim grabs you. We have learned ways to identify distress and to effect rescues of surfers, bodyboarders, and divers. We have learned about fugitive retrieval and special considerations for the rescue of persons attempting suicide. We have learned about the difficulties presented by fog and darkness, and ways to overcome them. We have learned about the hazards presented by rocks, jetties, and piers, and ways to successful effect rescues from them. We have learned about rescues of boats and their occupants. We have learned about rescues of persons from vehicle and aircraft crashes in water. We have learned about flood rescue, ice rescue, and cliff rescue. And we have learned about the rescue of victims of shark bites.

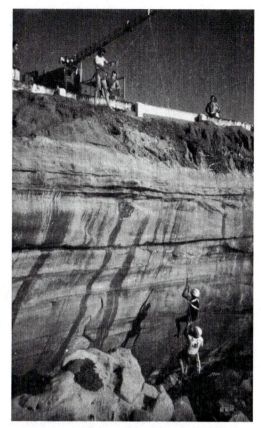

The San Diego lifeguard special rescue vehicle, with crane deployed, hoisting a victim.

Credit: B. Chris Brewster

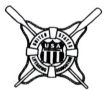

Discussion Points

- What are some techniques that can be employed to use the power of a rip current to your advantage?
- In cases of multiple victims who are spread out, how might you decide which victim to attend to first?
- If you must make a rescue without equipment, what are some considerations?
- If a panicked victim grabs you, what is your immediate goal and why?

- What are some indications of a surfer in distress?
- What are some clues that a diver may be a novice?
- What are indications of a diver in distress?
- What are some similarities between rescues of fugitives and rescues of persons attempting suicide?
- What are some ways to protect yourself during a boat rescue?
- In what ways might you be able to gain access to occupants of a submerged vehicle?
- What factors make swiftwater rescue so dangerous?
- What are some items that might be improvised for use in ice rescue?
- What are some steps lifeguards can take to prevent shark bites?

References

Brewster, B. C., Burgess, G. H., Gallagher, T., Gould, R., Hensler, M., & Wernicki, M.D., P. (2002). United States Lifesaving Association position statement shark bite prevention and response. Huntington Beach, California: United States Lifesaving Association.

Lifesaving Society (1988). *Ice: the winter killer, a resource manual about ice, ice safety and ice rescue.* Ottawa, Ontario: Lifesaving Society.

Vann, Ph.D., R. & Uguccioni, MS, D., Editors (2001). *Report on decompression illness, diving fatalities, and project dive exploration.* Durham, NC: Divers Alert Network.

Chapter 16

Emergency Planning and Management

In this chapter, you will learn about ways to ensure that responses to emergencies, both large and small, can be handled smoothly and efficiently, regardless of the number of responding personnel or agencies. You will learn about the incident command system and about pre-planning your emergency response. We will also present some tips about managing emergencies lifeguards commonly face.

CHAPTER EXCERPT

The *incident command system* (ICS) was created to promote effective coordination of diverse emergency resources. The incident commander, is the person ultimately responsible for overall management of the incident.

The Incident Command System

Successful resolution of any emergency requires a cooperative and coordinated response of all emergency resources. A rescue of a single swimmer may be handled routinely by a single lifeguard. If there are multiple victims involved though, several lifeguards may respond. At the most elemental level in this example, each lifeguard is an emergency response resource. Those resources must work in a coordinated manner if the rescue is to be completed successfully. If they all respond to the same victim, other victims are left without assistance. While they may work intuitively, they may also work under the direction of a lifeguard in charge who directs each of the other lifeguards to the victims. In the language of emergency response, this rescue is an *incident* and the person directing resources is the *incident commander* (IC).

As emergency incidents increase in complexity, additional resources (including both personnel and equipment) will be needed. Allied public safety agencies may be involved. For a lifeguard agency, this may involve summoning police officers, firefighters, ambulances, the U.S. Coast Guard, etc. Each will need to know what is expected of them. For example, consider a water rescue in which three victims suffer complications and need advanced medical treatment. Ambulances will be summoned, perhaps police for crowd control, patient information will need to be gathered, relatives will want to know to what hospital their family members will be going, and all the while there will be a need to ensure that those still recreating in the water and on the beach are protected. Coordination and direction are needed. The goal in these instances is to utilize all available resources in the most efficient manner possible to successfully resolve the emergency.

The *incident command system* (ICS) was created to promote effective coordination of diverse emergency resources. The incident commander, is the person ultimately responsible for overall management of the incident. The IC is usually a member of the agency most directly responsible for the emergency. The IC need not be the most senior member of a given agency. Initially the IC is the first emergency responder on-scene who is not directly involved as a rescuer and who is able to take charge. It could be the head lifeguard, a ranking police officer, or a fire department supervisor. Prearranged emergency operation plans will determine how the responsibilities of the IC are transferred as supervisory personnel and responders from allied agencies arrive at the scene of the emergency. Regardless of who the IC may be, members from the IC's agency and those of all other responding agencies ultimately report to the IC for assignment. This requires that agency pride be put aside in favor of achieving a common goal. At major incidents, a liaison system is arranged which allows a representative from each agency involved in the emergency to expeditiously communicate pertinent information to and from the IC.

The incident command system is designed to begin developing from the time an incident occurs until the emergency is resolved. The incident command structure can be expanded or contracted depending upon the changing conditions of the incident. It can be seen as a pyramid with the IC at the top. In its most rudimentary form, if two lifeguards respond to a reported drowning, one will usually take charge and make the decisions. This person is in command of the incident—the IC. At more complex emergency incidents, the IC may be ultimately responsible for hundreds of emergency responders. As the incident expands in size, the responsibility for acting as IC is typically pushed higher up the chain of command. Each lifeguard agency must designate its own protocols, but under the incident command system, the first lifeguard on-scene who is not directly involved as a rescuer is the incident commander until relieved by a higher authority from the lifeguard's own agency or a representative of another agency who has jurisdiction. This concept helps clarify the question of, "Who's in charge?" Even if you are not a supervisor, for a period of time, it may well be you.

The basic principles of the incident command system are easy to understand. They are an outgrowth of the concept of chain of command, but applied more broadly. Training is available online from the Federal Emergency Management Administration (FEMA)—*www.fema.gov.* Other possible sources of training include local colleges or fire and police organizations. The training is easily adapted to any public safety work, including lifeguarding. USLA recommends that all lifeguard

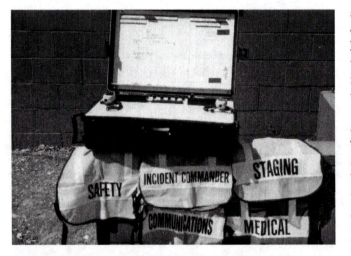

An incident command kit with vests to help identify those assigned to lead roles.

Credit: Dan McCormick

agency supervisors complete the incident command system orientation course (I-100) and the basic course (I-200). Intermediate (I-300) and advanced (I-400) courses are appropriate for lifeguard supervisors at agencies which regularly interact with allied public safety agencies at emergency scenes.

Incident Command Responsibilities

- Assess incident priorities
- Determine strategic goals and tactical objectives
- Develop or approve and implement the incident action plan
- Develop an incident command structure appropriate for the incident
- Assess resource needs
- Order, deploy and release needed resources
- Coordinate overall emergency activities
- Serve as the ultimate incident safety officer; responsible for preventing injuries
- Coordinate activities of outside agencies
- Direct information release to the media

Emergency Operation Plan Development

A vessel grounds on a rock off the beach with 23 victims aboard, some with serious injuries. What emergency resources will be responded? A plane with three persons aboard loses power and the pilot ditches in the water 100 yards from on-duty lifeguards. Who should be notified? Five people are swept offshore in a rip current. They are rescued, but all have aspirated water and need immediate advanced medical care. How will they be treated and transported to the hospital?

Most emergency operations involving lifeguards are routine. In these cases, standard response methods should be very effective; but major emergencies, by their nature, are not routine. They may call for numerous responders from different agencies and specialized rescue equipment. Critical decisions must be made throughout the incident. Because of the complexities of major emergencies, important options and resources can easily be missed. For these reasons, professional public safety agencies prepare an *emergency operation plan* (EOP) for each of the types of emergencies they expect to face.

Effective EOPs should be developed in consultation with all agencies likely to be involved considering all possible resources and courses of action for a given emergency. They usually include a menu of options to help ensure that no viable alternative will be missed in the heat of the moment. An EOP helps to utilize all resources in the most appropriate way.

Emergency operation plans are based on worst case scenarios. They utilize the emergency personnel who can reasonably be expected to be available. They are designed to expand or contract depending on the extent of the emergency. Some subjects of lifeguard emergency operation plans are:

- Drowning Persons
- Missing Persons
- Major Medical Emergencies
- Scuba Emergencies
- Fire
- Severe Weather

- High Surf
- Law Enforcement
- Dangerous Marine Life
- Environmental Disasters
- After Hours Emergencies
- Automobile/Aircraft Crashes

Emergency plans are sometimes drafted in the wake of a major emergency for which the agency was unprepared. This approach should be avoided. Preventive lifesaving includes anticipating worst case scenarios and preparing to handle them professionally.

Creating the Plan

Development of an effective emergency operation plan is usually begun with thorough consultation among lifeguard staff members, particularly those with experience in major emergencies and those with special skills. Various emergency scenarios are considered with best possible response modes and alternatives considered. If it becomes clear that a given type of emergency will require members of other agencies, they should be consulted and asked to provide input during the planning process. This not only provides expertise, but hopefully a buy-in to the plan which is ultimately devised. Once goals are set, representatives of each affected agency should be designated. They should then meet to prepare a draft plan. In doing so, they should consider the following list of items to facilitate an effective, coordinated response.

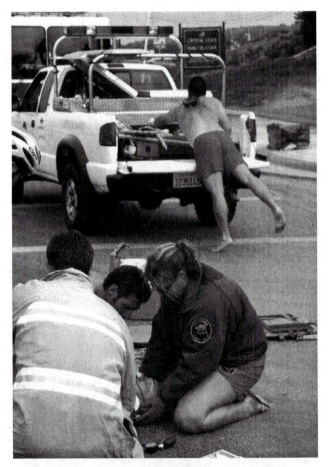

- *Skills Assessment*—What skills do members of each agency have that might contribute to successful management of the emergency? A skills list should be developed by each agency and shared among the planners.
- *Rescue Resources and Assets*—What resources and assets do each agency have that might contribute to successful management of the emergency. A list of rescue resources and assets should be developed by each agency and shared among the planners.

Lifeguards provide medical aid at an accident on the street.

Credit: Ken Kramer

- *Identify Standard Operating Procedures*—Each agency will have standard operating procedures in place, whether formal or informal, that may have an impact on the plan. For example, might the area that one agency's vehicles typically park conflict with access of responding vehicles of another agency? Creating a plan involves reducing the potential for actions by one agency that might impact response of another.

- *Lead Agency*—What agency should be the lead agency and assume incident command?

- *Communication*—How will the various agencies communicate during the response? Are there shared radio frequencies that can be used? If so, what will the protocols be to ensure that radio traffic is organized? Can a dispatcher from one agency handle communication among all agencies? If radio communication is not practical, what alternatives are there? How will primary agency representatives be identified on-scene?

- *Command Post*—Depending on the length of the emergency, it may be valuable to have an on-scene command post. This could be an office, a mobile command post, or simply a designated location for the respective agency representatives. Agreeing upon this in advance avoids the problem of trying to find representatives of the agencies at the scene.

- *Crowd Control*—Major incidents draw crowds. These crowds must be managed to prevent interference with emergency responders and to prevent spectators from becoming victims. Who will handle this responsibility?

- *Staging Areas*—Staging areas are places that personnel and equipment gather in advance of being committed to specific tasks, or in between those assignments. By designating staging areas, you can prevent the problem of having all emergency responders show up at the same location, which can create congestion and confusion.

- *Safety Officer*—The intense pressure on emergency responders, particularly at major emergency scenes with spectators involved, can cause agency supervisors to lose focus on personnel safety. Emergency response carries inherent risks, but those risks should be managed to ensure that all involved are protected to the greatest extent possible. Designating a safety officer, who stands aside and observes with a role of making recommendations to the incident commander about safety, helps reduce to possibility of unnecessary risk and unexpected injury.

- *Witness Statements*—In major emergencies, it is always a good idea to gather witness statements. These statements can help explain what happened, which may help in emergency response, and help make a record of the incident later. Responsibility for gathering witness statements should be designated.

- *Family Liaison*—Whenever someone is imperiled or injured, friends and family are inevitably concerned. They may have many questions. Part of an effective emergency response involves ensuring that someone is made available to answer their questions and address their concerns.

- *Media Liaison*—Major incidents inevitably draw attention of the news media. They have a desire to garner factual information about the incident. By designating a *public information officer* (PIO), the media can be provided with necessary information while rescuers handle immediate needs of victims without undue interference. For long-term incidents, briefings should be planned and an area designated for the media to gather.

Once the plan is developed in draft form, it should be circulated to staff members and leaders of allied agencies involved in the plan for comment. Comments should be incorporated as appropriate, and the final plan produced. It should then be provided to all involved parties. Each agency will have a responsibility to ensure that the plan is immediately available to key personnel who will be primarily responsible for its implementation.

Developing Checklists

Checklists are valuable adjuncts to emergency plans. A checklist helps ensure that basic steps are not forgotten when an emergency occurs. Checklists should include all of the likely sequence of procedures required, worst case in a specific emergency. The incident commander can select which steps in the sequence will be taken depending on the circumstances of the emergency, but the checklist helps to ensure that major options are considered. An example checklist for a submerged swimmer scenario (Code X) can be found in *Appendix B.*

Checklists are particularly valuable for dispatchers and scene commanders. For example, in a submerged swimmer emergency the dispatcher can simply be advised via radio to follow the submerged swimmer checklist, which may include summoning of an ambulance, arranging dispatch of a dive team, requesting police for crowd control, summoning additional personnel for the search, and so forth. In this way, the on-scene supervisor doesn't have to remember to advise the dispatcher of each step to take or tie up radio traffic. In addition, the task is accomplished sooner. Checklists for dispatchers can be written in such a way as to require clearance prior to taking a particular step, but they still help to remind all involved of the need to consider certain actions.

Training

Once emergency action plans are developed, all personnel who will be expected to implement them must be trained. Initially, this will include senior staff members likely to take charge or to play key roles. Since the most senior staff members may be off duty the day of a major emergency, training should also include any staff members likely to have a lead role in an emergency. Once persons at this level are trained, remaining staff should be familiarized with the plan. Although most lifeguard agencies operate under a chain of command system, in which subordinate lifeguards are expected to execute directions quickly and without unnecessary questioning, when employees have an understanding of the reasons for their actions and are able to anticipate likely roles they will assume, they are more likely to be prepared to act in accordance with expectations.

Conducting Drills

Once an EOP has been developed and training has been provided, drills should be conducted to test the integrity of the plan, to provide practice to those involved, and to identify areas that may require modification. This begins with the tabletop drill. An example scenario is developed and designated representatives of all agencies involved in the plan discuss their roles. Example scenarios might be a water rescue with missing victims and a search underway or a nearshore boat collision with multiple trauma victims.

How many personnel would be sent? Where would they go? To whom would they report? Each agency representative explains what they would do on a step by step basis. A good tabletop drill includes a few unexpected elements. For example, if the scenario involves a boat collision offshore with multi-

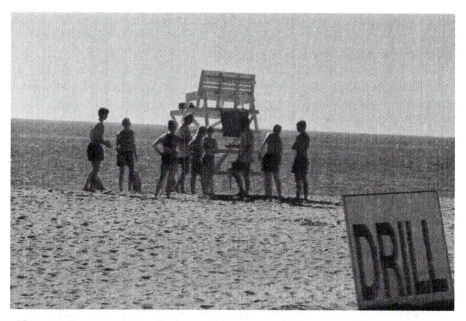

Lifeguards preparing for an emergency drill.

Credit: Michael Slattery

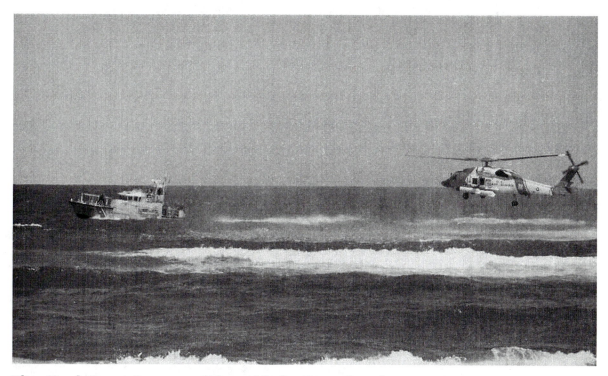

Kitty Hawk Ocean Rescue training with the Coast Guard.

Credit: Derek Boutwell

ple trauma victims, partway through the tabletop drill, it may be stated that one of the boats is now sinking or has caught fire. How would things change? This process is intended to get everyone thinking about their roles and how they can best contribute.

The next step is a walkthrough drill. This is a preplanned practice operation utilizing members of the responsible lifeguard agency to literally walk through a rescue scenario in coordination with members of assisting agencies who would be expected to be called to the scene. The focus is on having those involved develop a familiarity and trust with members of other responding agencies, as well as with their own roles.

The final step is a live drill. This involves an actual run-through of the designated scenario, with the goal of having the rescue operation seem as real as possible, albeit with an understanding that it will not mirror the real thing. A live drill happens only after the EOP has been finalized and personnel from each agency have received training in the plan. This step is intended to reinforce proper response protocols among all responders, and to prepare them for their roles when the inevitable happens. Live drills should not be a one-time event. Rather, they should be scheduled in a frequency that avoids unnecessary disruption, but that helps responders keep a fresh sense in their mind of what their roles will be.

Managing Common Lifeguard Emergencies

Missing Persons

Large crowds and an abundance of activity make reports of missing persons very common in the beach environment. Once a person is discovered to be missing, family and friends, particularly if a small child is involved, inevitably fear that the missing person has drowned. A crucial question in these cases is, *"Did you see the person submerge?"* In the vast majority of cases, a person reporting someone missing is very fearful that a person has died by drowning, but in fact the missing person is later found on the beach.

If a credible person reports *witnessing* a submersion, a water search should be initiated immediately. Conversely, if a person is simply reported to be missing and last known to be going swimming, a full water search may be inappropriate. In this case there is no *last seen point* at which to initiate the search, nor any certainty that the missing person is even in the water. Consideration should be given to the fact that committing lifeguard personnel to an extensive water search in this instance could unduly detract from safety protection provided to other water users.

The most difficult decision for a lifeguard in charge of a beach comes when the report of a missing person falls into the gray area between a witnessed submersion and a simple loss of a person on the beach. For example, how should the case be handled if a mother last saw her teenage son in the water, but turned away for a minute and upon trying to find him again couldn't do so? In this case, the son may well have left the water or be lost in the swim crowd. On the other hand, he may have submerged.

It is essential that lifeguard agencies develop procedures for such cases to assist lifeguards and to protect the agency from criticism for a failed response. Emergency action plans and checklists can help. Ultimately though, judgment decisions will have to be made based on the unique facts in each case.

In-water search procedures are covered in the chapter entitled, *Underwater Search and Recovery*. General management of shore searches for missing persons should include the following:

1. Elicit a full description of the missing person including:
    - name
    - age
    - height
    - weight
    - hair color
    - skin color
    - clothing description
    - swimming skills
    - medical problems
    - likely beach hangouts
2. Find out the last seen location and direction of travel.
3. Notify all agency staff in the area.
4. Check likely locations, such as bathrooms, snack bars, arcades and so forth.
5. If available, a public address system may be used to summon the missing person or to broadcast a description to elicit assistance in the search from beach patrons.
6. Regularly check the "towel area" (i.e., where the group located themselves on the beach). The missing person may return while you are searching elsewhere.
7. Check the car if the group drove to the beach.
8. Consider calling the home or hotel telephone number if nearby.

During a check of beach facilities, the reporting person should be kept at the lifeguard facility until the incident is resolved or should be allowed to join in land-based searches only in the company of a lifeguard with communications gear. This policy ensures reunification once the lost person is located. It also prevents situations where the reporting party locates the lost person and disappears into the crowd without telling lifeguards that the problem has been resolved. This could cause lifeguards to search endlessly. All other witnesses should be isolated from the general population and interviewed as soon as possible.

Any local law enforcement or clean-up crews who happen to be on the beach

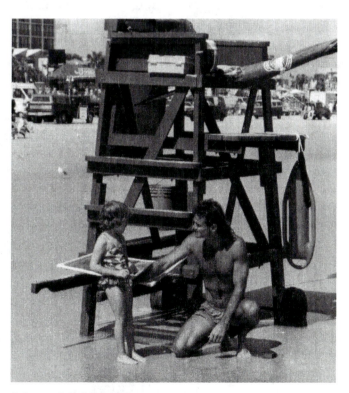

A lost child found.
Credit: Mike Hensler

should be notified. If a missing person is not located expeditiously, a formal notification to police should be made. The actual timeframe for this notification should be set by agency protocol. A missing person report form, which may be helpful in missing person cases, can be found in *Appendix B*.

Major Medical Emergencies

Depending on beach activity, some lifeguard agencies must summon an ambulance daily for transportation of an injured person to the hospital. At other agencies, this may happen only once or twice in a season. Regardless of volume, lifeguards should be prepared to expeditiously summon needed assistance in a medical emergency. This includes having proper telephone numbers and radio frequencies readily available.

Depending on remoteness of the beach area and availability, helicopter evacuation may be necessary in some cases. Pre-planning will involve consultation with the helicopter provider to determine the cases to which they will respond. It will also involve considerations for appropriate landing areas.

Medical emergencies on the beach can draw crowds which tend to obstruct efforts of emergency medical personnel and make the patient very anxious. Some agency protocols call for summoning police assistance for crowd control in any serious medical emergency.

Multiple trauma victims are a tremendous challenge to any medical aid provider. Boating accidents and car accidents are typical causes. Lifeguard agencies should be prepared to triage and treat several injured persons at the same incident. This includes knowing how to summon additional ambulances and other emergency resources for backup as necessary.

Law Enforcement Emergencies

Law enforcement emergency action plans may be initiated whenever the assistance of police is needed on the beach. In the case of a simple property crime, lifeguards may respond by calling for a police officer, while keeping the victim nearby to await the officer's arrival. More serious incidents however, may require additional emergency action.

Some lifeguards are trained and authorized to enforce the law. They may carry firearms or other weapons and act as primary sources of law enforcement for the beaches they serve. Lifeguards without special training, authority, or equipment should avoid attempting to diffuse or confront violent activity. Instead, the agencies they serve will usually advise them to react to violence by calling for emergency police assistance and taking steps to protect themselves and others. All lifeguards should make reasonable attempts to protect beach visitors by helping to move them away from scenes of violent criminal activity and to rescue and treat injured beach visitors, if it can be done with a reasonable degree of safety.

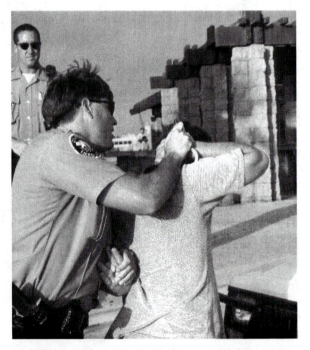

California State Lifeguard making an arrest.
Credit: Ken Kramer

Lifeguards should inform police of criminal activity and update them as the circumstances change. For example, police are understandably anxious to know if they are being summoned to an incident in which weapons are involved, as well as the type of weapons.

One area in which all lifeguards can provide invaluable assistance to law enforcement is through observation and documentation. Criminals often forget that lifeguards have a commanding view of the beach and may attempt to hide in plain view of lifeguards.

An impediment to law enforcement is that witnesses often forget details of the description of those involved in criminal activity. This information can be critical to capture of the perpetrator(s) and ultimate prosecution. Lifeguards should attempt to thoroughly document the descriptions of those observed to be involved in criminal activity and a description of their actions. Witnesses to a crime or victims should be contacted when it is safe to do so and asked to wait for police. Their names and addresses should be documented so that if they leave the scene, the witness information can be provided to police upon arrival.

Severe Weather

As explained earlier in the chapter on weather, lifeguards assist beach visitors by monitoring weather conditions, by warning beach visitors of approaching severe weather conditions, and by assisting beach visitors in the event of sudden, severe weather. When such weather conditions approach beach areas, emergency operations plans for severe weather are initiated. At small beach facilities, these plans may be initiated by the tower lifeguard after recognizing threatening weather patterns. At larger facilities, EOPs may be initiated by a supervisor.

The goals of any severe weather EOP are to:

- Alert the public to threatening weather conditions.
- Warn beach visitors who may be reacting to threatening weather conditions with unwise actions.
- Ensure the safety of lifeguard staff.
- Protect beach facilities.
- Assist with protection of adjacent beach property.

Severe weather warnings are best made using public address systems. Alerts can also be sounded using long blasts from whistles or other alarm devices. Gestures can be used to call people in from the water and warn them of weather conditions. Flags can be flown if their meaning is widely understood in the area. An important goal is to avoid issuing warnings in a manner that could cause panic.

Most people will recognize threatening weather and move toward reasonable shelter on their own. Some visitors, however, may react to threatening weather by attempting to wait the storm out on the beach or may gather in the unsafe shelter of tree groves or other areas. Lifeguards can watch for this behavior and warn visitors to move to adequate shelter, offering suggestions of areas or facilities that have been determined or established as storm shelters. Since beach patrons may attempt to return to the beach before it is safe, stay alert after providing a severe weather warning.

Lifeguards themselves should also take safe shelter. In many areas, lifeguards are ordered out of towers during lightning activity, since certain tower designs may not offer adequate protection from lightning strikes. These policies are to be taken seriously, since lifeguards have been killed during electrical storms at beach facilities.

At some agencies, lifeguards are recognized and trained as special rescue responders during times of severe weather incidents. Lifeguards may be called to stand by and respond to rescues in floods, hurricanes, tornadoes, and other storms. That type of rescue response requires special training, beyond the scope of this manual.

Fire

Emergency plans for fire usually involve the summoning of fire services and the establishment of crowd control measures to protect beach visitors. Lifeguards can also establish and maintain access for incoming fire fighting equipment. In the case of injuries, lifeguards should be prepared to provide medical aid to persons injured by the fire. At beaches in wooded areas, lifeguard EOPs should include evacuation procedures for personnel and the public if a wildfire should threaten beach areas or public access routes.

Chapter Summary

In this chapter, we have learned about the incident command system and how all lifeguards play a part in this system. We have learned about the importance of emergency operations planning to help prepare lifeguards, lifeguard agencies, and allied agencies to work effectively in major emergencies. We have also learned about some common emergency situations lifeguards face and how they can be effectively resolved.

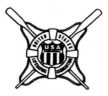

Discussion Points

- What are some circumstances under which the incident command system might be helpful?
- What are some responsibilities of an incident commander?
- Why is it valuable to develop emergency action plans?
- Who should be involved in developing emergency action plans?
- What are some values of drills in emergency action plan development?
- Why is important to keep the reporting party nearby in cases of lost persons at the beach?
- What roles might lifeguards take in law enforcement emergencies?
- In issuing warnings about severe weather, what are some important considerations?

Chapter 17
Underwater Search and Recovery

In this chapter you will about the steps to take if a victim submerges and is lost beneath the water. This includes searching for the victim, recovering them, and what to do afterward. This is a rare occurrence, but search and recovery of lost victims are essential functions of a lifeguard. They must be conducted quickly and efficiently if the victim is to have a chance of survival.

CHAPTER EXCERPT

If a lifeguard onshore observes a submersion or receives a credible report of a submersion, the alert to other personnel is essential. Extensive backup should be immediately responded.

When a victim submerges and is unable to return to the surface, the final stage of the drowning process begins. Breathing is no longer possible. Fresh oxygen is no longer available. Death is imminent. In some cold water instances, persons have survived for an hour or more underwater and have fully recovered. These cases though, are extremely rare and usually involve very cold water which lifeguards rarely patrol. In water where recreational swimming takes place, the submerged swimmer rapidly suffocates. Without freshly oxygenated blood, the heart will cease functioning. Brain death usually begins in three to six minutes after adequately oxygenated blood stops circulating. This oxygen starvation is why immediate resuscitation efforts, ideally with use of supplemental oxygen, are so critical for a submerged victim who is recovered. (Please see the chapter on *Drowning* for more information on the pathophysiology of drowning.)

The standard practice for search and rescue of victims who have submerged underwater in water of a temperature normally used for swimming is to continue an *emergency search* for one hour. The term *emergency search* refers to the period during which personnel and equipment are heavily committed in an effort to recover a victim who can be successfully resuscitated. During this period of time, if the victim is recovered, resuscitation procedures are normally attempted. Once this one hour period has ended, the emergency portion of the search is typically terminated, although efforts to find the body of the victim may be continued. For several reasons, this one hour standard intentionally involves a period of time far greater than a successful resuscitation is typically likely. One reason is the extremely remote possibility of a successful resuscitation up to one hour after submersion. Another is the possibility of an error in the time submersion is estimated to have occurred. Lifeguards must also consider the concerns of family and friends of the victim, who may find it extremely difficult to accept a brief emergency search.

The need for a reasonable emergency search period must also be balanced against the importance of protecting other beach users. Lifeguards have an ongoing responsibility for persons continuing to use the water area for recreation. Considering that a human being is presumed lost underwater, it is fully appropriate to devote significant resources in an attempt to recover and resuscitate the victim, but all beach users need protection. If a second person is lost while lifeguard resources are diverted in an effort to recover the first, the tragedy is compounded. This is a primary reason that many lifeguard agencies clear the water during a search effort.

Despite the one hour standard for emergency search and resuscitation efforts, USLA believes that in open water, there is a *two minute window* of enhanced opportunity for successful recovery and resuscitation of submerged victims. During the initial two minutes, responding lifeguards may be able to make quick dives at the last seen point, bring the victim to the surface, perform initial in-water ventilation, and retrieve the victim to shore for further medical assistance. After the two minute window has closed, the chances of successful recovery and resuscitation decline rapidly. Water currents and surf can quickly move the body, poor water visibility can begin to greatly deter the recovery attempt, and the last seen point of the victim can be obscured on waters with no immediate landmarks. In the flat water environment, some of these factors may not enter the equation, but successful recovery of a viable vic-

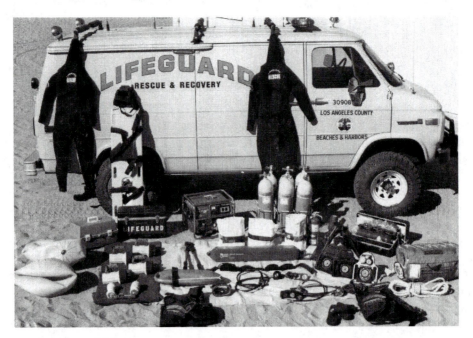

Credit: Conrad Liberty

tim remains very challenging. This brief opportunity is yet another reason that prevention is such a critical aspect of open water lifesaving. Nonetheless, all lifeguards must be prepared to instantaneously and effectively implement search and recovery procedures.

Certain equipment is essential to conduct effective search and recovery. Under USLA guidelines, all beach areas must have masks and snorkels readily accessible to mount an underwater search and rescue, and all must have marker buoys readily accessible to mark the last seen point. Swim fins are of great value when searches must be conducted.

Reports of missing persons do not always call for an in-water search. Often the missing person is simply lost on the beach. The chapter entitled *Emergency Planning and Management* provides guidelines for interviewing people reporting a missing person and determining whether an in-water search is appropriate. This chapter is intended to detail search and recovery procedures once it is determined that a full emergency search should be conducted for a reportedly submerged victim.

Search

In the chapter entitled *Emergency Planning and Management* we explained the importance of the incident command system, emergency operations plans, and checklists. All of these are needed in the case of a missing person who is believed to have submerged. An apparently valid report of a submerged swimmer should immediately trigger an existing emergency operation plan and implementation of steps on a checklist designed to help to ensure that all normal steps are considered by the incident commander in a logical, priority order. This should include automatically sending backup personnel to the scene for assistance, along with any available search equipment. Lifeguards from adjacent beaches and allied agencies may also be summoned.

The estimated time of submersion should be established and documented as soon as possible. This information is critical to determining the time available to summon additional personnel for the search and ultimately for determining when to conclude the emergency portion of the search. If available, it is a good practice to summon ambulance personnel at the start of a search for a submerged victim. In this way, advanced life support will not be delayed upon recovery of a victim. In addition, police may be useful to provide crowd control.

Initial Search

If a lifeguard onshore observes a submersion or receives a credible report of a submersion, the alert to other personnel is essential. Extensive backup should be immediately responded. If a victim submerges as a lifeguard approaches in the water, lifeguards onshore can be alerted by the lifeguard in the water using the USLA approved arm signal of a submerged victim. The lifeguard looks toward shore and crosses both arms overhead in the form of an X (the Code X signal). As with all arm signals, lifeguards ashore should respond with the same signal to show that the signal has been received and understood.

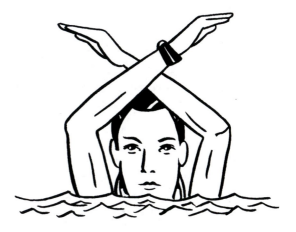

Perhaps the most critical task in initiating a search for a submerged victim is to fix a *last seen point*. Without landmarks, the surface of the water can make it virtually impossible to fix a specific point. The best executed searches will be foiled if the place the victim was last seen prior to submersion is not initially correctly fixed or if it is not marked in a manner to ensure that it is not forgotten. Extensive resources are normally devoted to missing victim searches and great care should be taken to ensure that they are focused on the proper location. If the submersion was witnessed by a non-lifeguard, the witness should be interviewed thoroughly, but expeditiously, in order to obtain an accurate last seen point. If the initial report by the witness is made away from the area of the reported submersion, the witness should be returned to the area and a lifeguard placed in the water to pinpoint the last seen point to the best recollection of the reporting party.

As soon as the best known last seen point is identified, bearings should immediately be taken to attempt to fix the point. Use cross bearings by lining up two stationary objects onshore in two separate locations, the imaginary lines for which form an X at the last seen point. The first lifeguard arriving at the last seen point should make several immediate surface dives in an attempt to locate the victim. The RFD can be left floating on the surface if it will impede diving.

The second lifeguard in the water should carry a marker buoy, along with a mask, snorkel, and swim fins. The value of a marker buoy cannot be understated. It is essential to keeping the search in the proper area. The buoy anchor should be strong enough to remain stationary in reasonably anticipated environmental conditions, but the cross bearings should be regularly checked during the search to ensure that the buoy has not moved. The second lifeguard drops the marker buoy at the last seen point and assists the first lifeguard in surface dives until the victim is found or a more organized search can be mounted. If a marker buoy is not immediately available, response of the second lifeguard should not be delayed while waiting for this equipment. The clock is ticking. The buoy should be placed as soon as it becomes available.

During the search, personnel allowing, at least one experienced lifeguard should be left ashore to act as the *incident commander* (IC) to coordinate the search and ensure safety of the searchers. As soon as possible, a safety officer should be assigned to focus solely on rescuer safety. For example, the safety officer ensures that any rescue boats summoned to the scene stay clear of swimmers and divers, and that all divers are accounted for. Communication must be maintained with arriving lifeguards and other public safety agencies.

Full Search

Prior to initiation of a full search, a search zone should be established by the IC or someone designated by the IC. This provides search personnel with boundaries. Ideally, the search zone should be marked to give search teams a reference point during water searches. Markers may include buoys or cross bearing landmarks. Like the buoy to mark the last seen point, these buoys, particularly when used in a surf environment, should be weighted heavily enough to keep them stationary in reasonably anticipated conditions.

Search Methods

In the flat water environment, if no currents are present, searches can concentrate on the last seen point with an expectation that the victim is most likely near this area if the last seen point is reliable. In the surf environment, or another environment with significant currents, submerged and inanimate victims may move significantly from the last seen point. Those overseeing a search in such conditions must make reasonable, educated guesses as to how the body of the victim might move underwater. In doing so, it is important to consider that currents beneath the surface of the water may be significantly different that those above.

There are three general search methods:

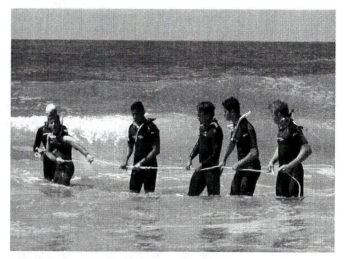

Lifeguards practice a missing person line search.
Credit: Ken Kramer

- *In-Water Search*—Wading and swimming lifeguards search the water. In shallow water, lifeguards may systematically wade back and forth along the shore in a line that extends perpendicular to the beach, searching the water with eyes, legs, and arms. In deeper water, lifeguards use face masks and snorkels, along with swim fins, observing from the surface. These searchers should make surface dives if the bottom cannot be seen from the surface.

- *Surface Search*—Lifeguards are deployed in boats or on paddleboards and use those craft as platforms from which the water is searched. Helicopters provide a superior vantage point for this purpose. EOPs and checklists for agencies with helicopters available should involve an immediate request for a helicopter. Since submersion victims normally sink, the value of a surface search is dependent on water depth and clarity.

- *Underwater Search*—Lifeguards equipped with scuba can dive below depths of skin divers and can stay down. Trained divers are extremely valuable during the emergency portion of a search, but only if scuba equipment is readily available. Advanced lifeguard agencies maintain scuba equipment at their beaches for this purpose.

Search Patterns

The IC or a person designated by the IC should establish a search pattern to ensure systematic coverage of the search zone. The three most common search patterns are the line search (also known as the parallel search), the circular search, and the fan search (sweep). The line search is the most effective option in the surf environment. Any of the three may be used effectively in flat water. Surface search teams may start in deeper water, working a pattern toward shore, while in-water search teams may work from shallow water deeper. Searchers using mask and snorkel should be spaced to maximize coverage, but close enough to see anything between them.

- *Circular Search*—In the circular search, a buoy is placed at the last seen point and an anchor guard holds a line at that point. Lifeguards then space out an appropriate distance from the anchor guard, holding the line, and swim a circular pattern. Once a full circle has been turned, the lifeguard furthest from center maintains position, while the other searchers move to points beyond on the line. The searchers then swim another full circle. This is repeated until the area is thoroughly covered or the victim is found. If the victim is not found at first, the pattern may be started over again.

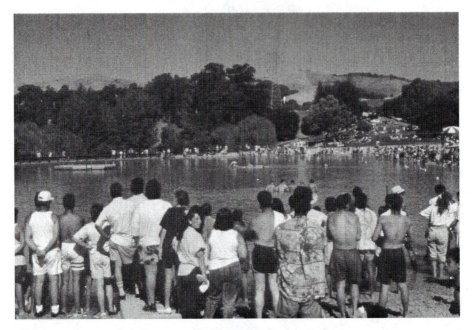

Lifeguards conducting a missing person search.

- *Fan Search*—The fan search is used with a line tender on shore or in a boat. Searchers on the line move back and forth in a fan pattern, extending outward as occurs in a circular search. The starting point of the search will be determined by the last seen point. As searchers complete each arc, the fan gets bigger.

- *Parallel Search*—In the parallel search (also known as the line search or grid search), it is best to start by marking off a rectangular area using buoys. A line of lifeguards, spaced appropriately, swim parallel to each other along one end of the rectangle, from one side to the other. They then move sideways along the side of the rectangle and swim back to the other side. This back and forth pattern can be continued until the area is fully searched. An option, depending on conditions, is use of a line, which searchers grasp to help ensure proper spacing and alignment. At this point the IC can order that the area be searched again, or create a new area adjacent to the area searched. Once the second area has been thoroughly covered, a new one can be created and so forth. It is a good practice to designate one offshore lifeguard to take charge of the search line. This helps ensure that order is maintained. If possible, this lifeguard should be on a rescue board or rescue boat.

To cover an area of limited water visibility more quickly, a team of lifeguards may use the following procedure to complete a parallel search pattern. Lifeguards are spaced in a line close enough to see, or touch, each other while on the bottom. Prior to each dive the team leader checks that everyone is lined up and ready, announces the dive count and starts the dive. For example, directions may go something like, "Everyone OK? Line up on me. Dive for a ten count, ready . . . go." Lifeguards then begin the dive while counting to themselves, "One and two and three," etc. They should dive straight down, while equalizing air pressure in their ears, and then begin their search along

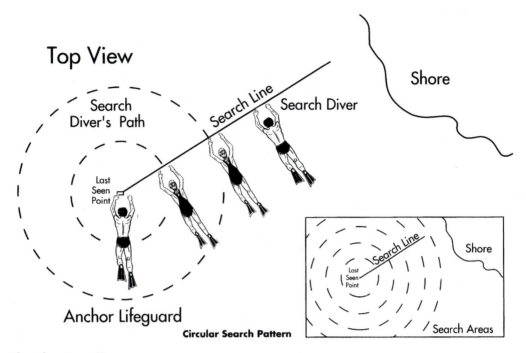

Circular Search Pattern

Circular Search

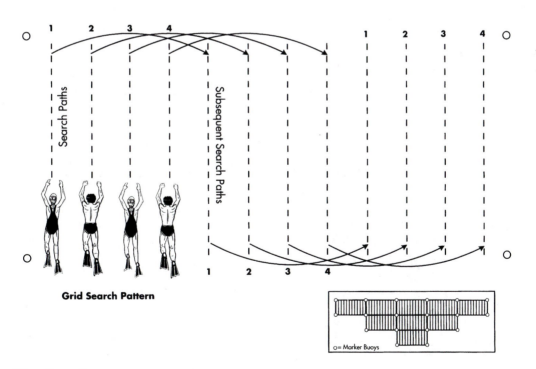

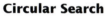

Grid Search Pattern

Line Search

the bottom. In water with zero visibility, searchers should touch hands as they feel along the bottom. Lifeguards should closely monitor each other while underwater, surfacing when the diver next to them does. This improves safety while minimizing the time spent on the surface reorganizing for the next dive. As lifeguards surface, they should identify who covered the least distance. The line should be reformed a few feet behind this lifeguard. On the leader's direction, dives should be repeated until the search area is covered or the victim is located.

Rescue boats are extremely valuable in searches and should always be used if available. They allow on-scene supervision, support of the searchers, and facilitate communication to shore. If a victim is recovered, rescue boats provide a rapid method of retrieval to shore. Some include a deck large enough for CPR, along with advanced medical equipment. When rescue boats are used, caution must be employed to avoid running over a submerged searcher.

The potential for success of a search is largely dependent upon water clarity and currents. In clear water, a few lifeguards can cover a large area in a short time. As water clarity decreases, the difficulty of mounting a successful search increases dramatically.

If the victim is not recovered within a one hour period, longer if so designated by the incident commander or agency protocol, the search may be changed from one of an emergency search to that of a body recovery. When the emergency portion of the search is terminated, lifeguard personnel can be returned to preventive lifeguarding duties, but it is a good practice to continue the search at a lower staffing level. While family members or friends of the missing victim may be able to understand the need to protect other swimmers, they are likely to view complete termination of the search as callous abandonment. A life has been lost and the shock can be profound for all involved. The investment of further time and resources is well justified if available.

Recovery

The goal of a search for a submerged victim is to recover a viable victim who can be resuscitated. This is not always achieved. Lifeguards must be prepared for either outcome.

Recovery of a Viable Victim

If a victim is recovered within an established time-frame after submersion (usually one hour) resuscitation efforts should be initiated. The most difficult decision in the case of a recovered, non-breathing victim is whether to first retrieve the victim to shore where well managed medical support can be provided or to initiate resuscitative efforts in the water. The pathophysiology of drowning dictates appropriate actions. The hypoxia caused by water aspiration from immersion or submersion, if not corrected, results first in respiratory arrest. The tissues of the body become starved for oxygen. If respiratory arrest is not corrected, it is followed by cardiac arrest within a variable, but short time interval, which is determined by physical condition of the victim, water temperature, previous hypoxia, emotional state, and associated diseases.

The Guidelines 2000 for Cardiopulmonary Resuscitation and Emergency Cardiovascular Care, upon which most current CPR standards are based, state, "The first and most important treatment of the [drowning] victim is provision of immediate mouth-to-mouth ventilation. Prompt initiation of rescue breathing has a positive association with survival." (American Heart Association, 2000a) The International Life Saving Federation Medical Commission (2001) recommends, "Whenever possible, if a victim is found in the water, the rescuer should immediately establish whether spontaneous breathing is present and, if it is absent, initiate artificial ventilation. Exceptions include threats to the safety of the rescuer and victim if immediate rescue is not initiated and cases of known submersion over 15 minutes." The primary author of this statement, in a five year study of lifeguards in Rio de Janeiro, Brazil found that providing in-water ventilation to a non-breathing victim resulted in a 3.15 times greater chance of recovery without lingering complications than waiting until the victim was brought to shore. (Szpilman, Orlowski, Brewster, & Mackie, 2003) While lifeguards may have concerns for mouth-to-mouth contact with a victim, the

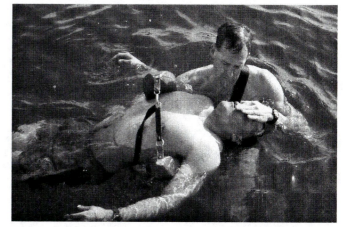

Credit: Sandra McCormick

Guidelines 2000 state, "The probability that a rescuer (lay or professional) will become infected with HBV or HIV as a result of performing CPR is minimal." (American Heart Association, 2000b) If a barrier device is available for the in-water ventilation effort and can be effectively used, it may be used, but this should not unnecessarily delay ventilations.

When a victim is recovered in deep water (overhead) lifeguards should take the following actions consistent with recommendations of the International Life Saving Federation Medical Commission (2001):

Position the victim face up, extending the neck to open the airway. This can be accomplished by a single trained rescuer with the aid of appropriate lifesaving equipment (a rescue tube, rescue can, rescue board, bodyboard, etc.) or by two or more trained rescuers without lifesaving equipment. In either case, swim fins are highly recommended and will greatly facilitate these procedures. If there is no spontaneous breathing, the rescuer should attempt to ventilate for approximately one minute (12 to 16 ventilations), and then proceed depending on circumstances. If ventilation is restored, proceed toward shore intermittently stopping to check that the victim is still breathing. If breathing is not restored after one minute of ventilation, the rescuer should consider if it is a long (over five minutes) or a short swim to a dry or shallow place. If a short swim, rescue the victim while ventilations are continued or stop every one or two minutes to ventilate again for approximately one minute (12 to 16 ventilations). If a long swim, continue ventilation one additional minute in place and check for movement or reaction to ventilation. If present, use the same procedures as with the short swim. If movement or reaction to ventilation is absent, the rescuer should bring the victim to shore without further ventilations.

When performed in deep water, this is a difficult procedure, requiring extreme fitness, swimming ability, a flotation device and prior training. Do not check victim's pulse or attempt compressions while in the water. These are difficult and inefficient, and will slow the rescue process. In case of a suspected back or neck injury the rescuer should check breathing before extending the victim's neck, then if there is no breathing, tilt the victim's neck backwards to check for breathing again. If there is no spontaneous breathing the rescuer should immediately start ventilations consistent with the rescuer's training protocol. Suspicions of back/neck injury should be greater in shallow water. The rescuer should always keep the victim under observation during the rescue, even if the victim is breathing spontaneously, since during the first 5 to 10 minutes the victim could again cease breathing.

Upon arrival onshore or in a rescue boat, appropriate resuscitation procedures in accordance with the lifeguard's training and information presented in the chapter entitled *Medical Care in the Aquatic Environment.*

Steps to Retrieval and Resuscitation of a Viable Victim

1. The victim is brought to the surface and the lifeguard signals to shore with the USLA approved arm signal for a resuscitation case—wave one arm back and forth several times.
2. The lifeguard turns the victim to a face-up position and thrusts one arm under both of the victim's armpits, behind the victim's back.
3. The lifeguard passes the RFD to the hand of the lifeguard's arm which is under the victim's armpits. The victim is now supported on one side by the lifeguard's body and on the other by the grasped RFD. The lifeguard's other hand is free.
4. The airway is opened and the lifeguard checks for breathing.
5. If there is no spontaneous breathing, the lifeguard should attempt to ventilate for approximately one minute (12 to 16 ventilations).
6. If breathing is not restored after one minute of ventilation, and the swim to shore is expected to be five minute or less, rescue the victim while ventilations are continued or stop every one or two minutes to ventilate again for approximately one minute (12 to 16 ventilations). It the rescue to shore is more than five minutes, continue ventilation one additional minute in place and check for movement or reaction to ventilations, then follow the same protocols as for a swim of five minutes or less.
7. If breathing is restored, rescue the victim to shore while carefully monitoring that spontaneous breathing continues. If spontaneous breathing stops, return to step 6.

Note: These steps should be followed for recent submersion victims who are recovered within 15 minutes of submersion in warm water or when total submersion time is uncertain.

Body Recovery

Agency protocols and individual circumstances will dictate a period of time after which an emergency search phase terminates and becomes a body recovery phase. The presumption of a body recovery search phase is that no resuscitation attempt on the recovered victim would be successful. At this point, priorities change. Concerns for rescuer safety and the safety of beach users is heightened. Some lifeguards may be released from the search to return to regular duties. Investigation of the facts surrounding the incident becomes a focus. These changes should be discussed with searching lifeguards. As well, friends and family members of the missing person should be informed carefully and sensitively.

Upon locating a body, depending on local protocol, lifeguards may be expected to make careful observations on land and underwater, collect evidence, and complete reports for those ultimately responsible for investigating the death. Body position, location, and water depth are three basic facts that will need to be recorded upon locating the body. Once the scene investigation is complete and actual recovery is to take place, consideration for the sensitivities of others at the scene should be addressed.

Body recovery requires preparation and discretion. Decedents should be handled with respect. To the greatest degree possible, the body should be protected from public view. Use of a body bag, blanket, or other covering is appropriate as soon as the body is removed from the water. (If feasible, this should occur prior to removal.) Crowd control is important, as is the sensitive treatment of family members and other people close to the deceased person who may be present at the recovery. Depending on local protocol, police, a coroner, or medical examiner should be summoned to accept custody of the body. Police officers often have experience notifying and working with next of kin of deceased persons. They can be a helpful resource in this area.

Crisis Intervention

In many communities, people are trained and assigned to help relatives and friends of deceased people cope with their loss. Some lifeguard agencies train designated lifeguards to perform this function. These services are of particular importance in unexpected deaths, especially those involving children. Part of an emergency operation plan for dealing with a submersion incident (as well as other incidents that might result in death) should include these resources. They should be summoned early in the recovery attempt, so that they are available as soon as possible. If such resources are not available, a lifeguard should be designated to provide any and all possible support to the family. This is true both for recovered victims who do not survive and in cases where the victim is not recovered and presumed to have died.

Debriefing and Counseling

Once search and rescue procedures are concluded, the incident commander should terminate command and return lifeguards to regular duty assignments as needed. Careful documentation of the event should be made for further investigation. In addition to standard incident reports, many agencies will require all involved lifeguards to prepare a narrative report and to participate in a debriefing session or operational critique. A major emphasis of this process should be development of ideas that will help do an even better job in the future. Any drowning in a lifeguarded area should be fully investigated.

Like all emergency personnel, lifeguards are susceptible to psychological trauma. Each person handles these situations in their own way. Supervisors should be prepared to offer support. Some agencies conduct a type of counseling called critical incident stress debriefing (CISD) as a routine following major incidents. Employee assistance programs, local crisis intervention services, and on-call psychiatrists may also be a source of assistance. Lifeguard supervisors should be careful to offer assistance to all employees and to watch for any unusual behavior that might suggest that a lifeguard is having particular difficulty in coping. See the chapter on *Lifeguard Health and Safety* for more on this topic.

Chapter Summary

In this chapter, we have learned about the steps to take when a victim is observed or reported to have submerged. We have learned the tremendous importance of a rapid search effort. We have learned some common aquatic search methods and patterns. We have learned the importance of in-water ventilations for a recovered victim and how to provide them. We have learned the importance of sensitively handling a recovered body and assisting relatives and families. We have also learned the importance of looking out for problems lifeguards may face in dealing with a death at their beach.

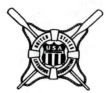

Discussion Points

- Why is the time available for recovery and resuscitation of a submerged victim so brief?
- Why is backup so important in responding to a report of a missing swimmer?
- What are some ways to fix and retain the location of the last seen point?
- What are some general search methods?
- What are some example search patterns?
- Why are immediate, in-water ventilations so important for a non-breathing victim?
- How should recovery of a body be handled when resuscitation is not appropriate?
- What are some steps that can be taken to address psychological trauma of relatives and friends of the victim?
- What are some steps that can be taken to address psychological trauma of lifeguards?

References

American Heart Association (2000a). Guidelines 2000 for cardiopulmonary resuscitation and emergency cardiovascular care. *Circulation, 102,* 8: II–234.

American Heart Association (2000b). Guidelines 2000 for cardiopulmonary resuscitation and emergency cardiovascular care. *Circulation, 102,* 8: I–51.

International Life Saving Federation Medical Commission (2001). *Statement on in-water resuscitation.* Leuven, Belgium: International Life Saving Federation.

Szpilman M.D., D., Orlowski, M.D., J., Brewster, B. C., & Mackie, M.D., I (2002). *In-water resuscitation—is it worthwhile?* World Congress on Drowning 2002. Amsterdam: Maatschappij tot Redding van Drnkelingen.

Chapter 18
Medical Care in the Aquatic Environment

In this chapter, you will learn some special considerations for providing medical care in the aquatic environment. These include recommended training and equipment, as well as general treatment guidelines and tips. You will learn methods for treating injuries from drowning, aquatic life, spinal trauma, and cold water. You will also learn about legal issues related to rendering medical care.

CHAPTER EXCERPT

Many of the back injuries a lifeguard will encounter involve people who walk up to the lifeguard complaining of neck or back injury sustained during water recreation, such as bodysurfing or a shallow water dive in which the bottom was struck. Recognition and immobilization are of tremendous importance to minimize further injury. The lifeguard should not assume that because the victim is able to walk, there is no serious spinal injury—there may well be injuries which could cause immediate, irreparable harm through one inadvertent movement.

The beach and open water comprise a natural, ever-changing environment with many dynamic forces at work. These forces, combined with the wide variety of physical recreational activities in which beach users participate, make injury and illness inevitable, even commonplace. Injuries which happen away from the beach, such as traffic or in-home accidents, typically result in the response of emergency medical aid providers to the scene, sometimes from significant distances; but when people are injured at the beach, lifeguards are an immediate source of emergency medical attention. Lifeguards are almost always the *first responders* to medical aid needs at the beach. It has therefore long been recognized that open water lifeguards must have adequate medical aid training to provide immediate medical care and to evaluate the need for further medical care.

In the case of minor injuries, the primary care rendered by lifeguards is usually adequate to fully resolve the immediate needs of the victim. These are the vast majority of cases handled by lifeguards. More serious injuries, such as difficulty breathing or loss of consciousness, require both the immediate care of lifeguards and assistance from providers with more advanced medical training and equipment. This will typically involve response of ambulance personnel and transportation to a medical facility; however, lifeguards must be capable of supporting life, sometimes for an extended period of time, until a higher medical authority can take over.

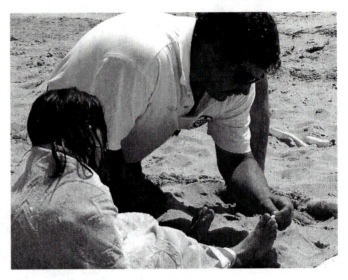

Lifeguard treats a bee sting.

Credit: Nick Steers

The information provided in this chapter and elsewhere in this manual regarding the treatment of injury and illness is intended to supplement approved courses in emergency medical aid. These courses usually do not go into great depth on issues specific to the aquatic environment. Lifeguards may find the information in this chapter a valuable supplement to other medical aid training they have received; however this is not a complete medical aid course and lifeguards should never practice any emergency medical aid technique beyond their level of training and qualifications.

Lifeguard Medical Training

To ensure that all open water lifeguards are prepared to perform at appropriate levels, USLA sets minimum recommended standards for emergency medical training. All open water lifeguards should be currently certified as having successfully completed a course in providing one person adult, two person adult, child, and infant cardiopulmonary resuscitation (CPR), including obstructed airway training. In addition to CPR training, lifeguards working on an hourly or seasonal basis should, at a minimum, have 21 hours of first aid training, including certification in a recognized course; however, USLA encourages that these lifeguards be certified in a course equivalent to U.S. Department of Transportation *First Responder*. For full-time open water lifeguards, the minimum recommended standard is *First Responder*; however, USLA encourages that these lifeguards be certified at the level of *Emergency Medical Technician*.

Lifeguard agencies should ensure that lifeguard personnel receive ongoing, in-service emergency medical care training, to supplement their basic training. This helps ensure that skills are maintained, that lifeguards can work as a team in an emergency, and that all established protocols are carefully followed. In-service training should also include top-

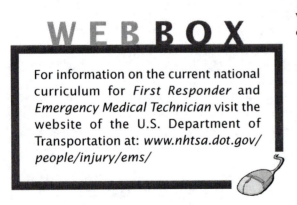

WEBBOX

For information on the current national curriculum for *First Responder* and *Emergency Medical Technician* visit the website of the U.S. Department of Transportation at: *www.nhtsa.dot.gov/people/injury/ems/*

ics relating to the local beach environment, use of oxygen, and automatic external defibrillators (AED), as needed.

Lifeguard Medical Equipment

USLA also sets recommended standards for medical equipment which should be made available to lifeguards. This includes:

- *First Aid Kit for Minor Injuries*—One at each staffed lifeguard post (including response vehicles).
- *First Aid Kit for Major Injuries*—One at each staffed beach area.
- *Oxygen*—Readily accessible at each staffed beach area, with all lifeguard personnel trained in its use.
- *Spinal Stabilization Equipment*—This includes a spineboard, head and neck immobilization devices, and fastening devices, readily accessible at each staffed beach area.
- *Cardiac Defibrillator*—One readily accessible at each staffed beach area, with personnel trained in its use. This is a requirement for lifeguard agencies seeking advanced level certification by USLA and recommended for all others.

First aid supplies and each first aid kit should be clean and properly stocked at all times. As supplies are depleted during the day, they should be immediately restocked as necessary. Oxygen and other medical equipment should also be inspected daily, and maintained in a ready condition at all times.

Providing Medical Care

Lifeguards should provide care in accordance with their training, policies, and any applicable regulations. Guidelines are available for lifeguards which address the fact that in many cases, they are asked to treat people for injuries and then to release them from care. This requires careful judgment to ensure that a person who might need further care, particularly at a higher level, is not released from care or left with the impression that no further assistance is needed.

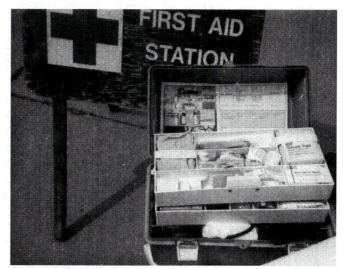

Levels of Injury

For purposes of classification and communication, injuries that lifeguards commonly encounter can be divided into three levels.

Minor Injuries

Minor injuries are conditions unlikely to require medical treatment beyond primary

Credit: Dan McCormick

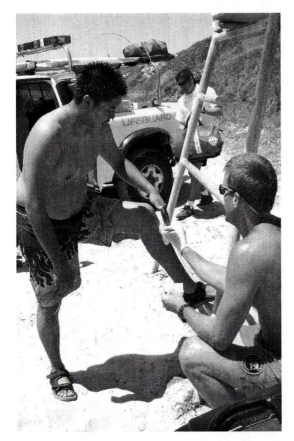

Credit: Ken Kramer

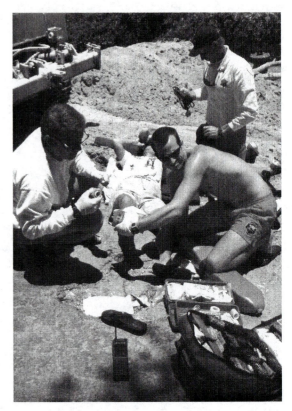

Credit: Ken Kramer

care. The vast majority of injuries sustained at beaches involve minor abrasions, cuts, and scrapes which can be quickly and effectively treated by lifeguards.

Intermediate Injuries

Intermediate injuries are those which are not immediately life-threatening, but which require further care at a medical facility. These are injuries like minor lacerations that require sutures, minor puncture wounds to the extremities, and other similar injuries. Intermediate injuries present a dilemma. Should an ambulance be called or should the victim be allowed to leave with only an admonition that a doctor be consulted? The best advice may be to err on the side of caution, encouraging that an ambulance be summoned, but accepting the fact that a conscious adult may decline this level of care. For minors however, release from care in the case of an intermediate injury is not recommended and may be prohibited by law or regulation. If an adult declines further care beyond what the lifeguard offers, lifeguards should first stabilize the injury to the greatest extent possible, then document both their recommendation for further medical care and the patient's refusal. See the chapter on *Records and Reports* for appropriate forms. Preprinted maps with directions to the nearest medical care facilities can be very helpful in these cases.

Major Injuries

A major injury is defined as any injury or illness requiring urgent care at a medical facility. This includes immediately life-threatening injuries, such as uncontrolled bleeding, as well as those which are not immediately life-threatening, such as a simple, closed fracture. The recognition and assessment of some major injuries will indicate the need to activate an emergency operation plan.

Treatment Guidelines

The following are some general guidelines for treating injuries and ailments, which may be modified in accordance with the severity of injury and general circumstances:

1. Determine whether the area where the victim is found is safe to enter without further risk to lifeguards or the victim, and mitigate any continuing threat to safety.
2. Summon necessary backup.
3. Use universal precautions for infection control.
4. Treat immediate problems according to level of medical training, including:
   A. Airway
   B. Breathing
   C. Circulation
5. Determine mechanism of injury.
6. Conduct a full assessment for any and all injuries.
7. Stabilize injuries according to medical protocol and level of training.
8. Avoid moving the victim until the full extent of injury is determined.
9. Monitor and record vital signs.
10. Protect body temperature.
11. Make the victim as comfortable as possible.
12. Recommend further treatment in cases that victim is not transported to the hospital. (See *Treatment Tips* below.)
13. Document your actions.

Treatment Tips

In addition to general guidelines for treating injuries, the following tips should help lifeguards address issues they will commonly encounter.

- *Prioritize Responsibilities*—Treating a minor injury that does not require immediate care may not take precedence over water surveillance. Ensure that drowning prevention activities are not unduly interrupted. If necessary, call for backup.
- *Inspect and Treat the Injury*—Beach users occasionally request medical supplies for self-treatment of minor injuries, without revealing the injury. This should be discouraged. Lifeguards are typically better trained and qualified to provide this assistance. Furthermore, a request for medical supplies is often, in reality, a veiled request for medical assistance. Lifeguards should offer to assist in treatment and take reasonable steps to ensure that the injury is no more serious than the person believes.

Direct treatment by the lifeguard helps ensure that wounds are treated properly and demonstrates the concern and capabilities of lifeguard personnel.

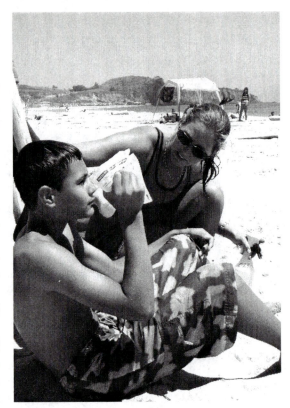

Credit: Ken Kramer

- *Assess Carefully*—The assessment of injuries requires good judgment and skills on the part of the lifeguard. The victim may be in a state of denial, but once lifeguard care is initiated, it is critical to conduct a thorough evaluation and to give good advice.

- *Treat Carefully and Thoroughly*—Whenever a lifeguard initiates medical treatment for an injury, the lifeguard undertakes a responsibility to treat properly. A carelessly treated laceration, for example, may become infected later, resulting in serious complications well beyond the severity of the initial injury.

- *Treat Minors with Care*—Even in the case of minor injuries, it is not a good practice to dispense medical supplies to minors in lieu of treatment. If there is a parent or an adult supervisor of the minor readily available, the lifeguard should make sure that the adult knows of the injury, preferably before treatment. If the adult wishes to treat the child using lifeguard supplies, it may be allowed. In the unusual event that a parent or guardian refuses treatment for a child who is clearly in need, a higher level of medical authority should be summoned. Police should also be summoned, as this may constitute neglect or abuse. If there is no adult accompanying the child, lifeguards will usually need to treat the injury, then take steps to make sure that a parent or legal guardian is notified.

- *Keep Bystanders Back*—A pushing crowd can aggravate the fear and anxiety of an injured person. Keeping onlookers away and calming bystanders can greatly assist the victim. In this effort, a courteous, but firm approach is best. Attempt to gain compliance if possible, but make it clear in a low key manner that compliance with the perimeter that has been established will be necessary. Police officers may be needed in some cases.

- *Maintain Control*—In a medical emergency, other beach visitors may offer assistance, suggest treatment, and try to take over care. It is not rare to have bystanders state, "I am a nurse," or "I am an EMT." These cases can be difficult. The lifeguard doesn't know the person or their actual level of training, but doesn't want to prevent care from a qualified medical provider with a higher level of training. Nonetheless, there are many examples of individuals professing to have high levels of medical qualifications who are later found to be impostors. While trained bystanders can often assist with stabilizing the victim, it is important for lifeguards to maintain control of the situation and keep treatment within the lines of established protocols.

- *Use Discretion*—The beach is a very public place. If treatment of a wound will require removal of clothing, it may be best to bring the victim inside, if possible. Privacy is a secondary issue in the case of a life-threatening injury, but it should be considered. When clothing must be removed or private areas of the body must be treated, it is best to try to have a lifeguard of the same sex as the victim handle treatment. If this is not possible, it is best to have another lifeguard present. While this may seem to create an additional violation of the person's privacy, it may be prudent to avoid a later complaint that liberties were taken.

- *Avoid Inappropriate Release from Care*—Lifeguards must be careful not to release a person whose status may quickly deteriorate. A person with blood loss from a head laceration, for example, might lose consciousness while driving to the hospital for sutures. It is therefore wise to establish guidelines to aid in this decision. (Please see the section on *Resuscitation of Drowning Victims* in this chapter for specific advice on release of drowning victims.) Some lifeguard agencies prefer to simply avoid such judgment calls due to the level of responsibility placed on the lifeguard. At these agencies, a higher level of care is *always* sought before the victim is released. Release of a minor from care without prior notification of a parent or guardian should be avoided. This must also take into account the extent of injury. As a general rule, minors with intermediate or major injuries should never be released after treatment. Either parents should be summoned to the scene or the minor should be turned over to an ambulance for transportation to the hospital. On the other hand, if lifeguards were required to summon a parent for every stubbed toe treated, lifeguard stations would be full of minors waiting for parents. In some areas, notification prior to release of a minor from care is a requirement of law.

- *Encourage Follow-Up Treatment*—For all but the most minor injuries, it is wise to recommend that victims follow up with their physicians. Even minor cuts can become major problems later.

- *Document Treatment and Advice*—The treatment provided, advice rendered, and all recommendations for further treatment of injuries should be carefully documented on medical reports. Example reports for this purpose can be found in *Appendix B*.

Resuscitation of Drowning Victims

Drowning victims may be conscious and alert or they may be unconscious. They may have a pulse with no respirations or they may have neither. To supplement the medical training of lifeguards, this section details some specific guidelines for treatment of drowning victims. If the victim is recovered in the water, follow guidelines for in-water resuscitation detailed in the chapter on *Underwater Search and Rescue*.

Positioning the Drowning Victim

On a sloping beach, the victim should be placed in a position parallel to the waterline, lying supine, so that the body is level. Do not position the victim head-down on the slope of the beach, as this will increase the likelihood of vomiting. Be sure to bring the victim far enough up the beach to avoid uprush, especially considering anticipated wave and tidal action. The first lifeguard takes a kneeling position on the side of the victim closest to the water. By leaning up the slope of the beach instead of down the slope of the beach while providing medical care, the lifeguard can work without falling forward over the victim, and can protect the victim from unexpected uprush. (International Life Saving Federation, 2003)

Oxygen

When a drowning victim is recovered from the water, the person is typically experiencing severe hypoxia. Immediate resuscitation efforts are therefore needed, ideally with administration of 100% oxygen and, if possible, positive pressure ventilation. (Orlowski & Szpilman, 2001) The administration of oxygen requires appropriate training, which all open water lifeguards should receive. You can provide oxygen in several ways, including:

- *Mouth-to-Mouth or Mouth-to-Mask*—Mouth-to-mouth and mouth-to-mask breathing, without use of supplemental oxygen, provides an approximately 16% concentration of oxygen.

- *Oronasal Mask*—By using a supplemental bottle of oxygen attached to an oronasal mask as you provide rescue breaths, you raise the oxygen concentration from 16% to as high as 50% or more.

- *Non-Rebreather Mask*—By providing supplemental oxygen through a non-rebreather mask to a person who is breathing spontaneously, you can deliver 60% oxygen or more depending on the delivery system.

- *Demand Valve*—By providing supplemental oxygen through a demand valve, you can provide 100% oxygen to a breathing or non-breathing victim. This method also provides positive pressure.

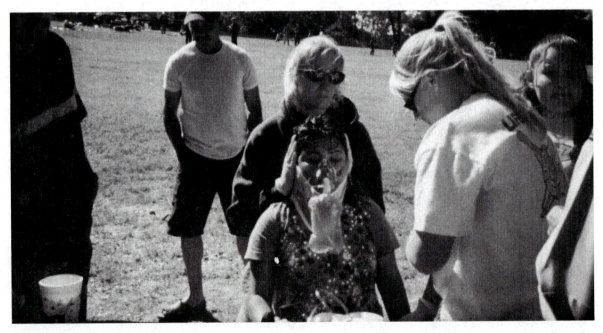

Non-Rebreather mask on a patient.
Credit: Dan McCormick

- *Bag-Valve-Mask*—By providing supplemental oxygen through a BVM, you can provide 100% oxygen to a non-breathing victim. This method also provides positive pressure.

Oxygen units require regular service whether they are used or not. If left unused, the equipment can deteriorate and leak. Equipment that is used or moved frequently can experience bumps, falls and other accidents that can cause mechanical problems. Oxygen cylinders should be visually inspected every time they are refilled and hydrostatically (pressure) tested every five years. Lifeguard agencies should maintain enough oxygen cylinders to ensure that there are always enough full bottles for reasonably anticipated demand. Empty bottles should be clearly marked and expeditiously filled. The oxygen regulator should receive an annual service check.

Abdominal Thrusts

Abdominal thrusts (the Heimlich maneuver) should not be used in resuscitation of drowning victims, except in cases that repeated repositioning of the airway suggests a foreign body obstruction (other than water). This maneuver will not remove significant amounts of water from the lungs. It may cause regurgitation and aspiration of stomach contents and other serious complications to resuscitation and recovery of the victim. (American Heart Association, 2000) (Orlowski & Szpilman, 2001)

Defibrillators

Automatic external defibrillators (AED) are becoming a common tool of lifeguards. They are primarily intended to correct problems associated with sudden cardiac arrest. AEDs can sometimes stop *ventricular fibrillation*, an uncoordinated beating of the heart. Ventricular fibrillation is rare in submersion victims. (Orlowski & Szpilman, 2001) (Morley, 2002) Most drowning victims have healthy hearts that simply cease to function due to hypoxia. The best approach in treating drowning victims is to prioritize immediate CPR measures, ideally with high flow oxygen. If available, an AED should be used, after appropriate training and in accordance with the manufacturer's instructions, in the relatively unlikely case the victim is experiencing ventricular fibrillation. AEDs have been shown to be safe for use in a wet (not immersed) environment.

Release of Drowning Victims from Care

Whenever a victim has aspirated water in a drowning incident, but is conscious, the lifeguard must make a determination whether further treatment is needed or the victim can be released from care. The International Life Saving Federation Medical Commission (2000) has developed the following guidelines to help lifeguards determine who should be sent to the hospital as a result of complications from drowning. Such determinations should be made with great care. If in doubt, consult a higher medical authority. As previously explained, minors require special consideration.

1. The following people should be sent to the hospital in most cases:
   - Any victim who lost consciousness even for a brief period.
   - Any victim who required rescue breathing.
   - Any victim who required cardiopulmonary resuscitation.
   - Any victim in whom a serious condition is suspected such as heart attack, spinal injury, other injury, asthma, epilepsy, stinger, intoxication, delirium, etc.

2. The following people may be considered for release from care at the scene if, after 10-15 minutes of careful observation, while being warmed with blankets or other coverings as required, the victim meets *all* of the requirements listed below. In such cases, it is unwise for the victim to drive a vehicle and the victim should be so advised. If any of these conditions do not apply or if the lifeguard has any doubt, then the victim should be transported to the hospital or advised to seek early medical attention.

   - No cough
   - Normal rate of breathing
   - Normal circulation as measured by pulse in strength and rate and blood pressure (if available)
   - Normal color and skin perfusion
   - No shivering
   - Fully conscious, awake and alert
   - An oxyhemoglobin saturation level over 95% (if a pulse oximeter is available)

3. There is always a risk of delayed lung complications. All immersion victims should therefore be warned that if they later develop cough, breathlessness, fever, or any other worrying symptom, they should seek medical advice immediately. It is preferable that these persons not return to a home environment where they are alone for the next 24 hours. Special care and observation should be given to child victims.

Injuries from Aquatic Life

Various types of aquatic life, discussed in the chapter *Aquatic Life and Related Hazards*, can cause injuries ranging from minor to major. This section includes specific treatment recommendations for common injuries from these sources.

Bites

If a swimmer is bitten by a predatory fish, it is crucial to get the victim out of the water. This will help prevent blood from entering the water, potentially provoking additional bites. (For shark bites, see the chapter on *Special Rescues*.) Minor wounds should be cleansed and disinfected. Major wounds require immediate transport to a medical facility. A tetanus shot should be recommended.

Stings

Lifeguard treatment procedures for wounds from stings may vary, based on the level of medical training, locally prevalent species, and local medical protocols. The victim should first be evaluated for any reaction that extends beyond pain and any bleeding controlled. Advanced medical care and transportation to the hospital should be carefully considered for more serious reactions or for stings to areas other than the foot or ankle. Procedures to protect against shock should be employed as appropriate.

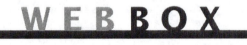

WEBBOX

You can read about marine stingers and best treatment for them at: *www.marine-medic.com/*

Jellyfish and Portuguese Man-of-War

For most jellyfish and Portuguese man-of-war stings in the U.S., unless there are medical complications beyond pain, the lifeguard's primary role is calming the victim and providing pain relief. First check to see if there are any tentacles remaining on the victim's skin. If so, they may contain nematocysts that have yet to sting. They should be washed off using seawater (freshwater will cause the nematocysts to sting), then removed with the fingers.

Ideally, the lifeguard should use a medical glove to remove the tentacles. If none is available, the pads of the fingers are thick and only a slight tingling will normally be felt. The lifeguard's hands must be washed immediately afterward though, because touching other areas of the body with the hands may produce painful stinging. Once this is accomplished, properly wrapped ice or an ice pack should be applied to the area of the sting until the stinging sensation fades.

Numerous solutions have been advocated over the years to treat these stings. They include urine, lemon juice, papaya, ammonia, vinegar, meat tenderizer, sodium bicarbonate, and commercial products, which are typically a derivative of these. None have been scientifically proven to work. (Williamson, Fenner, Burnett, & Rifkin 1996) Often the logic used in advocating these solutions is that they will stop the nematocysts from further stinging, but if the lifeguard properly removes tentacles and rinses the area with seawater, there should be no remaining nematocysts. Therefore, at this point, the only concern is to treat the pain of the sting, not to prevent further stinging.

As in all cases of medical aid, the victim's condition should be monitored closely. Special precautions, which may include transport to a medical facility, should be considered for those with a history of reactions to insect bites and stings. Any person with extensive stings or stings to the face, particularly in the case of children, may require hospital transport.

Stingray

In some areas, stingray envenomation is a regular occurrence. Lifeguards in these areas routinely treat and release persons who have been stung in the foot or ankle, and who display no unusual complications. The wound is first checked to make sure that the sheath and barb are completely removed. Otherwise, envenomation will continue. Thereafter, the injury site is immersed in water as hot as the victim can tolerate without producing further injury to the tissue.

In most cases, hot water reduces the pain dramatically. The affected area is then left in the hot water until it can be removed without the pain returning. This sometimes takes an hour or more. During treatment, as the water cools, add more hot water to maintain temperature. In remote areas, where hot water is unavailable, hot sand or hot packs have been used with some success. Hot water from outboard and inboard engines, collected in a bucket, has even been used in some cases, but the victim's immersed limb should be protected from petroleum products in the water. Once pain subsides, the wound is dressed and bandaged, as appropriate to the lifeguard's medical training and presentation of the wound.

Penetrating wounds often become infected due to retained venom. The lifeguard should counsel a victim who is released from care to see a physician and to watch for any signs of infection. A tetanus shot should be considered, as death from tetanus after stingray envenomation has occurred. (Rathjen & Halstead, 1969)

Scorpionfish

Stepping on the spines of a scorpionfish can cause immediate and severe pain. Generally, this can be treated in a manner similar to that for a stingray; however, serious complications are more likely.

All victims of scorpionfish envenomation should be monitored closely for reactions and should be referred to a doctor. The doctor may need to remove remaining parts of the spine and provide a tetanus inoculation.

Sea Urchins

The spines of sea urchins cause penetrating wounds, and the spines often break off beneath the skin. More severe reactions to urchin wounds include weakness, loss of body sensation, facial swelling, and irregular pulse. Rare cases involving paralysis and respiratory distress have occurred.

Treatment for urchin wounds differs from agency to agency, but often includes the application of hot compresses or soaking the affected area in hot water. Follow-up with a doctor should be recommended, particularly if spines remain in the skin or infection develops. A tetanus shot may be appropriate.

Mollusks

The shells of a variety of mollusks can cause abrasions and lacerations. The wound should be cleansed and a sterile dressing applied. Serious cases may require transport to a medical facility. In cases where the victim is treated and released, the victim should be advised to seek further medical care if infection develops and to ensure current tetanus inoculation.

Coral

If necessary, coral cuts should be rinsed with seawater, as stinging nematocysts may be left on the skin and freshwater may cause them to sting. These cuts often become infected, requiring a physician's care and antibiotics. The victim should be counseled about this. A tetanus shot may be appropriate.

Snakes

Toxic signs, appearing within twenty minutes, can include malaise, anxiety, euphoria, muscle spasm, respiratory problems, convulsions, unconsciousness, and all signs of shock. Treatment appropriate to the presentation and immediate transport to a medical facility is generally appropriate.

Leeches

Many agencies on beaches with leech problems provide lifeguards with equipment to help detach and dispose of leeches. A common practice is to simply place salt directly on the leech, which typically causes it to release. Treatment for minor bleeding is usually sufficient.

Spinal Injuries

Trauma that involves significant force can result in damage to the spinal cord. This can lead to permanent quadriplegia (four extremity paralysis) or even death, depending on the specifics of the injury. If the victim survives a spinal cord injury, the impact can be devastating, both to victims and their families. Future lifelong care and tremendous medical expenditures will be required. Thankfully, many more people suffer damage to the spine (vertebral column) without spinal cord damage, thus without nerve damage or paralysis. Careful rescue, immobilization, and transportation of victims suspected of having sustained spinal injury is crucial, because slight errors can greatly worsen the victim's outcome. Open water lifeguards should be thoroughly trained in spinal immobilization techniques and practice them only in accordance with their training.

The first step in treatment of spinal injury victims is recognition. Any neck or back pain after injury (even trivial injury) or head trauma needs to be treated appropriately. Numbness, pins and needles, or weakness, even if temporary, are all serious signs of possible spinal injury. Maintaining airway, breathing, and circulation (ABC) takes precedence over spinal immobilization, but efforts to avoid spinal flexion in the process are appropriate.

If possible, the most experienced lifeguard available should direct the stabilization and rescue process. Unless the victim is in imminent mortal danger and must be moved quickly, all actions should be taken slowly, carefully, and in unison. The lifeguards' ultimate goal is to successfully immobilize the victim on a spineboard and rescue the person to a point where

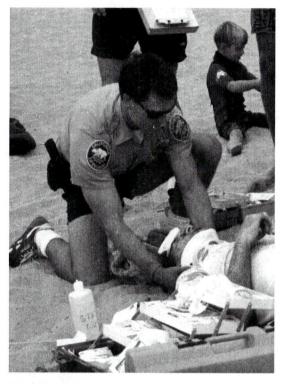

Credit: Ken Kramer

an ambulance can transport to the hospital, while doing no harm. The interim steps between recognition and transport are where the lifeguards' training and techniques most importantly come into play. The aim is to stabilize the spine and maintain the neck and back from further motion, usually in a neutral (straight) position or in the position of comfort. Proper immobilization will protect from further damage, and facilitate moving the victim. It will allow for efficient, more permanent immobilization. Specifics on strapping and movement should be taught and regularly practiced.

The best methods to use will depend on several factors:

- *Location*—Onshore or offshore, deep or shallow water, surf or flat water, distance from shore
- *Available Lifeguards*—Strength, training, and numbers
- *Victim*—Size and condition (i.e., walking or sitting, face up or face down, breathing or non-breathing, other injuries)
- *Available Equipment and Transportation*

Beach Presentation

Many of the spinal injuries a lifeguard will see involve people who walk up to the lifeguard complaining of neck or back injury sustained during water recreation, such as bodysurfing or a shallow water dive in which the bottom was struck. Recognition and immobilization are of tremendous importance to minimize further injury. The lifeguard should not assume that because the victim is able to walk, there is not serious injury to the spine—there may well be injuries which could cause immediate,

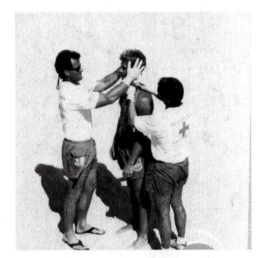

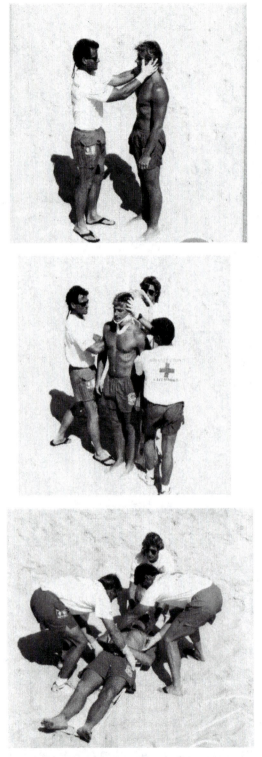

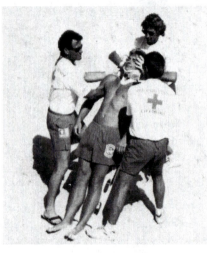

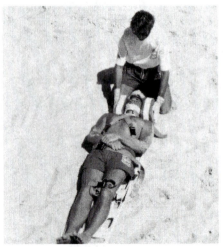

Standing backboard technique.

Credit: Mike Hensler

irreparable harm through one inadvertent movement. The very fact that the person has consulted with the lifeguard suggests significant concern. This victim should not be allowed to lie down. Instead, the *standing backboard technique* should be used.

One lifeguard moves to the rear of the victim and stabilizes the head and neck with one hand on each side. A second lifeguard applies a cervical collar. While the first lifeguard maintains neck stabilization (after application of the cervical collar), the backboard is slid in between the first lifeguard and the victim. At least two other lifeguards then stand facing the victim and grasp opposite sides of the spineboard through the victim's armpits and gently lower the board to the sand. Standard protocols for securing the victim to the spineboard are then followed.

Water Presentation

Victims found in the surf or floating in shallow water, or those seen diving, need appropriate precautionary care for possible spinal injury. Upon approaching a victim in the water with suspected spinal injury, avoid unnecessary turbulence. If the victim is not breathing, the face needs to be carefully removed from the water and rescue breathing begun as soon as possible, using appropriate techniques. The modified jaw thrust or jaw thrust maneuvers are the recommended airway methods. They allow the lifeguard to maintain the neck in as neutral a position as possible.

Recommended in-water spinal immobilization techniques involve one of three maneuvers. It is best to be skilled in more than one. Some are better under different conditions and none fit all circumstances ideally. Although names for these maneuvers vary, one or more are used by almost all lifesaving agencies throughout the world. For purposes of standardization, the names used in this section should be used for each technique.

Spineboards which float have been available for many years. Lifeguard agencies are encouraged to acquire these devices, since they can improve the quality of victim care by allowing full stabilization of the victim, even in deep water.

Vice Grip

The lifeguard approaches from the victim's side, places the lifeguard's dominant arm along the victim's sternum, and stabilizes the chin with the hand. The lifeguard's other arm is then placed along the spine with this hand cupping the back of the victim's head. The arms are squeezed together forming a vice which provides stabilization. Care must be taken to avoid excessive pressure on the airway. If the victim is face down, the vice grip is applied as described and the victim is slowly rotated toward the lifeguard.

This method is quickly and readily applied by any size lifeguard to any size victim. It works in deep or shallow water. It leaves the lifeguard in a good position to check respiratory status and carry out rescue breathing.

Body Hug

The lifeguard approaches the face-up victim from behind and partially submerges. The lifeguard then places the lifeguard's arms through the victim's armpits from the back and places the lifeguard's hands over the victim's ears, thus stabilizing the head. The lifeguard's face is placed next to the victim's head.

For a face-down victim, the technique is applied in a similar manner. The lifeguard reaches over the back and through the armpits of the victim and places the lifeguard's hands over the victim's ears. The lifeguard then rolls the victim toward the lifeguard, with the lifeguard submerging momentarily and then surfacing in the position described for a face-up victim. In this way, stabilization is maintained while the victim is turned to a face-up position.

This method provides exceptional immobilization. It may be impractical in shallow water though. It may not be applicable if there is a significant size mismatch between lifeguard and victim. A lone lifeguard cannot adequately perform rescue breathing using the body hug, although some modifications are used by some agencies. A change in the immobilization method is required before placing the victim on a spineboard.

Extended Arm Grip

Of the three methods, this is probably the most unique and complex method. The lifeguard takes a position at the victim's side and grabs the victim's arms just above the elbow right to right and left to left. The lifeguard then carefully raises the victim's arms above the victim's head pressing them together against the ears. This immobilizes the victim's head and neck. This head grip can be maintained by the lifeguard with only one hand holding the victim's two arms together. Further stability can be obtained if the lifeguard uses two hands with the lifeguard's thumbs supporting the back of the victim's head. A face-down victim has the method applied as above. The victim is then gently glided head first and slowly rolled toward the lifeguard, thus positioning the victim in the crook of the lifeguards arm.

This method can allow the lifeguard a free hand to support the body or to check for respirations and

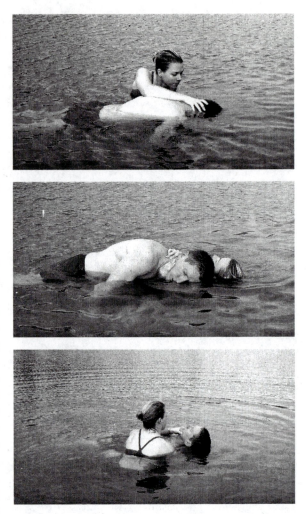

Vice Grip.
Credit: Sandra McCormick

begin rescue breathing. It can even allow a free arm for side or back stroke to assist in moving the victim toward shore or recovering the victim from a submerged position. It works in deep or shallow water and is arguably the only method for a single lifeguard to roll a victim in the surf zone or extremely shallow water. This is done using one hand to apply the overhead arm pressure and the other to roll the victim's hips. It further allows for easy transition to a spineboard. There may be some concerns about the degree of immobilization provided with this method, especially toward flexion forces.

Rescue to Shore

If in deep water and if a floating spineboard is available, carefully submerge it under the victim and secure the victim to it with the least amount of movement possible. If not, the victim should be carefully moved toward shore or a rescue boat. As a last resort, the lifeguard could place a rescue tube under the lifeguard's armpits and continue the immobilization until further help arrives, possibly kicking toward shore in the meantime. Each lifeguard agency should have all lifeguards practice coordinated transition from these methods to spineboard stabilization. All appropriate equipment needs to be readily available and frequently checked, including straps and C-spine immobilization.

Placing a victim on a spineboard is not possible with one lifeguard and difficult with less than three. More are helpful. The victim should be kept in shallow water until further help and equipment arrive, unless waves or cold water preclude this option. When holding or moving a victim in surf conditions, attempt to keep the victim's body perpendicular to incoming waves, in order to limit movement.

Cold Water Injuries

All cold water immersion victims should be quickly rescued. Those victims who have been in cold water for a considerable time, and who are breathing, should be rescued in a near horizontal attitude, if possible, to prevent a potentially adverse fall in blood pressure. (Golden, Hervey, & Tipton, 1991) Those whose airways are threatened should be rescued by the quickest method, regardless of body attitude.

Victims who are not in need of resuscitation and who are not severely hypothermic should have wet clothing removed and replaced with dry clothing, if available. They should then be wrapped in warm, dry blankets, making sure that their airways

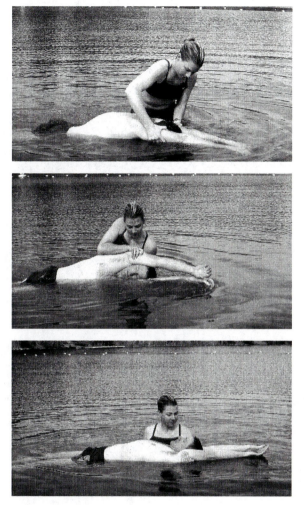

Extended Arm Grip.
Credit: Sandra McCormick

are clear and supported. Conscious shivering survivors will usually rewarm themselves reasonably quickly, but the process can be accelerated by immersion in a bath of warm water or a warm shower. When recovered, they should be removed from the bath to avoid overwarming. In cases of severe hypothermia active rewarming should be avoided until the patient is in a hospital setting.

In case of unconsciousness or apparent cardiac arrest, the airway should be cleared and appropriate procedures should be employed according to CPR protocols. It may be difficult to assess whether the unconscious victim of hypothermia has a heartbeat, because the heartbeat may be extremely slow and a pulse hard to assess. Check carefully for a carotid pulse for at least 60 seconds to ensure that cardiac compressions are not used unless the heart has stopped. Since drowning victims are typically starved of oxygen, pay particular attention to ventilating the victim, ideally with oxygen. Arrange rapid transfer to the hospital.

In those who are apparently dead, avoid a hasty diagnosis. The maxim *no one is dead until they are warm and dead* is appropriate provided you are not too remote from medical support. Follow resuscitation protocols and arrange rapid transport to the hospital. People, especially small children, who have been submerged for up to an hour in ice-cold water have been successfully resuscitated in the hospital. (Bolte, Black, Bowers, Kent-Thorne, & Correli, 1988) People who have experienced serious hypothermia, even if successfully revived, should always be sent to the hospital to be checked for pulmonary complications. (Modell, 1971)

One very rare complication of contact with cold water is *cold urticaria*. It can occur in water as warm as 60 degrees, perhaps warmer. This condition is an allergy-like reaction to contact with cold water, as well as other sources of cold. (Bentley, 1993) Within minutes, the skin may become itchy, red, and swollen. Fainting, very low blood pressure, and shock-like symptoms can present. In cases of apparent cold water urticaria, removal from the source of cold is essential. Treatment is similar to that for any allergic reaction, with priority being given to maintaining breathing and circulation. (Bentley, 1993) (Mathelier-Fusade & Pascale, 1998)

Legal Issues

Providing medical care in the aquatic environment, like anywhere else, involves certain responsibilities on the part of those providing this care. They are expected to act in an appropriate manner. Determining appropriate care is sometimes a matter of law and legal precedent.

Standard of Care

Standard of care is a legal term. In medicine, it generally refers to the care a person being treated has a right to expect based on common standards of medical practice. For example, a doctor who fails to provide a patient with important information about possible outcomes of a surgery the patient is considering might be found to have breached the accepted standard of care, particularly if most doctors in a similar situation would have provided this information. Since lifeguards provide medical care, they too must perform according to the standard of care. For example, medical aid courses lifeguards typically undergo instruct that bleeding can be controlled in several specific ways. If a lifeguard treats a person with uncontrolled bleeding and fails to attempt all of the methods the lifeguard has been taught, the lifeguard may be found to have breached the standard of care. That is, most lifeguards in the same situation would have implemented all of the common steps for controlling bleeding in the proper order.

In some cases, standard of care is set by law or regulation. In other cases, it is a concept based on common practice and reasonable expectation. Failure to meet the standard of care sometimes goes unnoticed. In other cases, particularly if the failure to perform to the accepted standard of care is believed to have resulted in unnecessary injury, legal liability may be found. In receiving emergency medical care, the victim typically places great trust in the actions of the person providing that care. It is important, both for moral and legal reasons for lifeguards to ensure that trust is well founded.

Each lifeguard agency should set limits on the emergency medical care that lifeguards are authorized to provide depending on local laws and policies. The provision and use of any special medical or rescue equipment should be restricted to those lifeguards who have received specific training in its use and who are specifically authorized.

Duty to Act and Abandonment

Because lifeguards are appropriately expected by the public to be knowledgeable in emergency medical care, visitors will look to lifeguards for advice and treatment. Lifeguards are considered to have a duty to act. Even when the lifeguard is confused or unsure about a particularly complicated injury or illness, it is important to follow through by carrying out the basic steps of care based on the lifeguard's level of training. In such situations, lifeguards should remember the medical credo, *do no harm*, as a reminder to be conservative and deliberate. Once treatment has begun for an injury, it should not be stopped until the situation is controlled, treatment is turned over to a higher medical authority, or consent is denied. Once CPR has begun, for example, it should not be stopped until the victim is revived or an authorized medical authority has determined that further attempts should be terminated.

One situation which can result in a charge of abandonment at a beach facility occurs when a bystander attempts to take over treatment and the lifeguard acquiesces, leaving the victim in the hands of the bystander. A lifeguard has no legal duty to relinquish control of a victim and should not do so until and unless it has been clearly established that the bystander is of equal or higher medical authority and willing to accept medical responsibility. Identification and documentation of the bystander's medical training is critical. In a major medical emergency, lifeguard personnel should maintain control of the situation until it can be turned over to the responding emergency medical service.

Consent

An adult has the right to refuse treatment. Exceptions may include people who are obviously delirious or otherwise unable to make reasonable decisions. In general, an unconscious person of any age is considered to have given implied consent for emergency treatment. If an apparently coherent adult declines treatment, it is best to ask the person to sign a waiver of treatment to help indemnify the lifeguard and lifeguard agency. Witness names should also be included. Most emergency medical services have special release forms that can help to absolve agencies of responsibility for refused treatment.

When treating minors, the most significant concern beyond treatment is the importance of gaining parental consent. Most lifeguard agencies establish strict policies regarding notification of parents before, during, or after medical treatment. In cases of life-threatening injuries, care should not be delayed for this purpose, but parents should be contacted as soon as reasonably possible. Parents and legal guardians may generally refuse treatment on behalf of minors, but at a certain point, this may border on child abuse or negligent care. If a parent refuses treatment for a minor in obvious and serious need, it may be prudent to contact police or a child welfare agency. Some states require emergency medical personnel to make notifications in any case of suspected child abuse.

Medications

Lifeguards should not dispense medication of any kind unless certified to do so and authorized in writing by an appropriate medical authority. Most lifeguard agencies establish policies prohibiting lifeguards from dispensing medications, including non-prescription remedies. This may include over the counter medications such as aspirin and aspirin substitutes.

Confidentiality

A variety of laws and regulations protect the confidentiality of people who receive medical care. The best advice is never to release any information regarding treatment provided to a victim or their medical status unless they specifically authorize (in writing) release of that information. Exceptions include people with a medical need and legal right to know. A paramedic arriving at the beach to take over care of the victim has both a medical need and legal right to be updated on the victim's status, history, etc. The same is true of the treating physician or an emergency room nurse. On the other hand, a news reporter has no right to medical information about a victim. Releasing such information may result in liability to the lifeguard and lifeguard agency. Similarly, while parents normally have the right to complete information about their minor child's medical condition and treatment, an acquaintance of a victim, even a close friend, generally does not. When in doubt, release nothing and consult with a supervisor.

Chapter Summary

In this chapter, we have learned the minimum medical training and equipment levels appropriate for open water lifeguards. We have learned to classify levels of injuries, along with some general medical care guidelines and tips. We have learned about resuscitation of drowning victims, including proper positioning, the value of oxygen, and when it is appropriate to release a drowning victim from care. We have learned about treating injuries inflicted by aquatic life, including bites, stings, and other injuries. We have learned about treatment of spinal injuries, both on the beach and in the water. We have learned how to treat victims of cold water injuries. And we have learned ways to ensure that medical care is provided in a manner consistent with legal requirements.

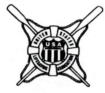

Discussion Points

- What are some reasons open water lifeguards should have strong CPR and medical aid skills?
- Why is it important to have medical aid equipment readily available?
- Why is it important to refer people who have been provided medical aid to their doctor for follow-up?
- What are some key points to remember in the resuscitation of drowning victims?
- Why is ice an appropriate treatment for jellyfish stings?
- Why is the standing backboard technique important for lifeguards?
- What are some considerations in stabilizing a spinal injury victim in the water?
- What are some warming techniques for conscious victims of cold water immersion?
- What are some considerations for lifeguards to ensure that they provide medical care in a manner consistent with legal requirements?
- Under what conditions would it be acceptable to release information about the medical treatment and care of a victim?

References

American Heart Association (2000). Guidelines 2000 for Cardiopulmonary Resuscitation and Emergency Cardiovascular Care. *Circulation, 102,* 8.

Bentley II, Burton (1993). Cold-induced urticaria and angioedema: diagnosis and management. *American Journal of Emergency Medicine, 11,* 1: 43–46.

Bolte, R. G., Black, B. G., Bowers, R. S., Kent-Thorne, J., & Correli, H. M. (1988). The use of extracorporeal rewarming in a child submerged for 66 minutes. *Journal of the American Medical Association, 260,* 377–379.

Golden, F. St. C., Hervey, G. R. & Tipton, M. J. (1991). Circum-rescue collapse: collapse, sometimes fatal, associated with rescue of immersion victims. *Journal of the Royal Naval Medical Service, 77,* 139–49.

International Life Saving Federation (2000). *Statement on who needs further medical help after rescue from the water.* Leuven, Belgium: International Life Saving Federation.

International Life Saving Federation (2003). *Statement on positioning a victim on a sloping beach.* Leuven, Belgium: International Life Saving Federation.

Mathelier-Fusade & Pascale (1998). Clinical predictive factors of severity in cold urticaria (correspondence). *Archives of Dermatology, 134,* 106–107.

Modell, J. H. (1971). *Pathophysiology and Treatment of Drowning and Near-drowning.* Springfield, Ill: CC Thomas.

Morley, P. (2002). Unusual rescue circumstances and considerations. *World Congress on Drowning 2002.* Amsterdam, The Netherlands: Maatschappij tot Redding van Drenkelingen.

Orlowski, J. P. & Szpilman, D. (2001). Drowning, resuscitation, and reanimation. *Pediatric Clinics of North America, 48,* 3.

Rathjen W. F. & Halstead B. W. (1969). Report on two fatalities due to stingrays. *Toxicon, 6,* 301–302.

Williamson J. A., Fenner P. J., Burnett J., & Rifkin J. (Eds.). (1996). *Venomous and poisonous marine animals: a medical and biological handbook.* Sydney, Australia. New South Whales University Press.

Chapter 19
Scuba Related Illness and Treatment

The development of modern scuba equipment has helped diving grow into one of the more widely practiced aquatic sports. Exploring the underwater environment however, is not without risk. In this chapter you will learn about risks associated with scuba diving and how scuba works. You will learn about diving illnesses, including why they occur, how to identify them, and how to treat them. You will also learn about proper reporting of diving accidents.

CHAPTER EXCERPT

Some very important information to convey to the receiving emergency room is the patient's dive profile. How deep for how long? How many dives in the last 24-hours? Was there a rapid ascent? If the diver is unable to provide this information, the diver's depth gauge or dive computer may provide it. The dive buddy is another excellent source. The lifeguard can then call the emergency room physician with this information. Since many doctors are unfamiliar with the Divers Alert Network, the lifeguard should advise of DAN's free medical consultation services and *provide the DAN emergency telephone number.*

Risks Associated with Scuba Diving

It is difficult to judge the rate of injury associated with diving because the number of participants is unknown. Most estimates of the number of active scuba divers in the United States easily exceed 1 million. Divers Alert Network (DAN), a nonprofit, membership association dedicated to the safety of recreational scuba diving, provides annual statistics based on the number of reported injuries and deaths associated with scuba diving. DAN, which is affiliated with Duke University Medical Center, collects this information primarily from hyperbaric chambers used to treat scuba related illness. Most of the statistical information in this chapter is provided by DAN.

Divers Alert Network (DAN) 24-hour emergency hotline number: (919) 684-8111

Each year, DAN is notified of over 1,000 cases of possible decompression illness and other dive related injuries. (Vann & Uguccioni, 2001) Additional cases certainly occur about which DAN is not notified. During the 1990s, DAN collected reports of an average 88 dive fatalities per year involving U.S. citizens. (Vann & Uguccioni, 2001) Death may occur due to a number of factors. Drowning is the reported cause of over 55% of diving deaths, with diving illness responsible for about 20% of diving deaths, and cardiac arrest responsible for about 5%. (Vann & Uguccioni, 2001) Many complications of diving underwater might result in death by drowning, including running out of air, entrapment or entanglement, equipment malfunction, or panic. More than half the scuba divers in a national survey reported experiencing panic or near-panic behavior on one or more occasions. This included both novice and experienced divers. (Morgan, 1995)

While fatalities show a gradual, uneven decline since 1970, the number of reported decompression illness cases treated each year is gradually rising. (Vann & Uguccioni, 2001) This divergent trend may be due to a higher frequency of decompression illness or increased awareness about the disease and resultant tendency to seek treatment. The tendency to seek treatment may, in turn, have helped to reduce the number of fatalities.

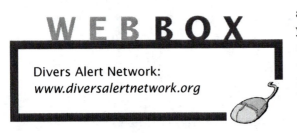

Divers Alert Network:
www.diversalertnetwork.org

Divers in the age range of 30 to 39 lead other age groups with dive injuries. Divers in the 40 to 59 year age range are most likely to be involved in fatal accidents. (Vann & Uguccioni, 2001) The experience of the diver is also a factor. Divers with two or fewer years of experience and divers with six or more years of experience make up the vast proportion of cases of injury and death. (Vann & Uguccioni, 2001)

How Scuba Works

Most scuba divers breathe air, which is compressed in two different ways—mechanically and by water pressure. Large amounts of air (not pure oxygen) are compressed into a scuba tank by a mechanical air compressor. This increases the air capacity of the tank. A regulator with a hose and mouthpiece attached is then used to breathe air from the tank. The regulator reduces the delivery pressure of the compressed air in the tank to ambient (surrounding) pressure, so that it can be inhaled normally without damaging the lungs.

Divers may also use mixed or altered breathing gases. These include nitrogen-oxygen (nitrox), helium-oxygen (heliox), or helium-nitrogen-oxygen (trimix). The use of mixed gases, which requires special training, generally allows the diver to avoid lengthy decompression stops when returning to the surface.

When air (or mixed gas) is made available through the regulator during a dive, it is inhaled at a pressure consistent with the depth of the dive. This is because as a diver descends, the ambient pres-

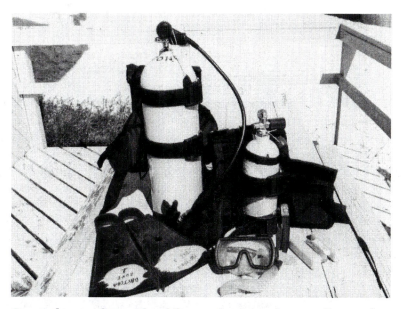

A regular scuba tank with regulator and a smaller tank, used by lifeguards for rapid search and recovery in shallow water.

Credit: Mike Hensler

sure becomes greater due to the increasing pressure of the water above. This pressure is expressed in *atmospheres*. Surface atmospheric pressure is 14.7 pounds per square inch (psi). This is known as one atmosphere of pressure. For every 33 feet a diver descends, an additional atmosphere of pressure is added. Therefore, a diver at 33 feet experiences two atmospheres of pressure, at 66 feet three atmospheres, at 99 feet four atmospheres, and so on.

As pressure of the water above increases, the volume of a given quantity of air decreases. For example, if a bubble of air at the surface were taken to two atmospheres (33 feet in depth), it would be reduced to one half its surface volume; at three atmospheres, one third its surface volume; at four atmospheres, one fourth its surface volume; and so on.

A diver at 33 feet in depth can breath normally through a properly functioning regulator, but the air is still compressed so that it is twice as dense as it would have been on the surface. However, the volume remains the same because regulators are designed to deliver air at the surrounding pressure. If this diver were to hold a breath while ascending to the surface, the volume of air in the lungs would double. Therefore, while the regulator reduces the pressure of compressed air from the scuba tank to a comfortable, breathable level, air breathed below the surface remains compressed by water pressure, compared to what its volume would be on the surface. For example, at 33 feet, air is two times (2X) as dense and at 66 feet, it is three times (3X) as dense.

Decompression Illness

Decompression illness (DCI), is the result of a bubble phenomenon which occurs in the body's tissues as the diver ascends to the surface, or at some point after the dive. There are two types of decompression illness: decompression sickness (DCS) and arterial gas embolism (AGE). The vast majority of scuba injuries involve decompression sickness, with AGE following at a much lesser frequency. (Vann & Uguccioni, 2001)

Decompression sickness, often called *the bends*, involves changes to dissolved nitrogen in the body. Nitrogen is an inert gas and plays no role in the body's metabolism. It makes up about 79% of the air we breathe and is carried through the bloodstream to the body's tissues as a normal process of circulation. As the diver breathes compressed gas underwater, the increased pressure during diving causes more nitrogen to be delivered to the body's tissues, thus, increasing the dissolved nitrogen content within the body's cells. As the diver slowly returns to the surface, nitrogen is eliminated by a gradual release back into the bloodstream where it can be eliminated by the lungs through respiration. If a diver ascends too rapidly to allow for the gradual release of nitrogen, bubbles can form in the bloodstream and body tissues, which can inhibit normal circulation. Decompression sickness most often occurs as a result of dives deeper than 80 feet and is strongly associated with repetitive, deep, and/or prolonged dives.

Dive tables were created many years ago to help scuba divers avoid decompression sickness. Through calculations based on these tables, divers can determine maximum depth and time profiles, as well as the number of dives they can make with relative safety in a day. *Dive tables* also help determine if in-water decompression stops must be made while ascending from various depths. These stops are intended to prolong the diver's ascent and allow the release of nitrogen from the tissues before it produces bubbles. This is known as *off-gassing*.

Many divers now use small, computerized gauges, attached to their scuba gear or on their wrists. Dive computers are known to interpret and calculate dive tables automatically and with more accuracy. Use of dive computers has been shown to reduce the likelihood of injury. According to DAN, "A diagnosis of AGE or barotraumas was two to three times more likely for divers who used dive tables and dive guides than for those who used dive computers." (Vann & Uguccioni, 2001) This is likely due to error avoidance in dive table calculations by divers and to ascent indicators found on dive computers that alert divers to an ascent that is too rapid.

Arterial gas embolism (AGE), also known as air embolism, occurs when compressed air is trapped in the alveoli—the small sacs in the lungs where exchange of carbon dioxide and oxygen take place. AGE most often results from a rapid ascent, which may occur when the diver runs low on air or is out of air. (Dovenbarger, 1992) In a panicked ascent, divers may hold their breath, which closes the airway, effectively trapping compressed gas within the lungs. As the diver ascends toward the surface, the decreasing ambient pressure allows gas to expand and over-inflate lung tissue. When a scuba diver ascends, the excess gas must be exhaled. Otherwise the lungs will progressively increase in volume until the elastic limit of the alveoli is exceeded, and rupture occurs. This process may force gas bubbles into the pulmonary circulation from the capillaries via the pulmonary veins to the left side of the heart, and then to the carotid or basilar arteries.

AGE can happen at any depth, although it is more likely to occur in shallow waters. Cases have been reported in water as shallow as four feet. In recent years, the percentage of AGE cases has been declining. DAN believes that this is due to slower ascent rates, better training, safety stops near the surface before exiting the water, and possibly the practice of spending the last minutes of the dive near the surface where divers are less likely to run out of air.

Symptoms of Decompression Illness

Onset of symptoms of decompression sickness (DCS) is usually somewhat gradual, although they may be present immediately upon surfacing. They may commonly include, in particular, pain in the joints and numbness or tingling. The pain is often described as a dull ache, perhaps slowly getting worse. Pain, when present, is most often felt first in the joints, such as elbows, shoulders and knees. Other frequently reported symptoms are dizziness, headache, extreme fatigue, weakness, nausea, visual disturbance, and difficulty in walking.

Divers tend to deny symptoms of DCS, which delays treatment. DAN reports that only 25% to 30% of symptomatic divers request assistance within four hours after symptom onset. This is a critical issue in treatment of decompression sickness because the longer the delay in providing proper treatment, the greater the likelihood of long-term health complications which may not fully resolve. (Dovenbarger, 1992) For this reason, *even a slight hint of decompression illness symptoms should be taken very seriously by the lifeguard.* Transport to the hospital should be strongly encouraged, as well as consultation with DAN.

Onset of symptoms of AGE is typically more rapid than those of DCS. They can be immediate and extreme. A diver who suddenly loses consciousness upon surfacing should be assumed to have AGE. (Kizer, 1992) Symptoms similar to an acute stroke can be one of the most serious results of AGE. (Kizer, 1992) These cases usually involve a dive profile with a very rapid ascent.

Treatment of Decompression Illness

Lifeguards need not spend extensive amounts of time deciding whether a diving case involves DCS or AGE. Both can be very serious. If either are suspected, the victim should be treated for ABCs, given *high oxygen concentrations (via either a demand inhalator valve or non-rebreather mask at 15 liters per minute),* and transported to an emergency room under care of trained ambulance personnel. DAN should be consulted.

At one time, emergency responders were taught to place divers in a radical head down position, perhaps on their side. *This is no longer recommended* and may actually worsen the problem. (Kizer, 1992) Instead the patient should be transported supine or in the recovery position. To position the patient in the recovery position, turn the patient onto either side and support the head, assuring the airway is open. Avoid crossing the extremities because circulation may be compromised for diving injuries.

Full resolution of a decompression illness generally requires treatment in a recompression chamber. A recompression chamber uses atmospheric air pressure to comfortably return the patient to a pressure environment while breathing 100-percent oxygen. Any remaining bubble growth may be reduced in volume and effectively diffused into the surrounding tissue where it can be off-gassed by the body's perfusion. The patient is then slowly reintroduced to normal surface air pressure.

Recompression chambers are not always readily available near a diving accident site. Even if a recompression chamber is nearby, it may be unattended or in use for other medical reasons. Therefore, in most cases it is important to transport the patient to the nearest emergency department for evaluation and stabilization, where the nearest recompression chamber can be notified as early as possible. In some areas, lifeguards call the recompression chamber immediately to advise them of the case, to inform them of the possibility they will be receiving a patient, and to elicit advice. Transport by helicopter may be necessary, depending on severity of the illness and the proximity of the recompression chamber. The aircraft should be pressurized to sea-level and fly at the minimum safe altitude, preferably below 1,000 feet. (Kizer, 1992) DAN will assist in coordination of evacuation of injured divers.

Some very important information to convey to the receiving emergency room is the patient's dive profile. How deep for how long? How many dives in the last 24-hours? Was there a rapid ascent? If the diver is unable to provide this information, the diver's depth gauge or dive computer may provide it. The dive buddy is another excellent source. The lifeguard can then call the emergency room physician with this information. Since many doctors are unfamiliar with the Divers Alert Network, the lifeguard should advise of DAN's free medical consultation services and *provide the DAN emergency telephone number*.

A diver with decompression illness symptoms who refuses treatment should be advised to seek further medical assistance, especially if there is any worsening of symptoms. One other important consideration in a decompression illness case is the dive buddy. If two divers have followed similar dive profiles and one exhibits complications, the other should be carefully evaluated. Even if symptoms are not readily apparent, they may appear within a short period of time.

Reporting Diving Accidents

The Divers Alert Network maintains a 24-hour diving medical emergency hotline. This hotline provides injured divers and health care providers with expert consultation and referrals. The DAN emergency hotline number is (919) 684-8111 or (919) 684-4DAN (collect). DAN also maintains a telephone information line to provide answers to commonly asked questions about scuba diving medicine, health, and safety. This number, (919) 684-2948, extension 222 and is answered between the hours of 9 a.m. and 5 p.m. Eastern Time, on regular business days.

All scuba diving accidents should be reported to DAN. This allows DAN to produce information aimed at increasing diver safety. Report forms are included in Appendix C.

Lifeguards and lifeguard agencies are encouraged to join DAN and help support this organization. Oxygen training courses are also available through DAN for lifeguards, divers and emergency medical personnel. Membership and training information is available by writing to: Divers Alert Network, Peter B. Bennett Center, 6 West Colony Place, Durham, North Carolina 27705 or on the Internet at: www.diversalertnetwork.org

Chapter Summary

In this chapter, we have learned about risks associated with diving, including drowning, diving illness, and cardiac arrest. We have learned about how surface air is mechanically compressed in scuba tanks and by the weight of water, and how a regulator allows divers to breathe compressed air. We have learned about decompression illness, including decompression sickness and arterial gas embolism. We have learned about the dive tables and how they help divers avoid diving injuries. We have learned some of the symptoms and treatments of diving injuries. And we have learned about reporting diving accidents.

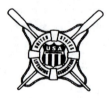

Discussion Points

- What are some circumstances that could lead to a diving death?
- What are some causes of diving deaths?
- What are the two ways that the air divers breathe is compressed?
- Why is it important for divers to follow the dive tables?
- What are some symptoms of decompression illness?
- What are some treatments for diving illness?
- What is some information it is important to gather about the dive of a victim of diving illness?
- Where can you telephone, 24-hours a day, for information on diving illness and treatment?

References

Dovenbarger, BSN, J. A. (Ed.). (1992). *1992 report on diving accidents and fatalities.* Durham, NC: Divers Alert Network.

Kizer, K. W. (1992). Undersea emergencies: treating barotrauma and the bends. *The Physician and Sportsmedicine, 20,* 8.

Morgan, Ed.D., W. (1995). Anxiety and panic in recreational divers. *Sports Medicine, 20,* 6, 398–421.

Vann, Ph.D., R. & Uguccioni, M. S., D. (Eds.). (2001). *Report on decompression illness, diving fatalities, and project dive exploration.* Durham, NC: Divers Alert Network.

Chapter 20
Lifeguard Health and Safety

In this chapter you will learn about ways to protect yourself. This includes recognition that lifeguards are athletes and therefore subject to a wide variety of related injuries. You will learn about protecting yourself from athletic injuries, protecting your skin, protecting your ears, and protecting yourself from infection. You will also learn about post-traumatic stress disorder.

CHAPTER EXCERPT

Skin cancer is highly curable if detected early and treated properly. Nevertheless, over 9,000 people die of skin cancer in the U.S. each year. Skin cancer can and has killed lifeguards, *even at a young age.*

The Lifeguard Athlete

Open water lifeguarding is, by its very nature, an athletic profession. The success of a lifeguard in carrying out critical tasks is highly dependent on the lifeguard's athletic skills. It is one of the few areas of employment, other than professional sports, where athletic skills are challenged on a daily basis. While some other professions, such as military service and firefighting, also require athleticism, none rise to the levels required for lifesaving. Like any athlete, the lifeguard is at risk for various types of associated injuries.

Lifeguard employment requirements include standard levels of training and health, but the lifeguard must also be able to successfully complete challenging physical activities. These include training drills, actual rescues, and other strenuous duties, such as moving heavy equipment. In any of these activities it is possible for the lifeguard to become injured, and just about any injury has the potential to prevent the lifeguard from performing the full range of duties required of a lifeguard. For example, if a lifeguard sustains a back injury while moving a boat, the lifeguard may be unable to participate in training or carry out rescues.

Lifeguarding involves several unique hazards. Although performing a rescue can require various skills similar to those involved in sports, such as jumping, running, swimming, paddling, and rowing, it may be impossible to perform them in the prepared, controlled manner of athletic competition. Lifeguards rarely have enough warning to be able to warm up and stretch prior to a rescue. They may have been sitting for several hours, and thus forced to make a *cold start*. The occupation also does not allow for certain activity controls of which most other athletes can take advantage during their sports or activities. For example, when proceeding on a rescue, lifeguards usually need to go all out and cannot be concerned with pacing themselves. In addition, lifeguards are unable to avoid their athletic activity. They cannot skip an event or a heat because they do not feel up to it. Lifeguards cannot come up short and drop out in the middle of their "event," since doing so might result in the death of someone in distress.

There are a wide variety of injuries that can be sustained in the course of rescue activity. They include death by drowning; trauma from the victim; trauma from equipment, such as rescue boards, boats, and ropes; trauma from environmental hazards, such as rocks, surf, inshore holes, aquatic life, and cold water; and a wide variety of orthopedic injuries to bones, joints, muscles, and ligaments. Statistics show that up to 40% of lifeguards sustain some type of lower back injury during the season and up to 20% of these have to limit their activities for the remainder of the season.

Most U.S. lifeguards are employed on a seasonal basis. This adds an extra layer of injury risk. Often, these lifeguards are less active in the off-season and their preseason conditioning may be less than ideal. The sudden increase in physical activity as the season approaches and gets underway, with training, rescues, and so forth, often leads to overuse problems. During the three to four months of the season, these lifeguards may be employed six to seven days a week. That compounds the physical strains to which they are subject. Full-time lifeguards can also be affected by varying levels of activity associated with the seasons.

Athletic Injuries

Athletic injuries lifeguards suffer are typically related to swimming, paddling, rowing, and running. In many cases they are standard overuse injuries in which the athlete has been trying to do something too often, too hard, for too long or incorrectly, thus over-stressing or straining involved muscles and tendons leading to their inflammation, pain, and decreased function. Many lifeguard activities involve shoulder and arm motion, thus compounding the overuse phenomenon.

The most common overuse injury of lifeguards is swimmer's shoulder, which represents a tendonitis of the inner shoulder muscles of the rotator cuff. Repetitive overuse, such as occurs in the standard crawl stroke, can lead to this condition. It can be further exacerbated by the fact that open water lifeguards are not merely swimming in a pool, but are fighting waves and currents, as well as pulling victims and equipment. This is one reason swim fins are recommended for most swimming rescues. With them, the lifeguard can greatly increase speed and strength, while easing strain on the shoulders.

Paddling and general use of rescue boards can cause shoulder tendonitis, but also neck and back strain, elbow problems—such as lateral epicondylitis or tennis elbow—and trauma from being struck by the rescue board. As compared to surfers, lifeguards typically use longer boards, which are paddled over greater distances, sometimes with a heavy victim aboard, thereby subjecting lifeguards to an increased rate of injury.

Since an integral part of lifeguard work involves running, lifeguards are susceptible to related injuries. These include runner's knee (knee cap discomfort), tendonitis, shin splints, plantar fasciitis (heel spurs), and numerous other injuries, mainly related to overuse. Lifeguards frequently train with running activities, but must also run on their way to rescues. Although, intuitively it might seem that running on the sand should be less traumatic than running on hard surfaces, this is not the case. Lifeguards en route to a rescue are usually attempting to keep their eyes on the victim, while running and donning rescue equipment. Due to the instability of the surface, irregularity of the contour, and lack of support, running on the sand can actually increase the rate of various injuries, including Achilles tendonitis, foot problems, sprains, and strains. It is therefore recommended to run on hard surfaces with appropriate running shoes when training.

Walking and running on the sand and beach environment can also lead to a significant number of lacerations and puncture wounds to the foot of a lifeguard. Up 79% of active duty lifeguards have sustained some type of foot trauma during their employment. These can be due to natural (e.g., shells, rocks) and human-made (e.g., glass, needles) hazards.

Another injury source is the lifeguard stand or post. For excellent reasons, related to effective surveillance, lifeguards are best located on an elevated post when scanning the water. When dismounting though, particularly en route to a rescue, lifeguards are susceptible to an injury known as *lifeguard's calf*. This involves a strain to the posterior calf muscles from jumping out of a high stand.

Lifeguards may also be injured while using motorized equipment, including watercraft and vehicles. In some areas of the country, lifeguard work includes rowing. Rowers are at increased risk for lower back injuries, which are a frequent injury for lifeguards. Surf adds greatly to the hazard that rowing presents and lifeguard rowers are frequently subject to lacerations, contusions, and even fractures.

These are just a few of the athletic injuries lifeguards can sustain in their daily work. Others, too numerous to mention, are well known to experienced lifeguards and their doctors.

Competition

Lifeguarding involves competition on many levels. During a rescue, the lifeguard competes against personal physical limits and the forces of nature. The lifeguard must sometimes contend with victims of varying sizes, strengths, and levels of anxiety. In these life and death struggles, failure could lead to disastrous results both for the victim and lifeguard.

In order to be employed as a lifeguard all agencies employ some type of competitive testing. USLA recommends a minimum swim standard of 500 meters in 10 minutes or less, which must be met and maintained throughout the course of employment. Many lifeguard agencies exceed this requirement. In some cases, employment opportunities may be related to how applicants for the job place in physical events as compared to other applicants. Once employed, daily training activities can involve inter-squad competitions to foster further improvement in skills and performance.

Considering the criticality of the athletic element of lifeguarding, which is essential to timely and effective rescue, it is perhaps inevitable that competitions among lifeguards have long been a part of lifesaving. These events have many benefits, both to lifeguards and lifeguard employers. They encourage high levels of fitness, create an incentive for lifeguards to practice lifesaving skills, and help lifeguards increase strength and stamina. All of these result in lifeguards who are better able to perform the physical duties of lifesaving. Competitions also foster improved teamwork and camaraderie. Many exchanges, which have resulted in notable improvements in lifesaving practices and equipment, have culminated from lifesaving competition.

These competitions can begin on a local level, where individuals compete to become part of a local competition team or on an individual basis. They may begin with a friendly town to town or county to county challenge. The next level is regional competition, sponsored by USLA. In August of each year the USLA National Lifeguard Championships are held, allowing lifeguard competitors to vie for national championship medals. Ultimately, every two years the International Life Saving Federation

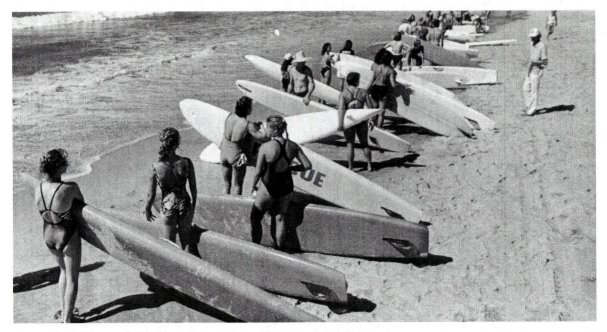

Lifeguard competitors line up.

Credit: National Park Service

sponsors the World Championships. Both a national team sponsored by USLA and local teams sponsored by USLA chapters, test their skills against others from around the world.

Lifesaving competition is recognized by the International Olympic Committee and lifesaving events have been featured in the both the World Games and the Goodwill Games. There are also professional competitive lifeguard competition series, both in the U.S. and at various sites around the world, where teams and athletes compete for prize money.

Like lifeguard training and rescue activity, competition related activity presents a source of possible injury to the lifeguard, both during the competition and also in training. Lifeguards are encouraged to clarify with their employer prior to competition whether they are considered to be performing a job related activity and, therefore, covered by worker's compensation, should they be injured.

Athletic Injury Prevention

Many of the injuries lifeguards experience as a result of the athletic nature of the job can be prevented. USLA recommends that all lifeguards receive a pre-employment physical, and then annually, whether on their own or through their agencies, lifeguards should obtain a preseason physical exam. This helps ensure that they have no medical conditions which would preclude strenuous physical activity. During preseason, lifeguards employed seasonally should gradually increase their training, beginning at least several months prior to starting work activities. An even better approach is to maintain a high level of fitness year-round, thereby avoiding a sudden increase in training and activities. This is certainly the best approach for full-time lifeguards, who may be called upon to employ their athletic talents at any time of year.

It is important that lifeguards acquire and maintain a high level of skills involving proper techniques in all the physical activities associated with the job, proper use of equipment, and appropriate ways of dealing with victims and the environment. Carrying out duties in the proper manner can greatly limit injuries. Workouts should include drills using all items of rescue equipment that will be used in rescue, including RFDs and rescue boards. This produces the combined benefit of physical conditioning and skill building. Rescue board launches and paddling drills should be included. If swim fins are used in rescue, they should be used in some workouts. Coaching and proper technique instruction should be emphasized in regular workouts.

Training programs should involve activities to help lifeguards keep up appropriate levels of fitness and strength. Equipment should be properly maintained to prevent damage, breakdown, or failure, which may result in injury. Knowledge of the environment, including location of hazards, such as rocks, jetties, piers, and inshore holes, will be invaluable in helping the lifeguard prevent injuries to themselves and others.

On a daily basis, lifeguards should engage in physical exercise, including cardiovascular workouts which stress the respiratory and circulatory systems. These activities should be carried out for periods greater than 20 minutes at a time and should significantly increase the heart rate to gain full benefit. This can improve speed and stamina.

Strength workouts should be carried out several times a week. This type of exercise is usually conducted with weights or machines and involves stressing individual muscle groups to increase strength. Strength exercises typically involve various groups including arms, shoulders, back, and legs. Several sets should be performed with between five and ten repetitions, using weights at levels just below maximum. If an athlete has increased strength, muscles will fatigue slower, perform better, and will be less subject to injury.

Each day lifeguards reporting for duty should carry out some type of warm-up and stretching activity. This will at least partly help to prepare for the sudden activity needed during a rescue. Appropriate warm-up and stretching should also be carried out prior to any exercise, including training and competition. An appropriate warm-up involves lightly using the muscle-groups involved to allow them to loosen, accommodate, and increase their temperature. Light jogging or calisthenics are appropriate ways of performing warm-ups for five or ten minutes.

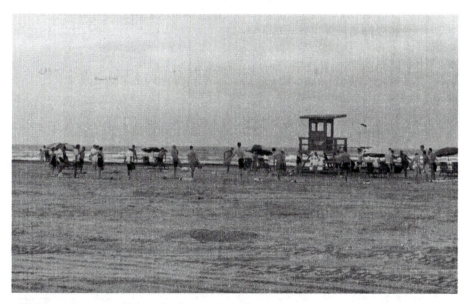

Lifeguards stretching before exercise.
Credit: Peter Davis

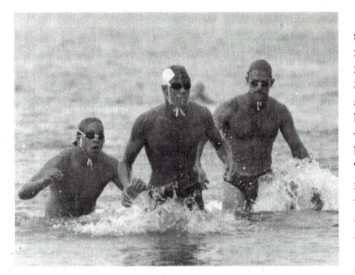

Credit: Mike Hensler

Once warmed up, muscle tendon units should then be stretched. This increases range of motion, allows for better performance, and may decrease injuries. Stretching should be carried out gradually, allowing the muscle group to be slowly brought to its full length. An example would be a hamstring stretch, where one bends over in attempting to touch the toes. This stretch should be held for approximately 5–10 seconds, released slowly, and then tension slowly reapplied. Bouncing and other ballistic motions should be avoided.

After activities are performed, an appropriate cool-down period should be allowed. When possible, the activities should not be stopped suddenly, but exercises continued at a lower level. For example, after finishing a run, walking is encouraged. This will prevent cramping, allow for a quicker recovery, and allow lactic acid, the byproduct of exercise, to be moved from the muscles quicker.

Lifeguard athletes are also advised to cross-train. They should not solely perform a single sport or exercise such as swimming, but also carry out other activities such as running and biking. The goal is to be able to continue to increase cardiovascular fitness and muscular strength, but to avoid using one body part or muscle set to the exclusion of others. This will greatly reduce the risk of overuse to these areas.

When carrying out activities about the beach, whether rescues, equipment movement, or training, proper ergonomics should be used. Heavy lifting should be accomplished using proper body mechanics in which one employs the legs and not the back to lift. Heavy weights should be moved by several individuals or using vehicles. These recommendations further extend to the moving of victims. Hazing and show-off activities involving movement of stands, boats, etc., are to be condemned.

The strained calf injury, known as lifeguard's calf, can be prevented by using ladders, stairs, or ramps from lifeguard towers, or by placing piles of soft sand in front of the stands to decrease the height. The time or expense involved in this is easily offset, not only by reduced injuries, but also by savings in worker's compensation costs.

To avoid foot injuries, lifeguards should always be vigilant about the state of the surface upon which they are running or walking, particularly in bare feet. The beach area should be checked on a daily basis and, if possible, footwear should be worn when ambulating about the beach. If injury to the foot occurs, proper wound care should be carried out as well as further treatment and follow-up as indicated.

With respect to injuries involving motorized boats and vehicles, the best approach is appropriate training, maintenance, and rules of use. Appropriate speed limits, designated areas of use, the use of helmets and other protective gear, seat belts in vehicles, and other measures are appropriate. In particular, lifeguard supervisors should take measures to ensure that motorized lifesaving equipment is not used for hot-dogging. This leaves a bad impression with the public and increases the likelihood of injury, both to the lifeguard and the public.

When on the beach, even while sitting still, but particularly when involved in heavy physical activity, lifeguards should maintain hydration. When involved in strenuous activity in hot weather, one can lose up to a quart of fluids in a half hour period. As one becomes dehydrated, performance decreases, judgment skills decline, and risk of serious injury increases. Fluid should always be available. Water is usually sufficient. If an activity is going to continue for a period of time greater than one hour, electrolyte replacement solutions may be needed.

Proper nutrition including a balanced diet high in carbohydrates and moderate in fats and proteins will help the lifeguard athlete perform at peak levels. Basic vitamin supplements will also help assure that the lifeguard does not have any deficiencies which may mar performance. Heavy off-duty consumption of alcohol deters health, performance, and preparedness to protect the public. True athletes avoid it.

Whenever an injury occurs, it should be reported, evaluated, and treated by a professional as necessary. Modified activities may need to be carried out by the lifeguard, such as light-duty or non-victim contact assignments, until the injury or problem has resolved. Lifeguards who have sustained injuries need to be appropriately cleared for duty to prevent reinjury to these areas.

Older lifeguards, who may have arthritic or other age related conditions, should be aware of their limitations, be sure they will not negatively affect their performance, and be especially diligent at keeping affected areas appropriately conditioned and strong. Lifeguards who follow recommendations in this section should be able to greatly lengthen their careers, but all lifeguards must be cognizant of the fact that it is more difficult to maintain high levels of fitness as we age and remember that the ultimate goal of lifesaving is the safety of the public served.

Once an athletic injury occurs, standard first aid such as rest, ice, compression, and elevation (*R.I.C.E.*) should be followed. If an area of injury worsens over time or does not improve quickly, appropriate activity avoidance and follow-up sports medicine care should be sought.

Protecting Your Skin

The skin is the largest organ of the body. It is a protective sheath, but in providing protection, it is susceptible to many types of injury. One of these is skin cancer. Skin cancer is the most common cancer, accounting for almost half of all cancers in the U.S. (American Cancer Society, 2002) Skin cancer is highly curable if detected early and treated properly. Nevertheless, over 9,000 people die of skin cancer in the U.S. each year. Skin cancer can and has killed lifeguards, *even at a young age.*

Lifeguards are particularly vulnerable to skin cancer because of the high levels of sun exposure they sustain and because of the strength of the sun's rays at the beach. The intensity of these rays can be tripled by reflection off the water and sand. The most serious threat comes from a spectrum of sunlight called ultraviolet (UV) light. There are two types of UV light which normally reach the earth—UV-A and UV-B. UV-B has a shorter wavelength and appears be the primary causation of sunburn.

UV-A, long thought to be the harmless, is now believed to present some significant hazards as well, including damage to DNA and development of melanoma. (Wang, Setlow, Berwick, Polsky, Marghoob, Kopf, & Bart, 2001)

There is no such thing as a safe tan. Even gradual tanning damages the skin. Exposure to UV rays adequate to produce tanning or burning actually harms the skin at the cellular level, causing direct injury to DNA. As the body begins a process of trying to repair

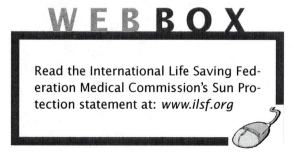

WEB BOX

Read the International Life Saving Federation Medical Commission's Sun Protection statement at: *www.ilsf.org*

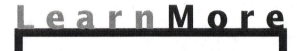

You can learn more about skin cancer on the website of the American Cancer Society at: *www.cancer.org*

the damage, it produces melanin, a protective pigment which darkens (tans) the skin. Most people's bodies can partially repair the damage; but the repair is never complete and long term injury accumulates over the years. Skin exposed to the sun ages at a significantly accelerated rate. Generally, people with darker skin color have more natural defense against sunburn than people with lighter skin. Darker skin however, only provides increased protection, not complete immunity from sun related skin damage.

Melanoma is the deadliest form of skin cancer and one of the most deadly of all cancers. If left untreated for an extended period, the cure rate is very low. Non-melanoma skin cancers include squamous-cell and basal cell carcinoma. Squamos-cell, like melanoma, can kill. Basal-cell carcinoma is the least threatening of the three and can usually be removed during an office visit to a physician.

If caught early, the deadly forms of skin cancer can usually be removed and their spread often stopped. USLA recommends awareness training for lifeguards, to help them better understand the problem and to check themselves for skin cancer, as well as annual evaluations by qualified medical experts.

Skin Cancer Symptoms

The following are some symptoms of skin cancer which should be evaluated by a physician:

- An existing mole which enlarges irregularly or takes on a notched border
- Red, blue, or white areas in a mole
- Itching or bleeding in a mole
- The appearance of a new mole in an adult
- A scaly or crusty raised area
- Raised hard red bumps with a translucent quality to their surface

According to the American Cancer Society (2002), "The best ways to lower the risk of non-melanoma skin cancer are to avoid intense sunlight for long periods of time, and to practice sun safety." One element of sun safety is use of sunscreen, which can reduce the chance of contracting skin cancer, help to avoid sunburn, and help to reduce skin damage caused by exposure to the sun. When selecting sunscreen, lifeguards should select those that protect from both UV-A and UV-B.

In an effort to describe the level of protection offered by different sunscreens, the *sun protection factor* (SPF) was developed. The theory of SPF is that a person who properly applies a sunscreen with an SPF of 15, for example, should be able to stay in the sun 15 times as long as if no sunscreen is worn and still receive about the same amount of skin damage. Lifeguards of all skin types should use a sunscreen with an SPF of at least 15. Beyond SPF 30 however, the value of increasing SPFs appears to be negligible.

The makers of sunscreen often include a variety of claims on their packaging. In 1999, the Federal Drug Administration proposed, "Cessation of unsupported, absolute, and/or misleading and confusing terms such as *sunblock, waterproof, all-day protection,* and *visible* and/or *infrared light protection*." It would therefore seem that relying on such claims or paying more for them is unwise. The best advice is to concentrate on the SPF and reapply regularly.

A concern of some dermatologists is that sunscreen may create an air of permissiveness about sun exposure. By using sunscreen, many people seem to believe they eliminate damage from the sun's rays and therefore do not have to worry about sun exposure. This may make them more likely to stay out in the sun. The reality is that there is damage to the skin even with sunscreen. Damage is simply less than it would be without any sunscreen.

Sunscreen should be applied to dry skin, 20 to 30 minutes before sun exposure. It should be used even on cloudy days because up to 80% of UV rays penetrate clouds. Attention should be paid to ensure an even distribution over all exposed areas. Particular heed should be paid to the lips, ears, nose, shoulders, and head, since these areas are highly susceptible to burning.

An excellent protection from the sun is the wearing of tightly knit, opaque clothing and wide brimmed hats. USLA recommends that all lifeguard agencies require their lifeguards to wear shirts and hats to help protect them from the sun, mandate use of sunscreen, and provide shade and protection. It has been demonstrated that mandating use of sunscreen and protective clothing by lifeguards reduces the incidence of skin cancer and related workers compensation claims. (Brewster, 1997)

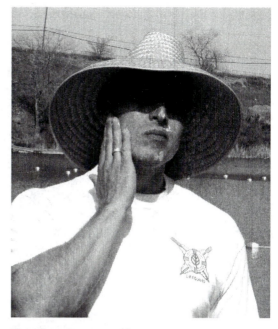

Good sun precautions protect a lifeguard's health.

Credit: Sandra McCormick

Eye Protection

Keen eyesight is essential to lifeguards and the swimmers they watch over. Unfortunately, eyesight can be seriously damaged by sun exposure. With proper protective steps however, the chances of eye damage can be significantly reduced.

Serious eye problems associated with sun exposure include:

- Cataracts: A clouding of the lens of the eye
- Macular Degeneration: Loss of central vision
- Photokeratitis: Damage to the cornea of the eye from exposure to intense light
- Pterygium: A callous-like growth that can spread over the white of the eye

Cataracts and macular degeneration generally occur over a period of years and primarily affect people later in life. They can cause full or partial blindness and require surgery. Pterygiums, caused by exposure to sun, wind, and dust, occur over a period of years and are often sustained by lifeguards. These three conditions typically require surgery. Photokeratitis can develop shortly after overexposure to intense UV light and can be very painful. Recovery occurs over several days and sometimes requires bandaging the eyes.

One study has found that those who do not protect their eyes from the sun triple their risk of contracting cataracts. Therefore it is clearly important to protect the eyes at all times. The best way to do so is through use of good quality (not necessarily high cost) sunglasses. The use of umbrellas, hats, and visors can also be of help. A wide brimmed hat greatly reduces the amount of UV rays reaching the eyes.

Selecting Sunglasses

Lifeguards need not pay high prices to purchase good quality sunglasses. Despite marketing claims to the contrary, many inexpensive sunglasses offer excellent protection. Lifeguards should insist on sunglasses which filter out 99 to 100 percent of both UV-A and UV-B light. UV protection is unrelated to darkness (tint) of the glasses. Even eyeglasses with no tint can be manufactured to provide full protection from UV light. However, wearing dark glasses that do not screen UV rays can actually cause more damage than not wearing glasses at all, since the screening of visible light causes the eyes to dilate, letting in more UV rays. The effects of UV light are cumulative. UV light can cause cataracts, retinal degeneration, and damage to the front surface of the eye.

In general, the best lens colors for lifeguards are gray, brown, green, or amber. Blue lenses should be avoided. Choose sunglasses of an adequate tint to allow observation of the water and sand without discomfort on days with bright sunlight. Lenses that block between 75 and 95 percent of visible light are probably a good choice. One rule of thumb is that if the eyes can be seen when looking in a mirror, the glasses are probably not dark enough, although if the glasses are too dark, vision may be inhibited.

Good quality lenses are generally made of high quality optical glass, plastic, or polycarbonate. Optical glass is more distortion free and resistant to scratching than polycarbonate or plastic, but glass is heavier and usually more costly. Polycarbonate lenses are more impact resistant, thus safer. Choose a design that covers as much of the area around the eyes as possible (wrap around sunglasses) without affecting peripheral vision. This helps protect from side light, and from the blowing sand that may cause growths on the surface of the eyes. Make sure the lenses pass the FDA requirement for breakage.

Polarized sunglasses dramatically reduce reflected glare—a major problem for lifeguards trying to watch a swim crowd. While tinted glasses darken glare, polarized glasses reduce glare with a filter in the lenses. Lifeguards should insist on polarized sunglasses to help reduce eye fatigue and improve observation.

USLA Buying Guide for Sunglasses

Feature	Recommendation
UVA Protection	99–100%
UVB Protection	99–100%
Lens Material	Polycarbonate
Lens Color	Brown, Grey, Green, or Amber Recommended
Screening of Visible Light	75–95%
Meets FDA Breakage Requirement	Required
Polarized	Highly Recommended
Wrap Around Style	Highly Recommended

Ear Protection

Chronic irritation and inflammation of the ear is a frequent problem for lifeguards and other swimmers. The most common afflictions are known as swimmer's ear and surfer's ear. The causes are similar. In both cases, the middle ear is affected.

A healthy ear is coated with earwax. This wax not only forms a water-repellent coating, it also contains antimicrobial substances. Unfortunately, continual contact with the water washes earwax away, removing the protection. This problem is exacerbated when people stick fingers or other items in the ear to remove water, scraping away the earwax.

Ocean swimmers, particularly surfers, are believed to have twice the ear problems of pool swimmers. (Schelkun, 1991) This is because the roiling ocean environment can cause sand and other debris to enter the ear canal. Bony growths (exostoses) within the ear canal can develop from prolonged exposure to cold water and wind. These further trap debris. In attempting to remove this debris, the lifeguard can traumatize the ear canal. These growths, in addition to increasing the risks of infection, can lead to decreased hearing. Often surgical removal is necessary.

The most common symptoms of these afflictions are pain, inflammation, and itching. Hearing loss may be experienced in some cases and there can be a fluid discharge from the ear. (Schelkun, 1991) Lifeguards with these symptoms should see a doctor.

Prevention of ear problems primarily involves keeping the ear canal dry and clean. Standard wax earplugs are not a good choice. Instead, use silicone earplugs. (Schelkun, 1991) Wearing tight fitting swim caps and wetsuit hoods can help reduce cold water induced injury and debris impaction. After swimming, tilting the head and jumping vigorously, as well as gently drying the outer ear with a towel are helpful. Lifeguards should make every effort to avoid reaching into the ear with anything. Physicians can recommend drying agents, as well as cleaning agents that help remove impacted debris.

Infection Control

Infection of a health care worker through exposure to the body fluids of another person (known as cross-infection) is very rare. Nonetheless, it can occur, particularly through exposure to blood and other bodily fluids. These secretions can carry *pathogens*—agents, particularly living microorganisms, which cause disease. Whenever medical aid is rendered by a lifeguard, contact with the victim's bodily fluids is possible. In some cases it is likely. The best way to avoid infection from bloodborne pathogens which the victim may be carrying is to employ *universal precaution.*

Universal precaution is an approach to infection control. According to the concept of universal precaution, all human blood and certain human bodily fluids are treated as if known to be infectious for human immunodeficiency virus (HIV), hepatitis

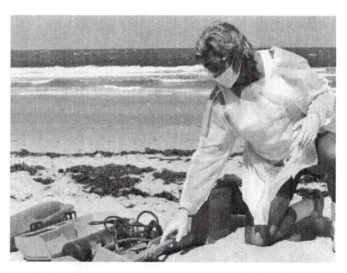

A lifeguard wearing universal protection including eye protection, a gown, a mask, and gloves.

Credit: William McNeely, Jr.

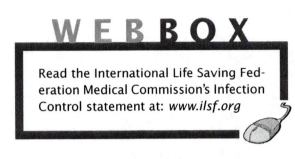

Read the International Life Saving Federation Medical Commission's Infection Control statement at: *www.ilsf.org*

viruses (including B & C), and other bloodborne pathogens. (OSHA, 1991)

Lifeguard exposure is most likely during treatment of open, bleeding wounds and during resuscitation attempts using mouth-to-mouth techniques. Mouth-to-mouth resuscitation provides an enhanced exposure to bodily fluids and sometimes blood. The most effective way to avoid this exposure and to provide the best possible resuscitation is through use of a mechanical resuscitator or a bag-valve-mask (BVM) device. Unfortunately, such equipment is not always available at the moment a drowning victim is recovered or a person collapses from a heart attack. For these circumstances, the so-called one-way mask may sometimes be an alternative.

The one-way mask is placed over a non-breathing patient's breathing passage, allowing the lifeguard to perform resuscitation while avoiding contact with the patient's breathing passage, saliva, vomitus, or blood. Many such masks are equipped with special ports to allow resuscitation supported by supplemental oxygen. At some agencies, masks are issued to every lifeguard and lifeguards are required to have masks with them at all times while on duty.

General Recommendations on Exposure

During Water Rescue of a Bleeding Victim

- Avoid contact with the victim if possible.
- Avoid contact with bleeding areas when removing the victim from the water.
- Wash off any blood as soon as possible.
- During in-water resuscitation attempts, wash any blood or body fluids away from the victim's mouth before contact. The rescuer's mouth should be washed out after contact.
- If possible, move the victim to dry sand to prevent further in-water exposure.

During Medical Treatment of a Victim Ashore

- Assume that all blood and other bodily fluids are infectious and treat them as such.
- Always use mechanical ventilation when possible.
- Use disposable resuscitation masks with a system that prevents body fluids from passing through the mask.
- Use oxygen delivery systems with disposable masks whenever possible.
- Wear occlusive gloves for handling bleeding victims.
- If the victim is bleeding profusely, especially from an artery, wear a mask, goggles, and an occlusive gown in addition to occlusive gloves.
- Wash the hands with soap and water after contacting blood, even if gloves are worn. Use diluted bleach or Betadine if blood directly contacts skin.

- Clean up blood and body fluids on equipment with a germicide containing household bleach and then air dry. Wear gloves while performing this task. Place used blades and needles in a disposable, puncture-proof container.
- Hepatitis B vaccination is recommended for all lifeguards. Hepatitis B immune globulin may be indicated after a documented exposure. Vaccine is also available for Hepatitis A (sometimes in combination with a Hepatitis B vaccination). The Centers for Disease Control and Prevention (2003) states that healthcare workers in the United States are not normally at increased risk of contracting this malady, but lifeguards may be at increased risk considering that one of the primary transmission routes is contaminated water. Hepatitis A vaccine should be considered by lifeguards working in or near areas where Hepatitis A is endemic, or when traveling to such areas. Check with your local health agency or the CDC about the prevalence of Hepatitis A in your area. No vaccine is currently available for Hepatitis C.

When Infected Items Are Found on the Beach

- Remove the items using universal precaution.
- Dispose of the items in a manner which avoids exposure to others, consistent with agency and regulatory protocol.

In Case of Possible Infection

- Lifeguards who are involved in contact with potentially infectious material should follow agency protocol. If no protocol exists, the lifeguard should contact a physician.
- Lifeguards exposed in a blood-to-blood inoculation with known or suspected fluids should follow agency protocol, which should include contact with a physician. Testing and drug regimens may be initiated.

OSHA Requirements

Under an employment rule established by the Occupational Health and Safety Administration (OSHA) in 1991 (29 CFR Part 1910.1030), certain steps must be taken by all employers to help employees avoid cross-infection. The OSHA rule specifically states, "This section applies to all occupational exposure to blood or other potentially infectious materials ... Occupational exposure means reasonably anticipated skin, eye, mucous membrane, or parenteral contact with blood or other potentially infectious materials that may result from the performance of an employee's duties." Lifeguards clearly fall under the requirements of this rule and USLA requires that all agencies seeking national certification provide equipment consistent with OSHA guidelines.

OSHA Requirement Excerpts

- *Hepatitis B Vaccine*—The employer shall make available the Hepatitis B vaccine

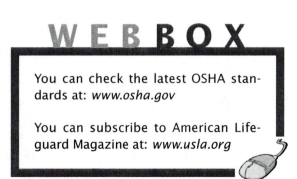

WEBBOX

You can check the latest OSHA standards at: *www.osha.gov*

You can subscribe to American Lifeguard Magazine at: *www.usla.org*

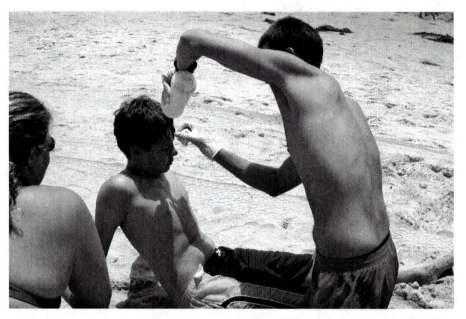

Credit: Ken Kramer

and vaccination series to all employees who have occupational exposure. There will be no cost to the employee.

- *Protective Equipment*—The employer shall provide at no cost to the employee and make readily accessible to the employee appropriate personal protective equipment.

- *Use of Protective Equipment*—The employer shall ensure that the employee uses appropriate personal protective equipment unless the employer shows that the employee temporarily and briefly declined to use personal protective equipment due to unusual circumstances.

- *Exposure Control Plan*—Employers must establish a written Exposure Control Plan designed to eliminate or minimize employee exposure.

The United States Lifesaving Association is closely monitoring development of procedures and techniques that can be used in minimizing lifeguard exposure to bloodborne pathogens. New developments in this area are frequently described in the USLA publication, *American Lifeguard Magazine*.

Post-Traumatic Stress Disorder

Like other public safety providers, open water lifeguards are regularly subjected to situations involving high stress. A rescue, for example, is a stressful event involving a person in mortal danger and an effort on the part of the lifeguard to save them from death; but even the frantic parent of a lost child can provoke great stress in lifeguards. These cases are normally resolved positively, and most lifeguards learn to cope with this level of stress as a part of the job. Occasionally though, events occur that are potentially much more troubling. Two examples include death or serious injury to a beach patron whom lifeguards have attempted to assist, particularly in cases where the circumstances are far removed from normal human experience.

Posttraumatic stress disorder (PTSD) is a psychiatric disorder which may occur after witnessing a life-threatening event. In the aftermath, people suffering from PTSD may have a number of troubling experiences. These can include nightmares, flashbacks, difficulty sleeping, and feelings of detachment. According to the National Center for Post-traumatic Stress Disorder (2003), "Most people who are exposed to a traumatic, stressful event

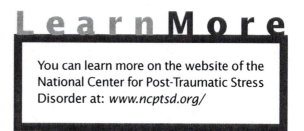

You can learn more on the website of the National Center for Post-Traumatic Stress Disorder at: *www.ncptsd.org/*

experience some of the symptoms of PTSD in the days and weeks following exposure. Available data suggest that about 8% of men and 20% of women go on to develop PTSD, and roughly 30% of these individuals develop a chronic form that persists throughout their lifetimes."

Public safety workers were once expected to simply deal with these stresses, but it has been learned that this is not always possible. It is now widely accepted that helping people deal with the high stress of public safety work is an obligation of employers, supervisors, and coworkers. PTSD can affect anyone. Some people are able to deal with terribly stressful circumstances for years without experiencing PTSD, only to suddenly and unexpectedly be affected. Others may have a reaction the first time they experience a highly traumatic, life-threatening event. Since it is impossible to know who will be affected and when, the best approach is to anticipate the problem and take proactive steps to address it.

After an event that might be expected to cause PTSD, particularly a highly stressful event that is significantly out of the ordinary for some lifeguards or for the organization, the best approach is to assume that a member or members of the team will be affected. Many public safety organizations address this first by conducting a *debriefing*. All people directly involved in the event are gathered to discuss it. Each person is provided a chance to ask questions and bring up concerns. Those with information about the event and a sense of perspective are expected to provide them. Debriefings are intended to be confidential, and all involved should be given a sense that what they have to say will be kept within the group. Moreover, debriefings should not be used to assign blame or point fingers. If something has been done improperly, it may well need to be addressed, but the debriefing process is intended to help people deal with stress, not to fix blame. It sometimes helps to focus on how the organization might better respond to a similar situation in the future. After all, every organization can always improve.

Depending on the circumstances and magnitude of the event, a more formal *critical incident stress debriefing* (CISD) may later be appropriate. These debriefings are normally led by mental health professionals, sometimes several days after the event. This allows for a more thorough approach by people whose expertise is in dealing with psychiatric issues and helping people cope with dramatic events in their lives.

Supervisors and coworkers are essential elements in helping manage PTSD. Recognizing and accepting that PTSD is a part of life in emergency services is an important step in avoiding stigmatizing someone who may be having difficulty dealing with an event, which could worsen the effects. It helps to make those affected comfortable with seeking assistance. Supervisors and coworkers should watch for unusual behavior among the persons involved and take actions appropriate within the organization to ensure that help is offered in a sensitive and caring manner.

Every lifeguard agency should develop protocols for dealing with PTSD. These can take into account available resources, such as counseling services, employee assistance programs, and mental health experts associated with the employer. Recognizing the existence of PTSD and developing standard ways to address it in the workplace is a fundamental aspect of maintaining lifeguard health and safety.

Symptoms of Post-Traumatic Stress Disorder

According to the National Center for Post-traumatic Stress Disorder, the following are some symptoms of PTSD. Those affected may experience some or all of them.

- Depression
- Despair and hopelessness
- Loss of important beliefs
- Aggressive behavior toward oneself or others
- Self-blame, guilt, and shame
- Problems in relationships with people
- Feeling detached or disconnected from others
- Getting into arguments and fights with people
- Less interest or participation in things the person used to like to do
- Social isolation
- Problems with identity
- Feeling permanently damaged
- Problems with self-esteem
- Physical health symptoms and problems
- Alcohol and/or drug abuse

Chapter Summary

In this chapter, we have learned that the lifeguard is an athlete who can be affected by injuries in a manner similar to other professional athletes, and we have learned ways to prevent those injuries. We have learned ways to protect our skin, particularly from skin cancer. We have learned about eye protection and how to select sunglasses appropriate for lifesaving. We have learned about ear protection. We have learned about infection control, including OSHA requirements. And we have learned how post-traumatic stress disorder can impact lifeguards.

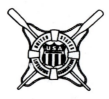

Discussion Points

- What are some similarities between lifeguards and people involved in professional sports?
- Why is it important for lifeguards to maintain a high degree of physical conditioning?
- What are some ways lifeguards can avoid injuries?
- How can lifeguards protect themselves from skin cancer?

- What are some considerations in selecting a good pair of sunglasses?
- How can the ears be affected the open water aquatic environment?
- What are some steps lifeguards can take to protect their ears?
- In treating others for medical problems, who should be assumed to be infected with a communicable disease?
- What are some steps lifeguards can take to protect themselves from infection?
- What types of inoculation are recommended for open water lifeguards?
- Who might be affected by post-traumatic stress disorder and why?
- What are some steps to take to address post-traumatic stress disorder among lifeguards?

References

American Cancer Society (2002). *Skin cancer facts.* Retrieved February 23, 2003 from the World Wide Web: *www.cancer.org/*

Brewster, B. C. (1997). *Lifeguard skin cancer protection, an approach to protecting health and promoting image.* International Medical-Rescue Conference Proceedings. San Diego, California: International Life Saving Federation—Americas Region.

Centers for Disease Control and Prevention (2003). *Viral Hepatitis A, frequently asked questions.* Retrieved February 24, 2003 from the World Wide Web: *www.cdc.gov*

National Center for Post-Traumatic Stress Disorder (2003). *What is post-traumatic stress disorder?* Retrieved February 23, 2003 from the World Wide Web: *www.ncptsd.org/*

Occupational Health and Safety Administration (1991). *Occupational exposure to bloodborne pathogens.* 29 CFR Part 1910.1030.

Schelkun, P. H. (1991). Swimmer's ear: getting patients back in the water. *The Physician and Sportsmedicine, 19,* 7, p. 85.

U.S. Food and Drug Administration (1999). *Sunscreen regulations finalized.* Rockville, MD: U.S. Food and Drug Administration.

Wang, S. Q., Setlow, R., Berwick, M., Polsky, D., Marghoob, A. A., Kopf, A. W., & Bart, R. S. (2001). Ultraviolet A and melanoma: a review. *Journal of the American Academy of Dermatology, 44,* 5, 837–846.

Chapter 21
Lifeguard Facilities and Equipment

In this chapter, you will learn about lifeguard facilities, including towers and main stations. You will learn about minimum and recommended lifesaving equipment that should be available at each beach area. You will also learn about daily tower preparation and maintenance.

CHAPTER EXCERPT

Like all emergency services, lifeguard agencies should have equipment available at a level adequate to allow a professional response to both the routine and major emergencies which can be reasonably anticipated.

Most emergency services operate from central stations—facilities designed to house the operations and equipment of the agency. This is true of police services, firefighting, and emergency medical services. Depending on size, some agencies also maintain satellite stations. Along with providing a gathering point for personnel and materiel, these stations serve as contact points for people requesting service, whether in person or by telephone.

Like the other emergency services, lifeguard agencies operate on the station concept by erecting lifeguard towers on beaches. Lifeguard towers serve as central points where lifeguard equipment is positioned for immediate use. Lifeguard towers are typically the most highly recognized features on a beach, often used by beach patrons as landmarks to meet each other. Beach patrons also look to the lifeguard tower for assistance, making it the focal point for summoning help.

Lifeguard Towers

Lifeguard tower design varies tremendously across the United States, from small portable chairs to large, enclosed units. They may also be known as stands, chairs, or perches, according to local custom. While towers were once typically made locally of wood or similar materials, prefabricated fiberglass towers are increasingly in use. These towers can offer a variety of beneficial features including an enclosed area protected from the weather, room for secure storage of equipment, a degree of privacy, and portability. All enclosed towers should have windows with an unobstructed view of the water. Certain features of lifeguard towers are common:

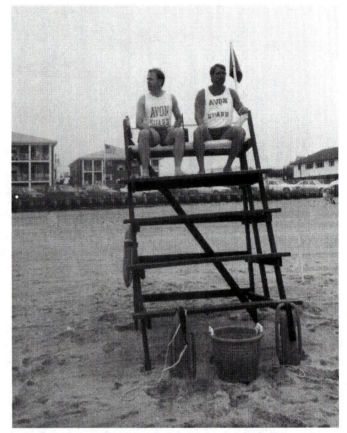

Two veteran lifeguards watch the water from a stand on a slow day in Avon-by-the-Sea, New Jersey. Note laundry basket with landline, which is used by lifeguard on right.

- *Elevation*—Towers provide lifeguards with an elevated position from which they can observe the entire area of responsibility, from the water to the beach. This elevation allows the lifeguard to look down on the water, which aids in recognizing hazardous conditions and facilitates observation of swimmers in heavily crowded swimming areas. Elevation of the tower also helps to make the station highly recognizable to beach users, should they need the assistance of a lifeguard.

- *Identification*—To assist the public in determining the status of lifeguard protection, many agencies have developed signs or symbols which are attached to lifeguard towers, indicating whether lifeguards are on duty. These signs may be locked into place when towers are closed, and include instructions for how emergency help can be summoned. It is a wise practice to devise and follow a system of notification to let beach users know when a tower is open and staffed, and when it is closed.

- *Numbers and Markings*—If there are several towers on a beach, it is recommended that they be numbered with large, easily readable numbers on all sides. This helps greatly in pinpointing reports of emergencies, particularly those received by telephone. Offshore rescue boats or helicopters responding to an emergency can be advised to work off a tower with a certain number. If helicopters are regularly used by police or other rescue agencies in the area, the tops of the towers (seats of open stands) should also be numbered. Another advantage of numbering is that it can greatly reduce the incidence of lost children. Since most towers on a beach look alike, visitors, particularly children, can easily become very confused. By numbering the towers, parents can advise their kids to "meet at Tower 5" if they become separated, for example. When lost children are found on a beach with a public address system, parents can be advised to claim their children at a tower of a certain number. Use of a numbering system also helps in directing beach users to appropriate locations. For example, water or beach use areas can be more readily identified when they are associated with a numbered tower. People meeting friends may agree to meet near a tower of a certain number. In addition to numbering, agencies may wish to consider unique symbols or icons on each tower. This adds to the ability of people, particularly small children, to remember where their group is located.

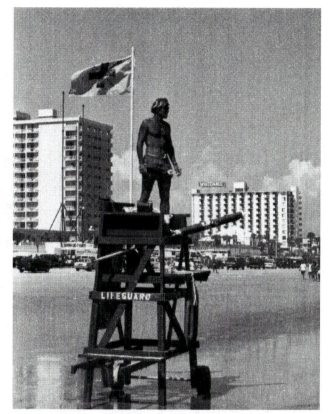

In Daytona Beach, Florida, lifeguard stands have wheels at the base to allow them to be continually moved in response to the wide tidal variation on this beach.

Credit: Mike Hensler

- *Equipment Storage*—Lifeguard equipment is normally kept at the lifeguard tower during duty hours. Tower design should therefore include places where equipment can be mounted or placed for immediate retrieval. While some towers require that lifeguards remove equipment for secure storage at the end of the day, other tower designs provide secure storage within.

- *Safety*—Until recently, many agencies designed lifeguard towers thinking only of economy of construction and resistance to vandalism. Today however, lifeguard agencies commonly design towers with features to protect lifeguards and beach visitors from possible injury. Ramps or stairs are replacing ladders, since experience has shown that lifeguards have been injured on the job by climbing up on or jumping down from towers. Lifeguard towers are often enclosed, to offer protection from the sun and weather. This provides two major safety benefits. First, as explained in the chapter on *Water Surveillance*, lifeguards exposed to the elements for long periods of time, particularly heat and wind, experience a marked reduction in their level of alertness, which can adversely impact vigilance, as well as physical preparedness to respond to emergencies. Second,

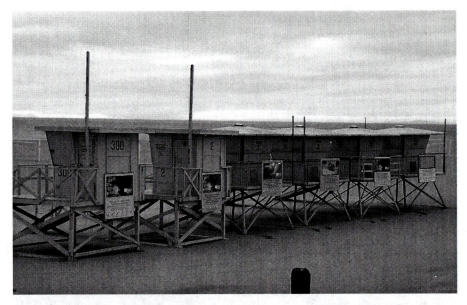

Los Angeles County lifeguard towers are stored for the winter. Newer fiberglass construction methods are used in the towers on the right.

Credit: Nick Steers

as explained in the chapter on *Lifeguard Health and Safety*, sun and wind exposure pose very real physical hazards for lifeguards.

- *Color*—Lifeguard towers should be of a color that is immediately recognizable to the public as a lifeguard facility. Consistent coloring is best. This is particularly important in an urban environment where the lifeguard station may tend to blend in with other buildings. Lifeguards sometimes forget that many beach visitors are there for the first time and in an emergency, need to know immediately where to go. Some agencies mark their towers with the simple word, *Lifeguard*.

- *Portability*—For lifeguard towers which are designed to be moved, the design should include features which allow movement without injury to lifeguards and protocols should be in place for movement in a manner that avoids injury. Back injuries are a major problem for lifeguards, partly due to efforts to move large objects.

Main Stations

While many smaller lifeguard agencies operate exclusively from moveable towers or stands, larger lifeguard agencies typically utilize permanent towers on their beaches, often referred to as main stations. These large, often multi-story structures are usually located at the waterfront, with direct access to and observation over the beach. The primary feature of these stations is a commanding view of the entire beach area. Under the Tower Zero system of water surveillance, described in the chapter entitled *Water Surveillance*, the observation deck is the first observation point staffed on the beach and the last to close. This system provides considerable operational efficiency, since the Tower Zero station can have telephone or radio contact with other towers, vehicles, and boats, while the high point of observation allows lifeguards in the tower to provide both direct surveillance and backup to lifeguards in the indi-

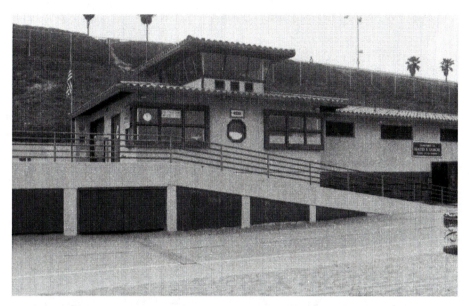

A main lifeguard station with offices, locker rooms, and an observation deck.

Credit: Rob McGowan

vidual towers. Main stations may also incorporate administrative staff offices, central communication and reception areas, first aid and recovery rooms, locker and shower facilities, training and apparatus rooms, maintenance shops, vehicle and equipment storage areas, meeting and training rooms, kitchen facilities, and areas to accommodate local police.

Equipment

At each beach where lifeguards will be assigned to the protection of swimmers, emergency equipment must be readily available. Like all emergency services, lifeguard agencies must provide emergency equipment at a level adequate to allow a professional response to both the routine and major emergencies which can be reasonably anticipated.

Minimum Equipment Standards

The following equipment standards should be met by all open water lifeguard agencies at each beach area:

- *Rescue Flotation Devices*—At least one rescue flotation device (RFD) for each lifeguard on duty.
- *Masks and Snorkels*—Mask(s) and snorkel(s) readily accessible to mount an underwater search and rescue, as appropriate.
- *Binoculars*—Binoculars readily accessible in the beach area, and in each main tower and emergency vehicle.
- *Marker Buoys*—Marker buoy(s) readily accessible for submerged victim search and rescue.

- *Swim Fins*—Swim fins for rescue purposes readily accessible to lifeguards as appropriate according to local conditions.
- *First Aid Kits*—A first aid kit adequate to treat minor injuries at each staffed lifeguard post and a first aid kit adequate to treat both minor and major medical emergencies at each beach area.
- *Personal Protective Equipment (PPE)*—Equipment to protect against bloodborne pathogens consistent with requirements of the U.S. Department of Labor Occupational Safety and Health Administration (OSHA).
- *Spinal Stabilization Equipment*—Spinal stabilization equipment, including spineboard, head and neck immobilization devices, and fastening devices readily accessible at each beach area.
- *Oxygen*—Oxygen readily accessible at each staffed beach area, with all lifeguard personnel trained in its use.
- *Public Communication Equipment*—Equipment for lifeguards to communicate with the public at a distance (e.g., public address system, bullhorn, whistles, megaphone(s), air horn(s), etc.)
- *Lifeguard Communication Equipment*—Equipment for lifeguard to lifeguard communication and equipment for lifeguards to immediately activate local emergency medical services (EMS).
- *Lifeguard Uniforms*—Readily identifiable uniforms for lifeguards to wear, denoting the lifeguard as a trained rescuer (e.g., *Lifeguard, Beach Patrol, Marine Safety*) and denoting the employing agency.
- *Sunscreen*—Sunscreen for all lifeguard personnel.
- *Sun Protection Equipment*—Equipment to protect lifeguards from sun exposure.
- *Report Forms*—A system for documenting lifeguard activities, consistent with USLA standards, with annual statistical data reported to the USLA statistics coordinator by March 1 of each year.

Recommended Equipment

In addition to the minimum equipment standards, USLA recommends the following:
- *Rescue Boards*—Rescue boards, readily available for use by lifeguards.
- *Rescue Boats*—Rescue boats, ideally motorized.
- *Boat Tow*—Boat tow for use by a swimming lifeguard in towing a boat offshore.
- *Positive Pressure Resuscitation Device*—An oxygen delivery device which provides positive pressure with 100% oxygen.
- *Cardiac Defibrillators*—Cardiac defibrillators readily accessible at each staffed beach area, with personnel trained in their use.
- *Blood Pressure Cuffs and Stethoscopes*—BP cuffs and stethoscopes for checking blood pressure and evaluating lung sounds.
- *Emergency Vehicles*—Emergency vehicles to transport lifeguards, equipment, and victims, in routine and emergency operations.

- *Posted Hours of Operation*— Hours of observation to inform the public of periods of lifeguard protection.
- *Public Information Board*—A board to inform the public of daily conditions, such as tides, currents, sunrise and sunset, etc.
- *Logbook*—An official logbook to record periods of operation, personnel assigned to water observation and periods of assignment, rescues, and other significant events.

Tower Preparation

At the beginning of each workday or shift, it is important that lifeguards make a thorough check of all equipment. Each agency should develop its own checklist for setting up the tower, including the following recommended points:

- *Initial Area Scan*—As the lifeguard enters the beach area, an immediate scan of the water and beach is conducted for any signs of trouble. This scan is repeated once the tower is staffed.

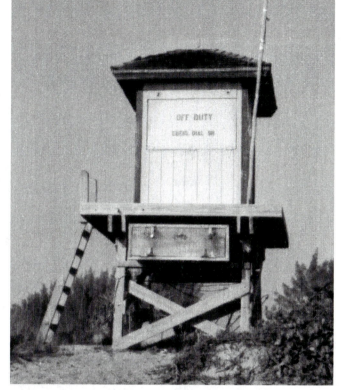

Lifeguard station with off-duty sign on shuttered windows.

Credit: Paul Drucker

- *Status Check*—The tower is checked for any damage or vandalism, which is reported immediately.
- *Tower Ready*—The tower is unlocked and equipment is readied. The first piece of equipment prepared for use is the lifeguard's RFD.
- *Open*—The tower is opened for service. Shutters may be removed or raised. Any *off-duty* signs are secured or stowed. Flags used by the agency are raised. Warning flags should be used in a manner consistent with USLA flag warning guidelines.
- *Communication Check*—Communication equipment is checked to see that it is functioning properly. Radio checks are made. If telephones are installed, checks include calls to dispatch centers followed by a callback to ensure that the telephone works in both directions.

WEBBOX

You can view a copy of USLA's Flag Warning Position Statement, which sets recommended standards for warning flags in the Lifeguard Library, at: *www.usla.org*

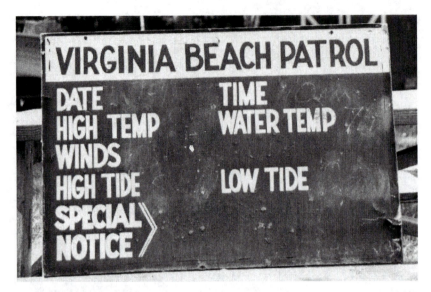

Credit: Dave Foxwell

- *Rescue Equipment Ready*—Lifeguard equipment is carefully checked and deployed. Each piece of equipment should be inspected for damage, wear, or improper maintenance. Once inspected, equipment is placed in predetermined positions for immediate retrieval and use if needed.
- *Medical Equipment Ready*—Medical aid gear and supplies are checked and deployed. Shortages of supplies are reported immediately so that they can be replaced. Oxygen tank pressures are checked.
- *Report Ready*—Supplies of report forms are checked. Completed forms that have not been turned in are submitted. Lifeguards ensure that there are suitable writing implements available. The lifeguard log is started for the day, including a listing of the time the station is opened and the personnel on duty.
- *Public Information Boards Updated*—Notice boards for public information are brought up to date with information that may include tide times and water/air temperature. Supplies of public education materials are checked.
- *Motive Equipment Ready*—If boats or vehicles are used, they should be thoroughly inspected. Motorboats and vehicles should be checked for gas, oil, and other fluids, as well as any unusual wear and tear.
- *Access-ways Marked*—As appropriate, runways formed of cones or rope may be placed to dissuade beach visitors from settling immediately in front of the tower. With respect to vehicle access-ways, see please see the chapter on *Special Rescue Equipment*.
- *Cleanup*—The tower is checked for cleanliness. Personal gear is neatly stowed.

At some agencies, checklists for setting up the station must be followed by each lifeguard, regardless of the number of employees assigned to a station. In areas where lifeguards work in shifts, agencies may require that second shift employees complete the checklist even though the same checklist was completed by a lifeguard on a previous shift. This system of redundancy helps ensure that in an emergency, all necessary equipment is fully prepared and readily available. There is nothing worse than needing an essential item in an emergency and finding it unavailable, depleted, or broken.

Tower Maintenance

During the workday, lifeguards must remember that the lifeguard tower is a public safety facility and treat it as such. The maintenance of a lifeguard tower will reflect upon the quality of service provided by the lifeguard agency. An agency that keeps well-organized and clean stations will be perceived by the public as an efficient, professional organization. Dirty, cluttered, and disorganized stations will leave the opposite impression.

Lifeguards must work to keep their stations tidy throughout the workday. This may include sweeping or washing the tower at regular intervals. Clothes and other personal items should not be hung or draped on or about the tower. During periods of low beach attendance, maintenance may also include minor repairs to towers and rescue equipment. During all periods the station is open however, surveillance over the beach and water should continue without interruption.

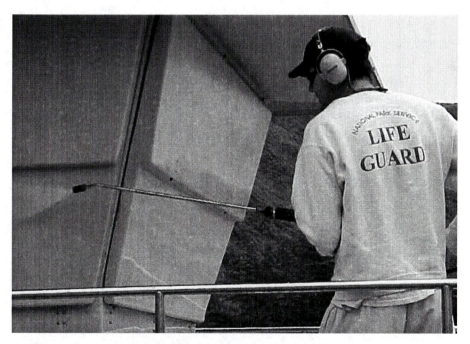

A lifeguard performs tower maintenance.
Credit: Steve Hills

Chapter Summary

In this chapter, we have learned about lifeguard towers, including main stations. We have learned about the minimum equipment standards recommended by USLA, along with additional recommended equipment. We have learned about the process of tower preparation and about tower maintenance. We have been reminded that during duty hours, beach and water surveillance should be maintained at all times.

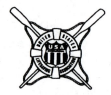

Discussion Points

- What are some benefits of enclosed lifeguard towers?
- What are some common features of lifeguard towers?
- Why might numbering of lifeguard towers enhance public safety?
- Why is the Tower Zero observation deck of a main station normally the first to be opened and last to be closed?
- What are some examples of minimum equipment standards for open water lifeguard agencies?
- What are some examples of additional recommended equipment?
- What are some of the steps involved in opening a lifeguard tower?
- What are some reasons to ensure that lifeguard stations are kept in a clean and tidy state at all times?

Chapter 22
Communication Methods

In this chapter, you will learn about methods lifeguards can use to communicate among themselves, with allied public safety agencies, and with the public. You will learn about electronic communication methods, including two-way radios, telephones, public address systems, and the Internet. You will learn about visual communication methods, including arm signals, signs, and flags. You will learn about audible signaling, including whistles and alarms. And you will learn about the 9-1-1 system.

CHAPTER EXCERPT

USLA strongly recommends that open water rescuers use two-way radios to communicate in the beach environment. Alternative methods, such as whistles and flags are not recommended as a primary method of rescuer to rescuer communication.

A fundamental measure of any emergency service is its ability to communicate quickly, broadly, efficiently, and effectively in a wide variety of conditions. It is the nature of lifeguard services that personnel are spread over large areas as they monitor and respond to problems in the beach environment. This creates a challenge for communication which must be met.

Communication Needs

All lifeguard services should have the capability of communicating effectively in the following three areas:

- *Internal Communication*—Communication among lifeguards is an integral aspect of two of the three points of a rescue. During the *recognize and respond* portion of a rescue, the alert to others requires immediate, effective communication. During the *signal and save* portion, the first step is a signal to other lifeguards indicating if further assistance will be needed. Effective communication is essential during periods of

325

emergency response, for maintaining effective coverage of supervised areas during normal operations, and for routine business in a work environment where lifeguards are necessarily widely dispersed.

- *External Communication*—Lifeguards must be able to communicate effectively with other emergency services, including neighboring lifeguard agencies, police, fire, rescue, and emergency medical services. In some areas, other services may also be of importance, such as the U.S. Coast Guard and any other source of rescue helicopters. For routine communication, lifeguards may need to contact animal control providers, tow trucks, child welfare workers, and so on.

- *Public Communication*—Lifeguards must have the ability to pass information efficiently and understandably to beach visitors in order to provide directions during emergencies or approaching weather, to move people out of dangerous areas (preventive lifeguarding), to help locate missing persons, and to provide important information about general beach conditions.

Communication Tools

There are three basic types of communication systems used by lifeguard agencies across the United States. The types of communication systems available depends largely on available funds for communication equipment and conditions under which communication is necessary.

Electronic Communication

The most effective form of routine and emergency communication is electronic communication. Electronic communication systems include two-way radio systems, telephones, and public address systems. Effective electronic communication systems allow for the transmission of a message over long distances with full clarity.

Two-Way Radios

USLA strongly recommends that open water rescuers use two-way radios to communicate in the beach environment. Alternative methods, such as whistles and flags are not recommended as a primary method of rescuer to rescuer communication. There are several reasons that two-way radios are a highly desirable tool for lifeguard communications. Like the telephone, the two-way radio allows for two-way conversation over long distances. While flags or whistles may allow some limited information to be transmitted over line of sight or audible range, the two-way radio can normally transmit well beyond this range and lifeguards using a two-way radio system can be very specific about their needs.

Unlike a wired telephone, when a lifeguard must leave the stand for a medical aid or warning to a beach visitor, the two-way radio allows a lifeguard to stay in communication at all times, able to request specific forms of backup if a problem develops. This is also helpful for supervisory personnel who can direct operations from a distance based on information provided.

A radio frequency serves as a constant conference call in which all members of the organization are immediately made aware of a message and can respond at will. For example, if a lifeguard sends a rescue alert, all adjacent lifeguards with radios are immediately made aware of this, as are backup resources. Attention is immediately directed to the area of need.

At agencies where radio traffic is high, multiple channels are recommended to segment radio traffic in geographic areas of the operation and to separate emergency radio traffic from routine business traffic. If possible, additional *tactical* channels can allow moving major incidents to a separate channel that avoids conflict with other operations. For example, in cases of a search and rescue operation for a missing swimmer, it can sometimes be helpful to move the responders to a tactical channel, thus allowing other lifeguards who are continuing to provide routine public safety needs to continue to communicate without distraction or radio interference.

The most effective radio systems include the ability to converse with other local emergency service providers. This can be of tremendous benefit in emergencies, allowing direct communication with responding resources and continual updates. It is particularly useful when the incident command system is invoked. Very inexpensive radios which allow direct communication with Coast Guard resources and private vessels are available from marine supply outlets.

The effective use of lifeguard rescue boats requires accessibility to direct communication with lifeguards ashore. Equipment has been developed which allows hand-held radios to be placed in watertight pouches for use by smaller boats. Some of these pouches even allow submersion of the radio without damage. Larger boats are normally outfitted with mobile radios designed for vehicles.

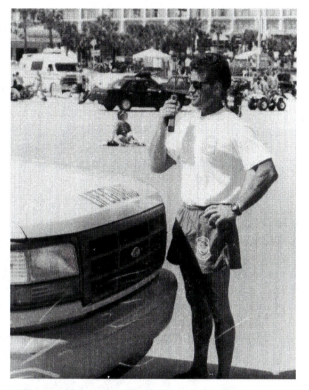

Lifeguard uses a portable radio for communication.

Credit: Mike Hensler

Some lifeguards use *codes* while speaking on the radio. Many people are aware of the radio code "10-4," which generally means an acknowledgment of a message received. This is one of the 10-codes, so-called because they start with the number 10. There are many others, which vary from agency to agency and from state to state. The concept of codes is two-fold. First, they can replace oft used phrases, thereby reducing the amount of time spent transmitting a message. This is particularly valuable in an emergency when seconds count and to limit radio traffic. For example, the term *Code 4* is used in some areas to mean, "no further assistance needed." In this case, a two syllable code replaces an eight syllable phrase. The second major value of codes is that they can help mask the meaning of transmissions to prying ears. For example, if an offshore rescue boat recovers the body of a missing swimmer, it is of immediate interest to all lifeguards, but by using codes, most beach patrons who might overhear the radio traffic would not know what the radio transmission means.

While these are valuable reasons to use radio codes, a downside is that they can be difficult to learn and remember. In addition, for lifeguard agencies that often communicate on the radio with other agencies, codes can be confusing. The U.S. Coast Guard, for example, does not use codes. Lifeguards used to using codes may have a difficult time transitioning between a conversation with an agency which uses codes and one which does not. The alternative to codes is known as *clear text*, i.e., simple language. Effective clear text requires that lifeguards carefully consider their words before transmitting and use the fewest words possible to get the message across as clearly as possible. For example, rather than stating, "I would like to ask for some additional lifeguard assistance here at Tower 4," the lifeguard could state, "Request backup, Tower 4."

Two-way radios can send and receive messages, but can only do one or the other at once. When one person is speaking, others normally cannot do so. Therefore, it is important that before a lifeguard transmits, it must be first confirmed that another conversation is not already taking place. Furthermore, the lifeguard should take great care to make transmissions brief and to the point, so that if a more urgent message must be broadcast by someone else, that person can break in and use the radio for the higher priority message.

Telephones

The first electronic communication method acquired by most lifeguard agencies is the telephone. All lifeguard agencies should have access to telephones for communication with outside resources, and to allow the public to call for assistance or with questions. Many lifeguard agencies also use telephones for communication among towers or stands. While it can be difficult to extend and maintain wired phones to temporary stands, this is a better form of communication than flags or whistles because a full explanation of a particular need can be transmitted using normal conversation and reception of the message is certain.

Cellular telephones allow for telephonic communication without the need for wiring. They can be a very useful tool for lifeguards and lifeguard supervisors, particularly in major emergencies and in areas where a wired telephone is prohibitively costly. In most beach communication among lifeguards however, the two-way radio is probably a better alternative because of the open broadcast of messages it provides.

Push-to-talk cellular service is a popular feature of cell phones. This feature allows predefined user handsets on a cellular network to behave in a manner similar to a two-way radio. In some cases, this may be an acceptable substitute for actual two-way radios, but agencies considering this option should carefully consider issues such as the need for immediate availability of airwaves and suitability of the devices in an aquatic environment.

Members of the public will sometimes observe emergencies or other incidents requiring lifeguard response at times or in places that lifeguards are not present. All lifeguard agencies which serve public swimming areas should have a published emergency telephone number to allow contact by the general public. This telephone number should be answered whenever lifeguards are on duty.

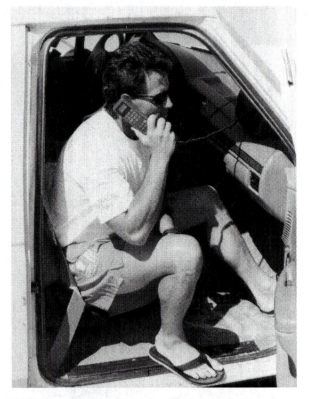

Cellular telephones can be a useful tool for lifeguards.

Credit: Mike Hensler

It is a good practice to arrange for emergency phone lines to be answered 24 hours a day. People reporting an emergency may have no idea of the hours of the lifeguard agency they are calling, and precious time can be wasted as they fruitlessly try to summon help for an emergency. Several major lifeguard agencies in the United States maintain 24-hour lifeguard response, along with 24-hour communications. Others use pager systems to allow them to be notified in after-hours emergencies. At a minimum, lifeguard agencies should arrange to transfer emergency telephone lines to another public safety provider, which can ensure an emergency response, or provide a recording explaining how to get help in an after-hours emergency.

Public Address Systems

Public address (PA) systems are electronic voice amplification devices used primarily to provide information or direction to beach visitors. PA systems can be installed along beaches, on towers, on vehicles or vessels, or can be carried as portable megaphones. Public address systems can be of great value in preventive lifeguarding. Persons in a rip current, even far offshore, can be advised of how to extricate themselves. Lifeguards offshore involved in rescue activity can be updated and directed. Beachgoers can be advised of approaching bad weather.

In searches for lost persons, the PA can be invaluable. A single broadcast of the description of a small child can immediately turn the entire beach crowd into a search team. If an area must be suddenly closed to conduct an emergency search or due to water contamination, the public address system conveys the message broadly and immediately. Public address systems are also used in some areas to remind beach users of general regulations in an effort to gain compliance without personal contact. At the end of the day, the PA system can be utilized to advise beach users, even those swimming offshore, of the departure of lifeguards.

One pitfall to avoid with the PA is overuse. People visiting the beach are trying to relax. They want to avoid some of the stresses of everyday life. Constant use of a public address system can be very annoying and can ultimately cause beach users to "tune out" the broadcasts, so that when a truly important message is broadcast, it is ignored. Lifeguard services with PA systems are wise to develop guidelines aimed at moderating use.

The Internet

The Internet allows lifeguards to provide a wide range of information to beachgoers and those considering beach visits. While few people at the beach bring a device for Internet access, many consult the Internet prior to a beach visit. This allows lifeguards to provide a wide range of information. Descriptions of beach areas, hours of lifeguard operation, safety hazards, safety tips, and regulations are all examples of valuable items of information. This can increase the likelihood that beachgoers will arrive informed and prepared to enjoy their experience safely.

The Internet can also be used for daily information, such as weather, rip current activity, surf size, etc. Many beach areas are covered by cameras that allow people using the Internet to actually observe current conditions. Overall, the Internet is just one more way that lifeguards can communicate with the public they serve and further disseminate messages aimed at promoting public safety.

Visual Communication

Arm Signals

The use of arm signals among lifeguards provides an essential form of backup communication when electronic communication is impractical. For example, a lifeguard swimming offshore usually lacks access to a two-way radio and certainly to a telephone. Basic arm signals approved by USLA are an essential component of a backup communication system. The very concept of the *signal and save* component of every rescue is that the swimming lifeguard will signal to other lifeguards whether the rescue is under control or further assistance is needed. The simple Code X signal can cause an entire search procedure to be commenced. These signals can be used on the beach as well. For example, a lifeguard's raised arm indicates a need for further assistance, regardless of where used. Limitations of arm signals include the fact that they must be observed to be effective and that they can convey only a simple message. USLA approved arm signals are covered in *Appendix A*.

Signs

Signs are used at many beaches to communicate with the public. Signs can explain rules and regulations, mark areas for special activities like surfing or boating, or explain the status of lifeguard protection, along with instructions for summoning assistance when lifeguards are off duty. Persons visiting an unfamiliar beach may be particularly likely to check signs to learn of unusual regulations with which they may be unacquainted. All lifeguard agencies should maintain inexpensive chalkboards or dry erase boards which can be updated daily with pertinent weather and safety information. Signs and bulletin boards are also used to provide beach visitors with general public education materials.

Flags

Some agencies also use flags to communicate among lifeguards. This is not a recommended method of communication, especially considering the relatively low cost of electronic communication options. A lifeguard who drops a flag or changes flags cannot be certain that other lifeguards have noticed. A flag system which depends on others to spot a flag change before assistance will be sent may leave the lifeguard on the rescue alone and without backup, due to lack of recognition of the signal.

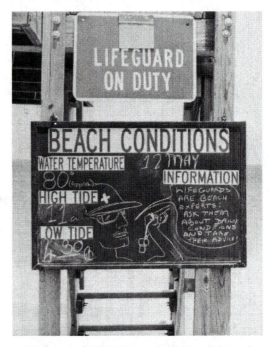

A lifeguard tide board with updated conditions and a safety message.
Credit: William McNeely, Jr.

In parts of the United States, as well as in other parts of the world, warning flags are sometimes flown to notify beach users of current water conditions. This form of public education is intended, in part, to help prevent drowning and other injury by notifying beach users of the degree of hazard and thus, the level of caution that may be warranted.

Flags, signs, and other public education efforts are not a substitute for the provision of lifeguards. Signs and flags may help some people avoid distress, but when a person encounters distress in the water, flags and signs cannot effect a rescue. That can only be reliably accomplished by trained professionals. Therefore, USLA strongly recommends that warning flags be used only as an adjunct to the provision of lifeguard protection, not as a substitute.

Where warning flags are flown, the public should be notified of their meaning via signs placed at multiple, conveniently located places. Examples might include beach access ramps, lifeguard towers, parking lots, and the flagpoles themselves.

Ocean conditions vary throughout the United States. Conditions that may be considered relatively mild in some areas, may be seen as a safety threat in others. Therefore, in each area where warning flags are employed, USLA recommends that specific local criteria be developed that provide objective, measurable criteria for posting the flags, and that the public be clearly notified of those criteria.

The first four flags listed below are intended to provide general notification of overall conditions for a beach area. That is, if it is decided that water conditions present a "moderate hazard" on a given beach, it should cover the entire beach, not a portion or area thereof. This does not prevent use of additional flags of the same warning level to accentuate the notification, but a single beach should not fly a green flag in one area and a red flag in another, for example.

Some or all of the flags listed below may be employed. It may be decided, for example, to adopt the first three, but none of the others. This is a local decision. However, USLA strongly discourages use of flags of similar colors that conflict with the meaning of those listed below. This would jeopardize the value of national consistency and confuse the public. In any case, with the exception of the double red, which indicates a closed beach, the first three should never be flown simultaneously.

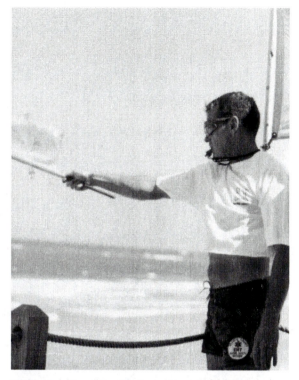

Lifeguard attracts the attention of swimmers with a whistle and gestures with a hand-held flag. Note that the lifeguard's patch indicates he is an EMT.

Credit: William McNeely, Jr.

Flag Color	Condition
Green	Low Hazard (small surf, light currents, and clean water)
Yellow	Moderate Hazard (moderate surf and/or strong currents)
Red	High Hazard (high surf and/or very strong currents and/or contaminated water advisory)
Red over Red	Water is closed to public contact. (One red flag flown above a second red flag.)
Purple	Marine pests present (e.g., jellyfish, stingrays, Portuguese man-o-war)—Note: This is not intended to be used to notify of the presence of sharks. If water is closed or hazardous due to the presence of sharks, use red flag(s).
Yellow with Black Ball	Surfing prohibited—Note: According to local regulation, this may include a variety of defined surfriding devices.
Black	Surfing permitted
Checkered	Use Area Boundary (example: boundary of a swimming and surfing area)
Red over Yellow	Protected Area

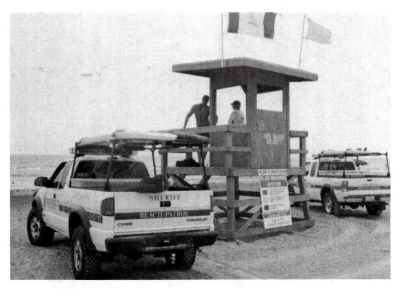

Credit: Peter Davis

Audible Signaling

Whistles

For years, whistles have been identified as communication equipment used by lifeguards. In many areas, whistles are used as attention-getting devices, followed by hand signals or other types of communication to impart messages or directions. Some agencies have developed complex whistle codes used for communication among lifeguards. Depending on the proximity of lifeguard towers, whistles may be a more certain method of communication among lifeguards than flags, in that the receiving lifeguard is alerted to the signal and can respond in kind. Nonetheless, the use of whistles should be seen as an ancillary form of communication which has limited application in the beach environment due to the restricted ability of whistle systems to convey complete messages with certainty.

Alarms

Audible alarms include air horns, bells, and buzzers installed at lifeguard towers. Like whistles, audible alarms are utilized in some areas as attention-getting devices, used to alert the public or other staff, and prepare them to receive directions or messages. Alarm codes may be developed for communication among lifeguards. Some agencies have installed alarms that automatically ring in at other emergency service agencies, triggering an immediate response.

The 9-1-1 System

The 9-1-1 system has created a national emergency telephone number for all emergencies. Unfortunately, some lifeguard agencies are poorly served by the system because it is generally designed to meet the needs of police, fire, and emergency medical services, not lifeguard services. Emergency calls for lifeguard services may actually be delayed or obstructed by the 9-1-1 system, unless steps are taken by lifeguard agencies to correct this situation.

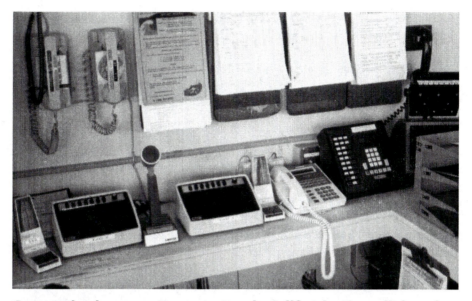

Communication area, Hermosa Beach, California. Note clipboards with answering protocols for 9-1-1 calls.

Credit: Rob McGowan

Prior to the advent of the 9-1-1 system, people summoning emergency assistance chose the emergency service they considered most appropriate to handle the emergency and called that agency's seven digit telephone number. Under the 9-1-1 system, people reporting emergencies no longer call directly to the responsible emergency service provider. Instead, they dial 9-1-1 and the operator who answers takes responsibility for conveying the information to the most appropriate emergency service provider. While this generally works well for police, fire, and emergency medical providers, 9-1-1 operators are not always familiar with lifeguard services and calls best handled by lifeguards can be misrouted to other emergency service providers, delaying response of lifeguards.

Once the 9-1-1 operator receives a call describing the need for response, conveyance of the information can generally take one of three forms: call transfer, call referral, or direct dispatch. The simplest system is direct dispatch. This is utilized by smaller communities with a central dispatch center for all emergency services. Under this system, the central dispatch center receives the 9-1-1 call, gathers pertinent information, and directly dispatches the emergency service provider.

Call referral and call transfer are used in areas where various emergency services maintain separate dispatching centers. Under call referral, the initial 9-1-1 operator elicits necessary information from the caller about the emergency, then calls the appropriate emergency provider by telephone and advises of the details. This system requires expertise on the part of the 9-1-1 operator about the details needed by each emergency service provider from callers.

Call transfer is a system under which the 9-1-1 operator makes a quick initial assessment, decides which is the most appropriate emergency provider, and immediately transfers the call to that agency. A dispatcher for the affected agency then has the opportunity to speak directly to the caller.

More advanced 9-1-1 systems include features known as automatic number identification (ANI) and automatic location identification (ALI). These features allow the 9-1-1 operator to see the location and call-back number of the caller on a computer screen. This can be particularly valuable for tourists unfamiliar with the address from which they are calling. Better 9-1-1 systems allow ANI and

ALI to follow a transferred 9-1-1 call to the destination agency. Unfortunately, technology to identify the location of cellular telephone callers, who are now a major source of reports of beach emergencies, has been slow to be implemented. Most 9-1-1 operators have no location information about cell callers, who may themselves be unfamiliar with the area from which they are calling. Without street signs or other types of landmarks that are recognized in computer mapping systems, it may be very difficult for operators who are not intimately familiar with the area from which the call is coming to direct emergency resources to the proper location. This technological gap has cost lives. It should be resolved over time.

Lifeguard agencies should take strong steps to make certain they are integrated into the 9-1-1 system to the fullest extent possible. Often monies for 9-1-1 are generated through surcharges on telephone bills and available to assist in implementation or purchase of equipment. Under any circumstance, lifeguard agencies should ensure that 9-1-1 operators are fully knowledgeable about the lifeguard service's area of responsibility and response capabilities, and that these operators have ways to immediately contact lifeguard agencies about reports of emergencies in areas under the supervision of lifeguards. This is of critical importance because misrouted 9-1-1 calls can and have resulted in unnecessary injury and even death.

Chapter Summary

In this chapter, we have learned value of two-way radios in lifeguard work, which is the preferred method of beach communication among lifeguards. We have also learned about use of telephones, including cellular telephones, public address systems, and public address systems. We have learned about arm signals, signs, and flags, including their relative benefits and detractions. We have learned about audible signaling using whistles and alarms. And we have learned about how lifeguards can maximize the value of the 9-1-1 system in receiving reports of aquatic emergencies.

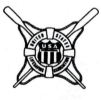

Discussion Points

- What are some reasons that two-way radios are considered the preferred method of beach communication among lifeguards?
- Why might a lifeguard agency choose to use codes or clear text in their radio communications?
- What are some benefits of public address systems?
- How might the Internet be used to enhance beach safety?
- What are some benefits and detractions in the use of arm signals?
- What are some things to remember with respect to the limitations of using flags to inform beach users of present conditions?
- What steps might a lifeguard agency take to ensure that it is notified of reports of emergencies received via the 9-1-1 system?

Chapter 23
Records and Reports

In this chapter, you will learn how to assemble and write a professional report. You will learn about some standardized reports commonly used by lifeguards. You will also learn about the importance of logbooks to record daily weather and activities.

CHAPTER EXCERPT

Lifeguard logbooks are legal documents, which may be publicly inspected or used in criminal or civil court cases. Lifeguards should limit their logbook entries only to information that is completely professional in nature and consistent with the information gathering needs of the lifeguard agency.

One important duty of a lifeguard is precise documentation of activities. Lifeguards, like other public safety providers, often view report routines as drudgery; but documentation helps justify appropriate levels of funding, staffing, and equipment. Documentation also provides the official records of an agency, which may be used in case of legal action. Few people can speak with certainty on the specifics of an incident which occurred in the distant past, without referring to reports taken at the time.

Report forms and required records vary from agency to agency throughout the United States, based on local or regional reporting requirements and laws. As a minimum requirement, however, most lifeguard agencies report on the topics covered in this chapter. A collection of generic lifeguard reporting forms can be found in *Appendix B*.

Nationally, the United States Lifesaving Association works to gather and report statistics from all open water lifeguard agencies in the US every year. These statistics are posted on the USLA Internet website *www.usla.org*. They are of tremendous value in helping inform the public about the important work of lifeguards. They are used for media reports and research. They also help justify the need for lifeguards. All open water lifeguard agencies are strongly encouraged to report their annual statistics to USLA. This is a requirement to maintain certification under the USLA Lifeguard Agency

Certification Program. To report annual statistics, consult the USLA website, where they can be easily entered and submitted electronically.

Report Writing

Well written reports are a positive reflection on the lifeguard and the lifeguard's agency. They help protect from liability based on speculation after the fact. They do so by depicting an accurate and complete record of the events. Good reports "stand on their own," telling a full story. They need no further explanations from the writer. The report should be understandable to a lifeguard or to a person with no lifeguard background whatsoever. Effective reports are concise, easily understood, in clear and correct English, and legible. They are factual, accurate, objective, and comprehensive.

Once the event has occurred, the report writer investigates the incident by interviewing witnesses (including lifeguards), observing the scene, taking measurements, and carrying out any other prudent actions needed to gather pertinent information. During this information gathering process, the lifeguard takes notes as appropriate. Taking photographs may be valuable, depending on the circumstances. Once this is complete, the report is developed. While many reports are very simple and brief, perhaps using standardized forms detailed later in this chapter, the following are some considerations in writing professional reports.

Report Writing Tips

- *Start Right Away*—Complete the report as soon after the event as possible, so that facts are not forgotten.
- *Keep Witnesses Available*—Ask witnesses to wait nearby until you can interview them. Otherwise, they may leave.

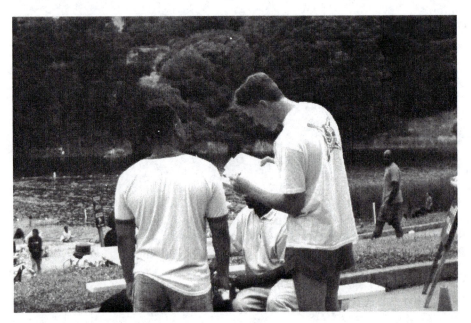

Credit: Dan McCormick

- *Interview Witnesses On-Scene*—It is usually easier for witnesses to remember and explain the circumstances and for you to understand them if you are at the scene of the incident.

- *Listen Carefully*—Within reason, let witnesses speak without interruption.

- *Don't Lead*—Witnesses should not be asked leading questions that imply a conclusion. Don't ask, "Is it true that this guy was showing off?" Ask, "What was he doing at the time this happened?"

- *Confirm Recollections*—Ask witnesses, "Did you see this happen?"

- *Include Details*—The report should include details of participants, like physical description, clothing description, personal data, last seen location, swimming skills, etc.

- *Companions*—Get information on any companions.

- *Medical Problems*—Ask whether the victim(s) had medical problems of any sort. Don't speculate on their contribution to the event, but state their existence.

- *Include Report Date and Time*

- *Include Date and Time of Incident and Key Elements*—Always record the time that key elements of the incident occurred, when that information is available. For example, "At 1030 hours, Lifeguard Dan McCormick, was on duty in tower #5. He states that he was contacted by a 35 year old female named Valerie Due, who advised that her five year old son, Matthew Due, was missing on the beach. McCormick states that he immediately contacted Lifeguard Supervisor Carl Martinez. At 1035 hours, Lifeguard Dave Shotwell made a general radio broadcast to all lifeguards, which was overheard by the writer of this report, including a full description of Matthew."

- *List All Responders*—Include the names of all officials (lifeguards, etc.) who responded to the incident. Include the rank of any referenced lifeguard, police, or fire official and the agency for which they work.

- *Include Addresses*—Include the name, address, and telephone number of every person in your report, other than an official associated with a named agency.

- *Investigate Contradictions*—In cases where the circumstances of the event are uncertain, interview several witnesses, if available. Separate witnesses, so that they don't color their recollections (whether intentionally or unintentionally) with what they hear from someone else.

- *Take Verbatim Statements*—Try to write down key elements of witness statements verbatim to the greatest degree possible, using quotes where appropriate. Have the witness slow down if need be. Read the statement back to them to make sure you got it right.

- *Use Chronological Order*—Report facts in chronological order, whenever possible.

- *Attribute Information*—Never state something as fact unless you personally observed it or know it to be a fact. Instead, attribute statements to the person who told you the information. Instead of stating, "Matthew had been told to stay beside tower #4," state, "According to Valerie Due, Matthew had been told to stay beside tower #4."

- *Be Concise*—Keep sentences short and to the point.

- *Use Simple Words*—Reports are not intended to display the education level of the writer or to challenge the reader's comprehension.

- *Avoid Jargon*—Codes, abbreviations, and lifeguard shorthand will make reports difficult to understand, particularly for non-lifeguards
- *Use Proper Spelling and Grammar*—Use a dictionary if you are uncertain of words and ensure that grammar is correct. A report with misspellings or grammatical errors can embarrass both the writer and the agency.
- *Measure*—When distances are cited, use actual, measured distances wherever possible. If you must estimate, explain the basis of your estimation.
- *Don't Speculate*—Reports are intended to be factual. If an opinion is needed, for some reason, make sure you state that it is your opinion and upon what facts that opinion is based.
- *Explain Conclusions*—If the report includes conclusions, explain how the writer arrived at them. Don't say, "Matthew had been sitting watching a volleyball game at tower #7 for over an hour." Say, "Information provided by witnesses Eric Bauer and Jerry Gavin suggests that Matthew had been sitting and watching their volleyball game at tower #7 for over an hour."
- *Write Legibly*—Printing is preferred.
- *Proofread*—Edit and proofread your report before submitting it.

Standard Reports

The following are some standard reports which lifeguards may be expected to complete. The forms may be generic (see *Appendix B*) or specifically designed for and by the agency.

Rescue Report

USLA defines a water rescue of a swimmer as any case in which a lifeguard physically assists a victim in extrication from the water when the victim lacked the apparent ability to do so without help. Even rescues considered routine by a lifeguard can represent the saving of a life which would otherwise be lost. This is a basic responsibility of lifeguards and should always be fully documented. USLA has developed a half page Incident Report Form for use in documenting rescues, medical aids, and other activities. It is included in *Appendix B* and may be reproduced by any lifeguard agency.

Medical Aid Report

Medical aids include all incidents in which medical care is rendered to a beach visitor. All medical aids should be documented. The level of documentation appropriate depends on the severity of the injury and disposition of the victim. For minor med-

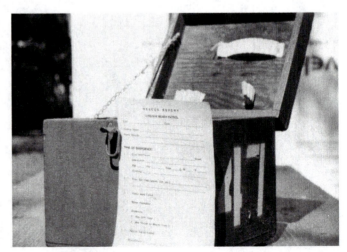

Credit: Dave Foxwell

ical aids and most intermediate medical aids, a brief report should usually be adequate. The Incident Report Form in *Appendix B*, for example, should suffice. Major medical aids, such as those involving life-threatening injury or illness, should be documented more thoroughly. An example Major Injury Report Form for this purpose can also be found in *Appendix B*.

Another form valuable in medical aid cases is the AMA form. AMA stands for *against medical advice*. In cases that a person refuses treatment when a lifeguard believes treatment is needed, it is a very good idea to have the person sign an AMA form, indicating that against medical advice of the lifeguard, the person is know-

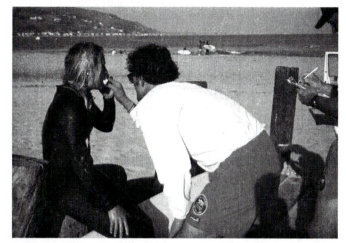

Credit: Ken Kramer

ingly refusing treatment. AMA forms can greatly reduce liability problems caused when people later accuse lifeguards of refusing to provide treatment or downplaying the nature of their injury. Attorneys should be consulted in creating an AMA form. Local emergency medical services are often good sources for language which meets local legal requirements.

Boating Assistance Report

Boat rescues include all cases in which lifeguards provide physical assistance to a vessel in apparent distress. While some agencies will record the rescue of boats using the same format as for the rescue of swimmers, other agencies require that a special form be completed. Usually, this report form will indicate the number of people rescued with the craft, and the estimated dollar value of the vessel before the rescue. The Incident Report Form in *Appendix B* can be used for most routine boat rescues.

Missing Person Report

Missing person incidents include situations where people, usually children separated from their group or parents, require assistance from lifeguard staff in being reunited. Missing person incidents are common emergencies at many beach facilities. Standardized report forms remind lifeguards to ask pertinent questions and allow ready dissemination of the information to others by reading from the report form.

While missing person cases are often seen as routine by lifeguards, there are situations in which missing persons are not found for days. In these cases, full documentation of the time and circumstances surrounding the initial report will be crucial to the continuing search. Since it can never be known upon the initial report whether the missing person will be quickly located, a thorough report should be taken in each instance. Taking a report also helps to demonstrate a sincere concern to anxious friends or relatives of the missing person. An example Missing Person Report can be found in *Appendix B*.

Death Report

Thorough reports should be completed whenever a death occurs in a beach area under the responsibility of lifeguards. In particular, a report should be completed whenever a drowning death occurs at or near a protected or unprotected beach. This report is usually required as part of a formal investigation into the drowning incident and may be required by law. Although police and medical examiners may also take reports, lifeguards should complete reports based on their information and involvement. The Major Injury Report Form in *Appendix B* can be used to report deaths.

Public Safety Program Report

Many lifeguard agencies are actively involved with programs given to the public at or away from the beach as a means of public education. Most agencies require that these programs be reported using special report forms, which usually indicate the estimated number of program participants.

Lost and Found Reports

Most lifeguard agencies provide lost and found services for the visiting public. People who have lost personal possessions can report their loss to lifeguards at stations or towers. People who have found items can turn them in. While operating a lost and found may sometimes be seen as routine, this service involves a significant degree of trust and responsibility. The person turning in the item(s) rightly expects honesty, integrity, and care on the part of the lifeguard, which must be fully satisfied.

Found items should be tagged and logged. Simple hang-tags may suffice. On them the receiving lifeguard should document the time the item was turned in, the place found, the name of the lifeguard, and the name and address of the person who turned it in. The item should then be logged on an appropriate form or in the logbook.

For cash, credit cards, or other valuables, a supervising lifeguard should take custody of the item and find an appropriate place to secure it. State or local laws, as well as agency protocols, may require that items of a certain value be turned over to police. In any case, it is important that these items be handled with great care and properly secured. When the property of others is entrusted to a lifeguard's care, the lifeguard and the agency immediately assume responsibility for its safekeeping and may be held legally responsible if the property is mishandled.

Narrative Reports

At times there is need for reports that do not fit into the standardized areas noted previously in this chapter. In other cases, there is a need to add further narrative descriptions or diagrams to detail the circumstances of an incident. *Appendix B* includes a sample Narrative Report form and a form for creating a diagram. Use of

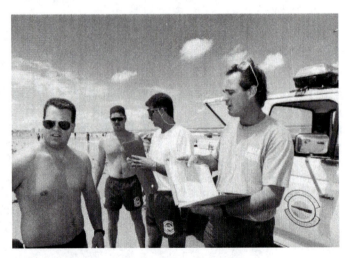

A lifeguard prepares to take a report.
Credit: Mike Hensler

report forms such as these can present a more professional image and ensure that important information about the author and incident are included.

Lifeguard Log

All lifeguard agencies should maintain a station or tower log, indicating, among other things, the weather and water conditions of the day, beach attendance, lifeguards on duty, workouts performed, rescues, and other key activities accomplished through the workday. Some agencies utilize simple hard bound datebooks. Others use photocopied forms. The daily log is used to document statistics for the lifeguard service's activities throughout the operational season or year. It also serves as a record of each day in case of inquiries at a later time. USLA affiliated agencies also use lifeguard logs to collect data used to report lifeguard activity statistics throughout the United States. Categories of lifeguard activities used for USLA statistics include:

- Beach Attendance
- Rescues Performed
- Preventive Actions
- Medical Aids
- Boat Rescues
- Drowning Deaths—Guarded Areas
- Drowning Deaths—Unguarded Areas
- Other Fatalities
- Missing Persons
- Public Safety Lectures

Lifeguard logbooks are legal documents, which may be publicly inspected or used in criminal or civil court cases. Lifeguard logbook entries should be concise, professional, and consistent with the information gathering needs of the lifeguard agency. Each entry should be initialed by the lifeguard making the entry. A sample of the statistical analysis form used for annual reporting to USLA is included in *Appendix B*. It includes the various categories of information which each agency should gather.

Chapter Summary

In this chapter, we have learned the steps required to develop a thorough and effective report. We have learned about standardized reports, including the rescue report, medical aid report, boating assistance report, missing person report, death report, public safety program report, lost and found report, and narrative report. We have learned about the value of a lifeguard logbook, what it should contain, and how it should be maintained.

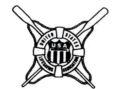

Discussion Points

- What are some considerations for completing a useful and understandable narrative report?
- What uses might there be for completed lifeguard reports?
- What daily events might be included in a lifeguard logbook?
- What are some uses for a properly completed lifeguard logbook?

Chapter 24
Public Relations

In this chapter you will learn about the importance of maintaining positive public relations. This includes all elements of lifeguard conduct, including public contact. You will learn about lifeguard uniforms, cultural diversity, and contacts with the media.

CHAPTER EXCERPT

Lifeguards are hired to protect and serve beach users. Tremendous courtesy and respect should therefore be paid to those asking questions, requesting assistance, or even filing a complaint.

Lifeguard operations are wide open to public view. It is often said that lifeguards work in a fishbowl, as they are constantly watched by beach visitors. On a busy day, just about every action of every lifeguard is probably observed by someone. Conversations are often overheard, despite assumptions to the contrary. How lifeguards conduct themselves is critical to garnering the respect and cooperation of the public. If lifeguards project an image of dedicated public safety professionals with an essential role of taking actions to protect the public, they are likely to engender great respect. On the other hand, if lifeguards project a cavalier image or fail to treat people fairly, public respect and support will be greatly diminished. An ongoing goal of lifeguards, in all activities, should be to enhance the image of lifesavers and the lifesaving profession. Each day and each public contact offer an opportunity to achieve this goal.

Principles of Lifeguard Deportment

Deportment is another word for behavior, but refers specifically to how one conducts oneself. Lifeguards are hired to protect and serve beach users. Tremendous courtesy and respect should therefore be paid to those asking questions, requesting assistance, or even filing a complaint. The fact that a beach user may seem rude is no license for the lifeguard to respond in kind. Becoming angry or confrontational is both unprofessional and counterproductive. A professional demeanor involves an even temperament and a helpful approach regardless of how the lifeguard may be treated by others. Professional conduct ensures a better outcome for the lifeguard and the lifeguard agency.

Another important reason for concern over lifeguard image involves the public perception of lifeguard services in general. If lifeguards wish to engender the respect and support commonly enjoyed by allied public safety providers, like police and firefighters, they must diligently cultivate a professional image. Professional lifeguards have worked hard to promote the image of lifesaving and to put aside negative stereotypes. Each lifeguard has a responsibility to all lifeguards to help maintain and further this image by conducting themselves as professionals *at all times*, whether on duty or off.

There are two major areas of lifeguard deportment: professional conduct and public contact. The following are tips for maintaining ideal levels of lifeguard deportment.

Professional Conduct

- *Maintain a Professional Appearance*—An alert, well-groomed, physically fit lifeguard in proper uniform immediately conveys a feeling of security to beach visitors. Male lifeguards are encouraged to report to work clean-shaven or with well groomed facial hair, depending on agency requirements. The wearing of jewelry should be avoided, both for safety reasons and to project a professional image.

- *Avoid Distractive Items*—Lifeguards should not keep items which create distractions in lifeguard stands or towers. Such articles may include musical instruments, reading materials unrelated to work, photographs, games, television sets, CD players, tape players, or toys.

- *No Games On Duty*—Lifeguards should not participate in beach or water games while on duty. Workouts and lifesaving drills however, are encouraged, in accordance with agency guidelines.

- *Don't Gambol*— Horseplay and pranks constitute unprofessional conduct.

- *Keep Stations and Equipment Neat and Clean*—Vehicles should be regularly polished. Assigned lockers should be tidy. Emergency equipment should always be in a ready condition, and positioned in an obvious and highly visible place. Unnecessary noise in and around the station should be eliminated. The public should not be permitted to use lifeguard stations as dressing rooms, checkrooms for valuables, or clubrooms. Only authorized personnel should be allowed in towers.

- *Keep the Area Clean*—Although lifeguards should not be assigned to general beach maintenance, when problems can be quickly and easily rectified, lifeguards should not avoid taking reasonable steps to help clean up. The beach should be regularly checked for general cleanliness and any potentially dangerous debris. If a condition cannot be rectified easily, appropriate maintenance personnel should be notified through proper channels. Lifeguards should never litter. They should inform the public about regulations on littering and use appropriate means to ensure compliance.

- *Face the Water*—Lifeguards should always attempt to position themselves so that the beach and water is in full view and face the water. Turning away from the water invites not only criticism, but also potential disaster. Lifeguards should learn to accomplish all essential activities facing the water, including holding short conversations.

- *Avoid Congregating*—While lifeguards need occasional breaks, when several gather in one place for an extensive period of time it can create the appearance of having nothing productive to do. If time is available, routine tower straightening and cleaning are alternatives. Workouts may also be appropriate or patrols of the beach, which can enhance lifeguard image and performance. After a significant rescue or medical emergency, it is natural, sometimes essential for lifeguards to come together for a debriefing, but this should be accomplished expeditiously and lifeguards should quickly return to their assigned positions. In these situations non-responding personnel are often spread thin and the system must be returned to normal status as quickly as possible.

- *Don't Leer*—Many people who come to the beach are proud of their physical fitness and appearance. They may seem to want to be viewed and appreciated. The skimpy covering provided by many bathing suits can easily attract attention. Lifeguards are not expected to completely ignore the appearance of others, but a glance is more than enough and extensive discussions about the appearance of a particular beach visitor are unprofessional. Such comments about the public or fellow lifeguards may constitute sexual harassment.

- *Use Binoculars for Lifesaving Duties*—Binoculars are an important lifeguard tool. It will be noticed however, if lifeguards use binoculars to view objects or people for reasons unrelated to their duties. Just as leering is inappropriate, using binoculars for this purpose only compounds the injury to a professional image.

- *Address Supervisors by Title*—Lifeguards should address lifeguard supervisors by their title (chief, captain, lieutenant, etc.) rather than by first names or nicknames, particularly when in the presence of beach visitors and other lifeguards.

- *Keep Disagreements Private*—Lifeguards should not engage in public disputes with fellow lifeguards or other emergency service providers. Problems should be worked out in a businesslike manner, with the assistance of supervisory personnel. If a dispute arises during an emergency, wait until afterward to work out differences of opinion, unless they must be resolved immediately in the interest of public safety. As Shakespeare wrote, the better part of valor is discretion.

- *Don't Pose for Unprofessional Photographs*—In the interest of public relations, many agencies will allow lifeguards to briefly assist with photography or pose for pictures. Lifeguards should always present a professional image in these cases, since they're likely to ultimately end up in somebody's slideshow. They may also show up in the media. A photograph, once taken, cannot be undone.

- *Enforce Rules Consistently*—Lifeguards should enforce all rules and regulations equally, with tact and diplomacy. Exceptions must sometimes be made, but they should never be made based on personal relationships or biases.

- *Keep Language Clean*—Lifeguards should never use foul language while on duty.

- *Don't Disrespect Other Lifeguards*—The best rule in any workplace is if you have nothing good to say about someone, don't say anything at all.

- *No Hazing*—Hazing has no place in a professional work environment.

Public Contact

- *Be Courteous and Polite*—Avoid approaches that start from a shout of, "Hey you," or similar words. Use sir or ma'am. Whenever possible, visitors should be approached personally and spoken to individually. The use of public address systems, whistles, and signals is good for general announcements, but is often embarrassing when used to address individuals. Such behavior will not achieve the goal of compliance.

- *Answer Questions Courteously*—Lifeguards should patiently and thoroughly answer all questions asked, unless it will interfere with public safety duties. When asked a question to which the lifeguard cannot supply an answer, the lifeguard should politely direct the visitor to a source where the information is available. When asked a question that seems to display ignorance on the part of the questioner, lifeguards should never display arrogance or disdain. Such questions offer the lifeguard an opportunity to educate the public. When speaking to a beach visitor, it is usually more polite to remove sunglasses.

- *Be Prepared with Answers*—Each day, beachgoers can be expected to ask similar questions. Examples are air and water temperature; times of tides (if any); forecast weather; the correct time; and conditions for swimming, surfing, diving, and other activities. Be prepared with answers. If the station has a bulletin board containing this information, the board should be updated regularly and neatly.

- *Don't Flirt*—Lifeguards should keep social conversation with non-lifeguards to a minimum. One negative stereotype of the lifeguard is of a person who uses the position to make social contacts. This appearance diminishes the public's perception of lifeguards. Conversations with beach visitors should be polite and businesslike. Reserve social conversation for after work.

- *Keep Electronic Communications Professional*—Public address systems and two-way radios should be used only for official matters. Lifeguards using them should realize that remarks made on these devices will be heard and judged by the public. Courteous

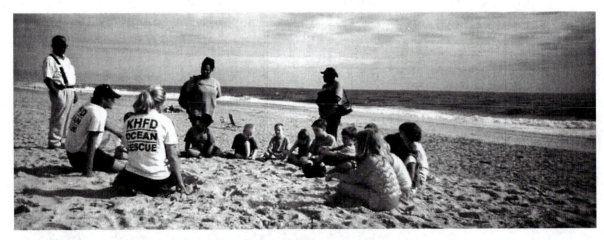

Lifeguards providing beach safety information.

Credit: Derek Boutwell

language is particularly important when the message will be heard by large numbers of people.

- *Don't Reprimand Victims*—The person who has been rescued has likely already learned a lesson. If a lifeguard considers it important to say something to help the person learn about the reason they were rescued and ways to avoid it in the future, the contact should be private and diplomatic. The egos of those who have been rescued are often bruised. Lifeguards should be aware that the public will side with them if they remain professional. Conversely, they will side against the lifeguard if it appears that the lifeguard is using a position of power to embarrass another member of the public.

- *Identify Yourself*—On-duty lifeguards should immediately provide their full name, position, and employer to any person requesting the information. The lifeguard who refuses to provide such information suggests a need to hide from a complaint that may or may not be valid. It is good practice to inform a supervisor of all complaints. This procedure provides the lifeguard's record of what transpired and eliminates the possibility of a supervisor being blind-sided by a complaint.

Uniforms

Most beach visitors will never actually speak to a lifeguard or even observe a rescue in progress. Their image of a lifeguard will be based on what they see and hear. Uniforms are a major part of that image. Uniforms are an effective and inexpensive way to establish a professional image for a lifeguard service. They are a valuable public relations tool which immediately identifies the wearer and shows authority. For example, when warning swimmers to move from one area to another due to a hazardous condition, the uniform itself lets people know that the lifeguard is someone who knows about these conditions and is authorized to move the public. Uniforms can be especially helpful in emergencies, since the public tends to defer to people in uniform. Properly designed uniforms also provide protection from the elements.

The most typical lifeguard uniforms are trunks for men and tanksuits for women, who may also be permitted or required to wear trunks over the tank suits. The color is most often red. Usually an authorized patch including the agency name and logo is sewn on one thigh (always the same thigh) of the trunks or the lower side of the tank suit. A T-shirt or collared shirt of consistent color and design is also typical. The low cost of silk-screening allows inexpensive creation of a uniform appearance.

Lifeguards are often seen from behind while watching the water or crouching over an injured victim. For this reason, some

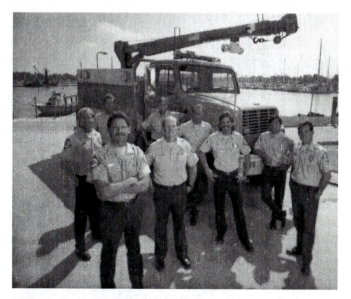

The San Diego Lifeguard River Rescue Team poses in front of their special rescue vehicle wearing "Class A" dress uniforms.

Credit: Dean Collins

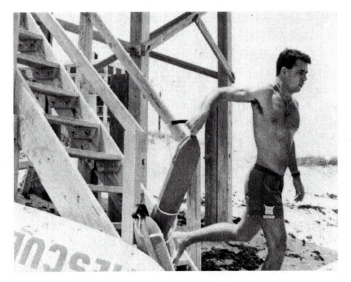

Credit: William McNeely, Jr.

lifeguard agencies make a point of silk-screening the word "LIFEGUARD" in bold letters on the upper back of the shirt, along with the name of the agency. The large wording immediately identifies the lifeguard to the public and to other arriving emergency responders. Uniforms may also include patches that identify advanced training that the lifeguard has received, such as *EMT* or *First Responder*. Other uniform items include hats, jackets, wetsuits, and so forth. In general, the more uniform lifeguards are and the neater the uniforms, the more professional the lifeguard agency will appear.

RFDs are not part of a uniform, but they have become symbolic insignias for lifeguards. Many agencies require that a lifeguard leaving a tower or stand carry a rescue device for identification and for ready use when needed. USLA strongly recommends this practice.

To be effective, uniforms should be identical or nearly so. Lifeguard agencies should issue policies to help in this regard. Few variations or changes from year to year should be permitted, so that uniformity is maintained and readily recognized by the public. In some agencies, lifeguards of different ranks may have different colored uniforms, but within ranks, they should be identical. Uniforms should always be neat and clean. Uniforms, such as faded or "salty" trunks or hats that are clearly past their useful life should not be permitted to remain in use. While lifeguards sometimes eschew uniformity in favor of comfort, this is counterproductive to maintaining a professional image. Lifeguards are part of a public safety team and should take appropriate steps to maintain the image of the team at all times.

The wearing of uniform items by off-duty lifeguards is no more professional than it would be for police or firefighters. The lifeguard image is perhaps more easily tarnished. For this reason, most agencies issue policies restricting the wearing of official uniform components during off-duty time. This policy should be strongly enforced, especially since the design of lifeguard uniforms makes this clothing particularly attractive for casual wear by off-duty employees proud to be lifeguards. Lifeguards should recognize that the image of the entire lifeguard agency can be compromised by the indiscriminate use of lifeguard uniforms while off-duty.

Cultural Diversity

The United States is made up of people from myriad cultures and ethnicities. Some are descendants of many generations of Americans. Others may be newer arrivals. Tourism draws people from around the world to U.S. beaches. Lifeguards must take great care to display evenhandedness and sensitivity to the users of their beaches.

From time to time disputes occur on the beach and lifeguards are placed in a position of being mediators. Nothing is more likely to incite anger than the appearance that one person's opinion is being valued over another's based purely on appearance or for similar subjective reasons. If all people are treated with a strong degree of fairness and equality, the lifeguard's decision, recommendation, or direction is much more likely to be accepted by all. By treating situations involving people of different cultures and lifestyles as learning experiences, lifeguards can broaden their professional and personal knowledge.

Media Contacts

Most lifeguards will not have direct communication with the news or entertainment media. This is typically a responsibility of supervisors. Nevertheless, the media has a high interest in beach activities and interviews of lifeguards are not uncommon. The media is generally very supportive of lifeguard services, but lifeguards can easily be unwittingly quoted in a newspaper report or on radio making a casual comment never intended for publication. Lifeguards should assume that anything they may say to a media representative may be quoted verbatim. This advice is particularly important in the aftermath of a death or other serious accident, or in regard to a controversial issue.

Lifeguard agencies should disseminate clear media policies that direct the media to designated contacts, whether supervisory personnel in general or specific media relations personnel. When being interviewed, lifeguards should take great care to state only facts, avoiding speculation. When being interviewed on-camera, it is particularly important to have a professional appearance. Confidential matters related to issues such as personnel discipline or the medical status of a victim should not be divulged, unless specifically permitted by rules or regulations. By maintaining a professional demeanor appropriate for any public contact, most media contacts will be positive.

Chapter Summary

In this chapter, we have learned some principles of lifeguard deportment, including elements of professional conduct and appropriate public contact. We have learned about the benefits of uniforms in projecting a professional image and identifying lifeguards. We have learned about the importance of being sensitive to issues of cultural diversity. And we have learned about some issues related to media relations.

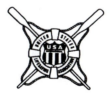

Discussion Points

- Why is lifeguard deportment so important in public relations?
- What are some guidelines for professional conduct?
- What are some guidelines for public contact?
- What are some examples of ways lifeguards can demonstrate respect for cultural diversity?
- What are some considerations in contacts with the media?

Chapter 25
Junior Lifeguard Programs

In this chapter, you will learn the history and purpose of Junior Lifeguard Programs in the United States. You will also learn about the components of typical junior lifeguard programs.

CHAPTER EXCERPT

Today, according to USLA statistics, there are well over 20,000 participants in junior lifeguard programs each year. Many current open water lifeguards and junior lifeguard instructors were themselves junior lifeguard participants at one time.

Junior lifeguard programs have become an important component of the services of open water lifeguard agencies. They help train young people about safe ways to enjoy the aquatic environment, serve as a recruiting tool, and offer a valuable summer activity. Junior lifeguard programs combine the fun of a summer camp with the physical and mental challenges of a lifeguard training program. In the course of a typical five to ten week program, participants can be introduced to the beach environment, educated about how to identify and avoid possible dangers, and grow in their confidence and ability to enjoy the beach. Most programs charge a fee intended to partially or fully offset program costs. In some cases, fees may be waived based on need.

History

During World War I, Chicago beaches faced a triple threat. The budget was tight, the war had caused a decline in lifeguard candidates, and the influenza epidemic made things even worse. Chicago was lacking in money for lifeguards and in people who could assume the responsibility. As one solution, the head of the city's beaches, Thomas R. Daly, decided to develop a junior lifeguard corps. Initially, this group was composed of boys who would add to the eyes of the regular lifeguards, notifying them of problems. In exchange they received T-shirts and the opportunity to practice with lifeguard equipment. Although they weren't supposed to be involved in rescue work, in 1924 six junior lifeguards rescued the 35-foot sailing vessel *Casmere*, which had run aground on a sandbar. As the Chicago program evolved, the numbers increased and the training became much more thorough. In 1926 there were 40 junior lifeguards. By 1939, there were 160. (Serb, 2000)

In other areas, the first junior lifeguard programs evolved decades later as a means for creating a pool of candidates for lifeguard jobs. Potential lifeguard candidates who showed promise, but were either too young or were not selected for a job were placed into a junior lifeguard program. Here, they would undergo a training process similar to that of a new lifeguard recruit, but without pay or assurance of future employment. In this way, lifeguard agencies would develop recruits for the next summer season.

Lifeguard agencies quickly realized that these summer training programs not only produced strong lifeguard recruits, but also provided a valuable public safety education opportunity and youth activity. By 1963, several California lifeguard agencies in Los Angeles, Orange, and San Diego counties had established junior lifeguard programs. The goal was to offer a fun, safe way for children to become oriented to the beach, as well as to learn lifesaving fundamentals, including CPR and first aid. This public education model had very positive results.

The first Junior Lifeguard programs were small by today's standards. For example, Huntington Beach, California's program was founded in 1963 with 24 participants and two instructors. Today, the Huntington Beach junior lifeguard program trains over 1,000 participants per year and employs about 50 staff instructors. Although it was 10 years before the Huntington Beach program accepted girls, they now make up about half of program participants.

Today, according to USLA statistics, there are well over 20,000 participants in junior lifeguard programs each year. Many current open water lifeguards and junior lifeguard instructors were themselves junior lifeguard participants at one time. Other junior lifeguards go on to take jobs outside lifesaving, but benefit greatly by the instruction they have received.

Junior Lifeguard Program Components

The content of junior lifeguard programs varies somewhat, depending on local needs and interests. This section covers some of the typical elements of these programs.

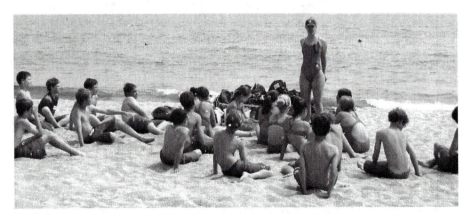

Credit: Eric Wayman

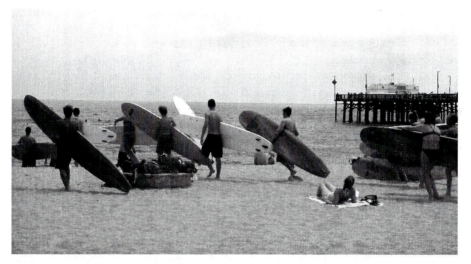

Credit: Eric Wayman

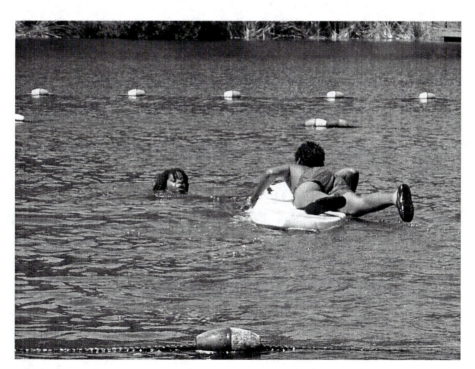

Credit: Stephanie Korenstein

Beach Orientation

Over the course of a summer session, a junior lifeguard is introduced to the beach environment. Depending on location, this may include information on subjects such as surf, piers, jetties, and aquatic life. Junior lifeguard programs also offer participants the opportunity to become acquainted with several areas to which the public does not readily have access, such as lifeguard towers, emergency response vehicles, and rescue boats. An emphasis on beach orientation is developing an understanding of the hazards present in the aquatic environment and how to enjoy the area safely. For example, junior lifeguards are taught about inshore holes, currents, and sandbars. They learn to read the water to determine the hazards that exist. They are taught how to react if they should find themselves in a dangerous position.

At surf beaches, junior lifeguards may learn the basics of bodysurfing and use of bodyboards. Many programs teach participants about the wealth of sea life in and around the ocean, as well as instructing them how to both avoid injuries caused by sea life. They are taught to respect the beach as a precious and fragile resource which can be and often is negatively impacted by careless human influence.

In addition to learning how to enjoy the beach and avoid potential dangers, junior lifeguards are introduced to the tools of the lifeguard trade. They are taught about purpose of lifeguard towers, the meaning of warning flags, how lifeguards work together as a team, how lifeguards use emergency vehicles and rescue boats, and how lifeguards use tools like RFDs and rescue boards.

The most important instruction involves teaching junior lifeguards how they can utilize these existing lifesaving resources when they visit the beach on their own. One of the golden rules for all junior lifeguards is the USLA admonition to *always swim near a lifeguard*. Though they may emerge from their junior lifeguard program feeling stronger, smarter, and more capable of enjoying the beach on their own, they will also be more aware of the fact that accidents can and often do happen, so they should use appropriate caution and select a beach with on-duty lifeguards.

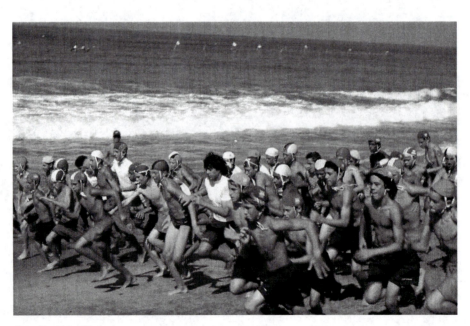

Credit: Eric Wayman

Skills Training

Junior lifeguards are constantly reminded that in case of an emergency, the best assistance they can offer is to call for help. However, many junior guard programs also attempt to provide their participants with skills training, so they will have additional options in the event of an emergency. The lifesaving skill most universally provided in junior lifeguards courses involves first aid. Depending on the program and age of the participants, this may be simple orientation to the basics of maintaining airway, breathing, and circulation. Some programs go well beyond, teaching recognized courses in CPR and first aid, and issuing appropriate completion certificates.

WEBBOX

You can find information on upcoming junior lifeguard events and download a copy of the rules for USLA competition at: *www.usla.org*

Junior lifeguard programs may also offer training in use of swim fins, mask and snorkel, RFD, and rescue boards. They may perform mock rescues or learn to spot victims in distress. They are usually provided sun protection tips, the importance of keeping themselves hydrated, and how to read a tide book.

The purpose of skills training is to prepare program participants to respond to the most common dangers or accidents that present themselves in a beach environment. It is not, however, intended to make these junior guards into self-sufficient lifeguards. In fact, one of the very first

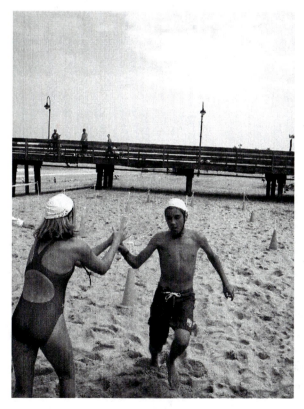

Credit: Eric Wayman

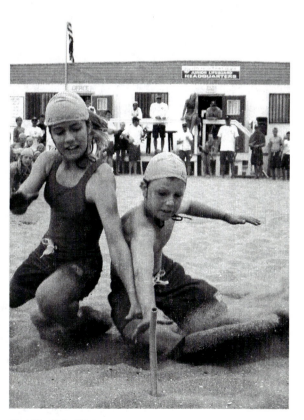

Credit: Eric Wayman

rules that junior guards are taught is *when in doubt, get help.* Junior lifeguard program instructors want to ensure that the confidence instilled in program participants will not cause them to over-extend themselves. A goal of any junior guard program is to prepare each participant to face every dangerous situation with a level head and calm rational thinking. This will help alleviate panic, which so often makes matters worse.

Physical Training

A valuable benefit that junior lifeguard programs boast over most conventional summer day-camp programs is physical training. While many 9-17 year-olds may spend their summer in front of a television or computer screen, junior lifeguard participants partake in a number of physically challenging events and competitions. Junior lifeguards participate in activities such as mock rescues, sand runs, rescue board paddling, and buoy swims.

Every event has some practical purpose for preparing a junior lifeguard to safely enjoy the beach or see what it takes to be a lifeguard. Beach runs and swims improve stamina as well as helping participants become more comfortable in and around the ocean. Games like beach flags and surf

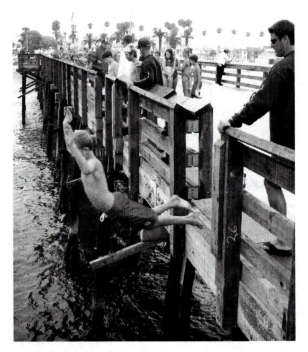

Credit: Eric Wayman

balls help a junior lifeguard locate and reach a potential victim. Ultimately, the goal of these events is to make junior lifeguard participants stronger, faster, and more confident in their physical ability.

Competition

Most junior lifeguard programs designate a competition day, on which junior lifeguards compete against one another. Competition events not only encourage each participant to push themselves physically, but also prepare them for the types of physical events that they might encounter in a lifeguard try-out or throughout lifeguard training. Although there are a number of universal events that most junior lifeguard programs run (e.g., soft or hard sand runs, swims, run-swim-runs, paddle-board races, rescue relays), each junior lifeguard program also offers its own unique, fun, and challenging events.

USLA regional and national competitions include a day of junior lifeguard competition, allowing representatives of these programs to compete in larger events and to meet other junior lifeguards from around the country. Competitors are divided into divisions by their age:

AA 16-17 years old
A   14-15 years old
B   12-13 years old
C   9-11 years old

USLA sanctioned competition events include: Distance Swim, Swim Relay, Run-Swim-Run, Distance Run, Beach Flags, Distance Paddle and Rescue Relays. Winners of each event can earn medals for themselves as well as competition points for their team.

Chapter Summary

In this chapter, we have discussed how and why junior lifeguard programs exist, as well as some of the physical training and lifesaving skills that a typical junior lifeguard program will offer. Ultimately, one of the greatest benefits of a junior lifeguard program is that, unlike regular summer camps which often act merely as baby-sitting programs for older children, junior lifeguard participants learn about the aquatic environment, are taught valuable lifesaving skills, and are challenged physically and mentally.

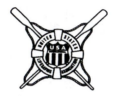

Discussion Points

- What are some of the ways a junior lifeguard program could help to improve public safety in a community?
- Beyond public safety, what are some additional benefits of a junior lifeguard program?
- What are some examples of appropriate activities for junior lifeguards?
- What are some important limitations that should be instilled in junior lifeguards?

Reference

Serb, C. (2000). *Sam's boys.* St. Joseph, Michigan: Imperial Printing Communication Company.

Chapter 26
The Responsible Lifeguard

In this chapter you will learn about what is involved in ensuring that lifeguards go about their duties in a responsible manner. You will learn about the influence of local laws, good Samaritan laws, immunity, and liability. You will also learn about professional responsibility.

CHAPTER EXCERPT

There is a tendency in the United States to focus heavily on the civil liability system. Unfortunately, the emphasis on liability tends to overshadow the real issue, which is that lifeguards, like all other public safety providers, need to live up to the tremendous trust placed in them by the public. Not because the law says they must, but because it is the responsible and right thing to do.

Many new lifeguards understandably have a great deal of pride at achieving their goal of working in the lifesaving profession. With that achievement comes a tremendous responsibility. Every day, people unknown to the lifeguard entrust their lives and those of their family and friends to the skill and vigilance of the lifeguard. Parents may still watch their children carefully, but they rely on presumption that if need be, the lifeguard will be there for them. This creates expectations, both professional and legal, that every lifeguard must meet. Each day, lifeguards have the opportunity to enhance their profession by rising to the level of trust placed in them by the beachgoing public. One inadvertent lapse though, may mean the difference between a happy day at the beach and the most profound tragedy of all—untimely death.

Legal Considerations

The expectation of the public and the legal system is that lifeguards will perform their job within the parameters of the training they have been provided. If another person or another person's property

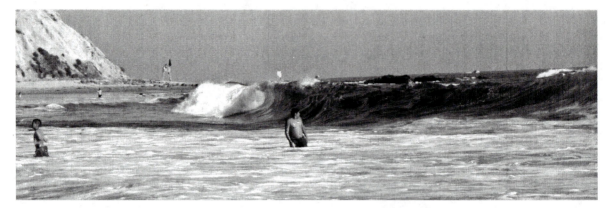

Credit: Ken Kramer

suffers injury due to failures on the part of the lifeguard to perform to appropriate standards, the lifeguard may be sued and found to be *liable* (responsible) for the injury. For example, the lifeguard who is distracted for no excusable reason when a preventable accident takes place may be successfully sued, along with the employing agency. Such a situation may also result in discipline and loss of employment. Lifeguards who do their job professionally, in accordance with their training, should have no inordinate fear of the civil liability system.

Discussions of legal points and case histories can fill an entire textbook on lifeguard management. The administrators of any well-organized lifeguard agency spend a considerable amount of time and effort studying the legal aspects of lifeguard services and developing appropriate protocols. These protocols are not only intended to protect and serve the public, but also to protect the lifeguard service and its employees from allegations of malfeasance. The training program provided by each agency is intended to reflect the protocols that have been established.

Collectively, the protocols developed will help to establish the standard of care provided by a lifeguard service. In legal terms, a safety provider found to have acted in accordance with a reasonable and accepted standard of care is without fault. This manual will not include extensive information on the various ways lifeguards may be held accountable for their actions. Instead, the following three generalizations are provided as yardsticks used to develop legal expectations:

- *Lifeguards Must Perform Their Duties*—Each lifeguard is given a special trust by the public as a guardian of safety at the beach. That trust requires constant vigilance during duty hours. Failure to act when actions are needed can be one of the most serious charges brought against a lifeguard; especially if that failure occurred because of distraction due to unprofessional conduct.

- *Lifeguards Must Perform Their Duties Consistently*—In addition to establishing policies and procedures for lifeguard duties, each agency establishes criteria for the performance of those duties (whether formally or informally), and a routine that lifeguards should follow during the workday. It is important to enforce rules and regulations and take preventive actions consistently, without making undue assumptions about conditions or abilities of beach visitors. Take for example the case of a beach where lifeguards consistently make a public address announcement at the end of each day to warn beach users that they are leaving the beach. One day, the announcement is forgotten and a swimmer dies by drowning soon after the lifeguard leaves. In addition to the tragedy of a death, this inconsistency of performance may cause a serious problem for the lifeguard and agency. Variations from normal protocol may be necessary in emergency work in special situations, but they should be considered carefully.

- *Lifeguards Must Perform Their Duties Properly*—During training, lifeguards are taught many procedures and techniques for use in rescuing and treating people who are the victims of aquatic accidents. These procedures and techniques are not advice to be considered, but rather directions and protocols to be followed. While judgment skills are important, lifeguards are expected to perform their duties following the established and authenticated procedures provided in training. Deviation may result in charges of malfeasance.

Conduct Checklist

The following checklist provides another way in which lifeguards can help ensure that their conduct is appropriate in a legal sense:

- Is it my intention to protect the health or safety of another person or property?
- In doing so, am I acting within the scope of my training and employment, either by handling the incident properly myself, or by handing it off to someone of equal or higher training?
- Am I exhibiting good faith as shown by behavior that the average, reasonable, trained person in my profession would exhibit under a scope of employment similar to mine?
- Am I providing medical care in accordance with the recommended standard of care?
- If I must make a judgment call due to a circumstance that is not covered by my scope of employment, am I doing so in accordance with what the average, reasonable, trained person in my profession would do in same or similar circumstances?

Local Laws

Each lifeguard agency falls under the jurisdiction of local or regional laws that have been established either to define the professional responsibility of an agency or employee or to limit liability. Because these laws vary from region to region across the United States, they cannot be covered thoroughly in this manual. Generally however, these laws fall into two categories:

Good Samaritan Laws

In many areas of the United States, Good Samaritan laws have been established to protect people who happen upon an emergency scene and stop to render aid to injured or distressed people. These people may be shielded from liability as long as they act in good faith and to the best of their abilities. In most areas, these laws are limited to protecting lay people who provide assistance and professional emergency providers (physicians, paramedics, lifeguards, etc.) who stop to provide assistance during off-duty time. In other areas, Good Samaritan laws also protect on-duty emergency personnel, but only under special stipulations and conditions.

Immunity Laws

In some areas, certain governmental agencies will be exempt from specific liabilities under governmental immunity laws or special provisions of constitutions. In other areas, the there is a ceiling to the amount of damages an agency can be forced to pay if found liable for injuries. Some states have laws which specifically define types of recreation as hazardous and thereby regulate claims which may be made as a result of injuries sustained in hazardous recreation. There can also be special tort claims laws which limit claims that may be made against agencies as a result of loss, damage, or injury.

Protecting from Liability

Most lifeguard agencies have access to the assistance of legal departments, corporate attorneys, district attorneys, city attorneys, or other legal experts in defending against lawsuits. Under some circumstances these legal departments may also represent or defend employees who are named in lawsuits as codefendants. Lifeguards should become aware of the level of protection which may be afforded them in a liability case. Even in frivolous lawsuits, where there is clearly no fault on the part of the lifeguard, significant costs may be incurred in mounting a legal defense.

Ultimately however, the best protection from liability is to perform all duties effectively, within the guidelines provided by the hiring agency. A lifeguard who stays alert, responds expeditiously as needed, and provides aid which meets a reasonable standard of care should have few worries or incidents. After all, liability arises only it is believed that errors have been made which could reasonably have been prevented by prudent action. By avoiding those errors in the first place, civil liability itself normally becomes a moot issue.

Professional Responsibility

There is a tendency in the United States to focus heavily on the civil liability system. Unfortunately, the emphasis on liability tends to overshadow the real issue, which is that lifeguards, like all other public safety providers, need to live up to the tremendous trust placed in them by the public. Not because the law says they must, but because it is the responsible and right thing to do.

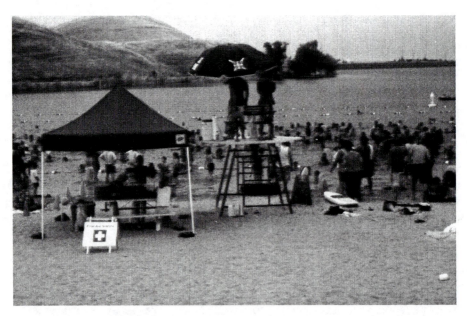

Credit: Dan McCormick

When a father comes to the beach with his three children, he is not thinking about suing the lifeguard or lifeguard service. He simply wants to go home with his family at the end of the day with all of them safe and sound. He may not ever speak with a lifeguard, but he nevertheless entrusts the safety of his family to that lifeguard. When a lifeguard is on the stand and is tired or distracted or otherwise less than fully attentive, the lifeguard would do well to remember that people are counting on that lifeguard—to protect their lives.

This manual, along with a training program which meets the minimum recommended standards of USLA, is intended to provide all lifeguards with the knowledge, skills, and tools needed to ensure

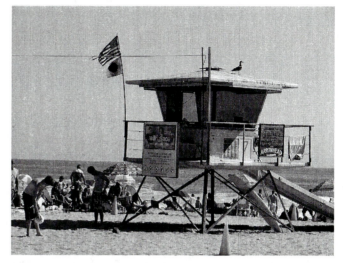

Credit: Nick Steers

beach safety. All the training in the world however, will be to no avail if a lifeguard fails to maintain a vigilant and professional approach to the job at all times.

Lifeguards are given the gift of a job which can provide an extraordinarily high degree of personal satisfaction. The work environment is unmatched and hundreds of lifeguards go home each day having saved the life of another person. Those who choose to accept this gift should take the public trust that comes with it and protect that trust by doing the best job they can every day.

Many people who work as lifeguards have stayed with the profession for years. Others go on to take other jobs; but they invariably look back longingly. "I used to be a lifeguard," they will often say, "best time of my life."

We think it will be the best time of yours, too. Good luck in your service.

Chapter Summary

In this chapter we have learned some of the elements of being a responsible lifeguard. We have learned about expectations of the public and the legal system, including local laws, Good Samaritan laws, and immunities. We have learned ways lifeguards can protect themselves from liability. And we have learned about the professional responsibilities of being a lifeguard.

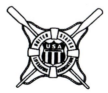

Discussion Points

- What are some circumstances that might cause liability for a lifeguard or a lifeguard agency?
- How can lifeguards limit the possibility of being found liable for an injury?
- In what kind of cases might Good Samaritan laws apply?
- What are examples of immunities?
- What are the primary reasons that all lifeguards should act in a responsible manner?

Appendix A

USLA Approved Arm Signals

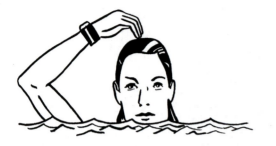

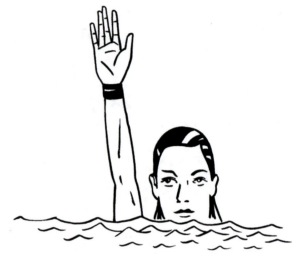

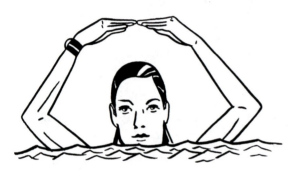

All Clear (OK)

Assistance Needed

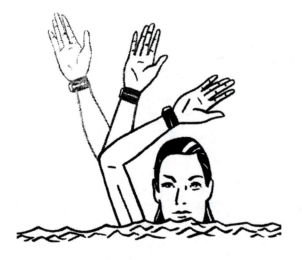

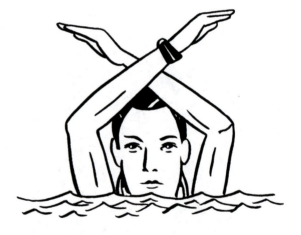

Resuscitation Case or Oxygen Needed

Submerged Swimmer

Appendix B
Report Forms

These forms are intended for photocopying.

United States Lifesaving Association
Incident Report Form

Lifeguard Agency: _____

Incident Location: _____

Incident Date: _____

Time: _____ ☐ AM ☐ PM

Incident Description

Water Rescue:
- ☐ Ocean
- ☐ Bay
- ☐ Lake
- ☐ River
- ☐ Other:_____

Medical Aid:
- ☐ Abrasion
- ☐ Laceration
- ☐ Burn
- ☐ Fracture
- ☐ Other:_____

- ☐ Lost Person
- ☐ Boat Rescue
- ☐ Cliff Rescue
- ☐ Flood Rescue
- ☐ Arrest
- ☐ Other:_____

Victim's Activity

- ☐ Swimming
- ☐ Floating
- ☐ Wading
- ☐ Surfing
- ☐ Body Surfing
- ☐ Non-Swimmer

- ☐ Boating
- ☐ Walking/Running
- ☐ SCUBA/Skin Diving
- ☐ Beach Activity
- ☐ Jumping/Diving
- ☐ Other:_____

Primary Cause

- ☐ Rip Current
- ☐ Large Surf
- ☐ SCUBA
- ☐ Drop-off
- ☐ Alcohol/Drugs
- ☐ Other:_____

Victim Information

Name: _____ Street Address: _____ City: _____ State: ____ Zip: _____ Phone: _____

Age: _____ ☐ Male ☐ Female ◆ Injury Description: _____

Incident Details

_____

Victim Disposition: ☐ Released ☐ Released to Parent ☐ Advised to see Physician ☐ Ambulance ☐ Police ☐ Other:

Responding Lifeguards: _____

United States Lifesaving Association
Incident Report Form

Lifeguard Agency: _____

Incident Location: _____

Incident Date: _____

Time: _____ ☐ AM ☐ PM

Incident Description

Water Rescue:
- ☐ Ocean
- ☐ Bay
- ☐ Lake
- ☐ River
- ☐ Other:_____

Medical Aid:
- ☐ Abrasion
- ☐ Laceration
- ☐ Burn
- ☐ Fracture
- ☐ Other:_____

- ☐ Lost Person
- ☐ Boat Rescue
- ☐ Cliff Rescue
- ☐ Flood Rescue
- ☐ Arrest
- ☐ Other:_____

Victim's Activity

- ☐ Swimming
- ☐ Floating
- ☐ Wading
- ☐ Surfing
- ☐ Body Surfing
- ☐ Non-Swimmer

- ☐ Boating
- ☐ Walking/Running
- ☐ SCUBA/Skin Diving
- ☐ Beach Activity
- ☐ Jumping/Diving
- ☐ Other:_____

Primary Cause

- ☐ Rip Current
- ☐ Large Surf
- ☐ SCUBA
- ☐ Drop-off
- ☐ Alcohol/Drugs
- ☐ Other:_____

Victim Information

Name: _____ Street Address: _____ City: _____ State: ____ Zip: _____ Phone: _____

Age: _____ ☐ Male ☐ Female ◆ Injury Description: _____

Incident Details

_____

Victim Disposition: ☐ Released ☐ Released to Parent ☐ Advised to see Physician ☐ Ambulance ☐ Police ☐ Other:

Responding Lifeguards: _____

Lifeguard Agency:

_____

☐ Non-Fatal
☐ Fatal

United States Lifesaving Association
Major Injury Report Form

Page 1 of _____

Report #: _____

Incident Date: _____ Time: _____ ☐ AM ☐ PM Exact Location: _____

Victim Information

Name:	Date of Birth: Age: ☐ Male ☐ Female
Street Address:	City: State: Zip: Phone:
Description: Hair Color:	Eye Color: Weight: Height: Ethnicity:

Apparel: ☐ Bathing Suit ☐ T-shirt ☐ SCUBA ☐ Other (describe): _____

Evidence of: ☐ Alcohol Consumption ☐ Drug Use ☐ if either, describe _____

Injury Description: _____

Witness Information

	Name	Street Address	City	State	Zip Code	Age	Telephone
1.							
2.							
3.							

Incident Details

☐ The area was not guarded ☐ The area was guarded by (lifeguard names): _____

The following lifeguards responded: _____

Equipment used: _____

Apparent reason for injury: _____

Medical aide rendered: _____

Primary Cause of Incident: ☐ Rip Current ☐ Surf ☐ Alcohol ☐ Drugs ☐ Ability ☐ Other: _____

Other responding agencies: ☐ Police ☐ Fire ☐ Rescue Squad ☐ Paramedic ☐ Coast Guard ☐ Park Ranger ☐ Other: _____

For Water Related Cases: Water Conditions ☐ Calm or _____ foot waves Water Temperature: _____ Water Depth: _____

For Submersion Cases: Search Time Start: _____ Search Time End: _____ ☐ Recovery Date: _____ Time: _____ ☐ None

Incident Narrative

_____
_____
_____
_____
_____
_____
_____
_____ ☐ Report Continued

_____   _____
Report Completed By   Report Approved By

United States Lifesaving Association

Missing Person Report

Date: _____

Time: _____

Lifeguard: _____ Station: _____ Report Number: _____

Missing Person

Name: _____ Age: _____ ☐ Male ☐ Female

Physical Description	Clothing	Last Seen

Height: _____ Swimsuit: _____ Time: _____

Weight: _____ Shirt: _____ Place: _____

Hair Color: _____ Pants: _____ Activity: _____

Hair Texture: _____ Shoes: _____ Direction of Travel: _____

Eye Color: _____ Hat: _____ Towel Area: _____

Race/Ethnicity: _____ Other: _____

Local Address: _____

Local Phone: _____ Car Location/Description: _____

Other Info: _____

_____

Reporting Party (RP)

Name: _____ Relationship: _____

Street Address: _____ Home Phone: _____

City, State, Zip: _____ Local Phone: _____

Local Address: _____

Beach Location: _____

Found

Date: _____ Time: _____ Location: _____ By: _____

Lifeguard Agency:	**United States Lifesaving Association**
	Search & Recovery Checklist

Page 1 of _____

Report #: _____

Date: _____

<u>Time</u>

_____ Submersion victim reported by: _____

Last seen point: _____

Last seen time: _____ □ AM □ PM

Victim description: _____

_____ Preliminary search commenced

_____ Incident Commander (name): _____ declares Code X

_____ All units advised of incident via □ radio broadcast □ telephone □ other: _____

_____ Search and rescue team summoned

_____ Full search commenced

_____ Rescue vessel(s) requested and dispatched

_____ Emergency medical services (EMS) ambulance requested to standby at scene

_____ Availability of search helicopter checked, Incident Commander advised

_____ Helicopter requested for aerial search from (agency): _____

_____ Medical evacuation helicopter placed on standby, Incident Commander advised

_____ Crowd control assistance requested from (agency): _____

<u>At Scene Times</u> • who? • what unit number? • how many?

_____ _____

_____ _____

_____ _____

_____ _____

_____ Emergency medical services (EMS)

_____ Search helicopter

_____ Medical evacuation helicopter

_____ Victim recovered (or) □ no recovery

_____ Search terminated on order of Incident Commander

_____   _____

Report Completed By   Report Approved By

☐ NARRATIVE REPORT ONLY	United States Lifesaving Association	PAGE
☐ CONTINUED FROM	**Narrative Report**	OF
		INCIDENT DATE

AGENCY	VICTIM	INCIDENT LOCATION

I was informed by... • The type of incident was... • I observed... • The witness/victim said... • I did... • The incident was resolved by...

_____

_____

_____

_____

_____

_____

_____

_____

_____

_____

_____

_____

_____

_____

_____

_____

_____

_____

_____

_____

_____

_____

_____

_____

_____

_____

_____

_____

_____

_____

_____

_____

_____

☐ Report Continued

REPORTING LIFEGUARD	REPORT APPROVED BY	REPORT DATE

Use Arrow and N to Show True North

Appendix C
Diver Accident Report Forms

These forms are intended for photocopying.

IDAN DIVING INJURY REPORT FORM (DIRF)

DAN Chamber Code   (*Diver Completes Pages 1 & 4*)   **Chamber Patient ID #**

Last Name _____

First Name _____ MI _____

Daytime Telephone # _____

Evening Telephone # _____

❑ Male ❑ Female

Date of birth (mm/dd/yy) _____

Height _____ cm or ft/in Weight _____ kg or lbs
                (circle)   *(circle)*

Are you a certified diver?   ❑ Yes ❑ No

If yes, year first certified _____

Highest certification _____

Number of dives in past 12 months _____

Number of dives in past 5 years _____

Are you a DAN Member?   ❑ Yes ❑ No

Are you a volunteer for *Project Dive Exploration*
or *Project Safe Dive*?   ❑ Yes ❑ No

Check all medications you currently take
❑ Decongestant/Antihistamine/Allergy
❑ None   ❑ Inhaler for Asthma
❑ Diarrhea   ❑ Oral Asthma Drug
❑ Motion Sickness   ❑ Pain Killer
❑ Anticonvulsant   ❑ Anti-Malarial
❑ Insulin   ❑ Other *(List in 'Comments')*

Check all current health problems
❑ None   ❑ Heart Disease
❑ Asthma   ❑ Back Pain
❑ High Blood Pressure   ❑ Joint/Muscle Pain
❑ Diabetes   ❑ Other *(List in 'Comments')*

Check all past health problems
❑ None   ❑ Ear/Sinus Surgery
❑ Treated for DCS/AGE   ❑ Asthma
❑ Back Surgery/Problem   ❑ Ear Barotrauma
❑ Lung Surgery/Problem   ❑ Other *(List in 'Comments')*

Cigarette smoking
Do you smoke cigarettes?   ❑ Yes ❑ No
If yes, how many packs per week? _____
How many years have you smoked? _____

For women
Menstruating during dive series?   ❑ Yes ❑ No
Do you take oral contraceptives? ❑ Yes ❑ No
Are you pregnant?   ❑ Yes ❑ No
Are you post-menopause?   ❑ Yes ❑ No

Where were you diving when you were injured?
❑ Ocean/Sea   ❑ Lake/Quarry/River
❑ Tank/Pool   ❑ Cavern/Cave
❑ Dry Chamber   ❑ Other *(List in 'Comments')*

Dive series (all dives or altitude exposures with less than a 48-hour surface interval)
Dive Site: Country _____ State/Province _____

Total # Days Diving _____ Total # of Dives _____

Last Dive Ended: Date _____ Time: _____

Max Depth in Series _____ fsw or msw *(circle)*

Max Depth of Last Dive _____ fsw or msw *(circle)*

Were all dives at sea level?   ❑ Yes ❑ No

If no, altitude of dive site _____ft or m *(circle)*

Altitude exposure between dives? ❑ Yes ❑ No

Did you make any safety stops?   ❑ Yes ❑ No

Decompression stops required (& made) by dive
table or computer?   ❑ Yes ❑ No

How did you conduct your dive when injury occurred?
❑ Dive Computer   ❑ Follow Another Diver
❑ Dive Table   ❑ Other *(List in 'Comments')*

Altitude exposure after diving
Within 48 hours of last dive?   ❑ Yes ❑ No

If yes, surface interval _____ hrs

Altitude (if known) _____ ft or m *(circle)*

❑ Commercial Fixed Wing   ❑ Mountain Travel
❑ Unpressurized Fixed Wing ❑ Helicopter
❑ Medical Evacuation Aircraft

Purpose of dive when injury occurred
❑ Recreational   ❑ Instructor/Guide
❑ Technical   ❑ Scientific
❑ Student   ❑ Military
❑ Other (specify) _____

Breathing apparatus when injury occurred
❑ Open-Circuit Scuba   ❑ Closed-Circuit Scuba
❑ Semi-Closed Scuba   ❑ Surface-Supplied
❑ Other (specify) _____

Breathing gas when injury occurred
❑ Air   ❑ Heliox % O2 _____
❑ Nitrox (EAN) % O2 _____ ❑ Other *(List in 'Comments')*

Diving dress when injury occurred
❑ Wetsuit   ❑ Swimsuit
❑ Diveskin   ❑ Drysuit
❑ Other (specify) _____

Problems during dive when injury occurred
❑ Out of Air   ❑ Nausea / Dizziness
❑ Rapid Ascent   ❑ Injury
❑ Missed Decompression   ❑ Cold
❑ Heavy Exertion   ❑ Short of Breath
❑ Equipment *(List in 'Comments')* ❑ Other *(List in 'Comments')*

	Signs, Symptoms and Findings *(see Recommendations in 'Instructions')* Verify Diver's reports from Page 4	Body Location	Onset Date (mm/dd/yy)
1			
2			
3			
4			
5			
6			
7			
8			
9			

COMMENTS *(use another DIRF for additional signs & symptoms, medications, parenteral fluids, etc.)*

EMERGENCY OXYGEN ON SURFACE *(See 'Instructions' for Method)*

Date & Time Started	Duration	% O2	Flow Rate	Method	Comments

RECOMPRESSION *(See 'Instructions' for Chamber Type, Protocol, Gas & Complications)*

Date & Time Started	Chamber Type	Protocol	Gas	Complications	Comments

MEDICATION *(See Instructions for Route. List additional drugs in 'Comments')*

Date & Time Started	Drug Name	Dose	Route	Comments

PATIENT EVALUATION AND TREATMENT *(For use by chamber personnel)*

Onset Time (hh:mm)	SEVERITY *(see 'Instructions' for recommended Severity Scores)*								
	After Emerg 02	At Admission	After 1st Recomp	After 2nd Recomp	After 3rd Recomp	After 4th Recomp	After 5th Recomp	Maximum Severity*	At Discharge

COMMENTS *(use another DIRF for additional recompression, etc.)*
❑ *Check here if another DIRF was used*

* *List time of maximum Severity*

DISCHARGE SUMMARY *(check all that apply)* **Discharge Date** _____   **Discharge Time** _____

Diagnosis	Summary Description			Discharge Status
❑ DCS-I	❑ Pain Joint	❑ Gait/Coordination	❑ Pneumomediastinum	❑ Complete Relief
❑ AGE	❑ Pain Muscle	❑ Vertigo	❑ Pneumothorax	❑ Improved but has Residual
❑ DCS-II	❑ Pain Girdle	❑ Hearing Loss	❑ SOB/Cough	❑ Unchanged
❑ DCI	❑ Sensory Nonspecific	❑ Constitutional	❑ Aspiration/Immersion	❑ Deteriorated
❑ Lung Barotrauma	❑ Sensory Joint	❑ Higher Function	❑ Otic Barotrauma	❑ Deceased
❑ Not due to Pressure	❑ Sensory Peripheral	❑ Dermatological	❑ Marine Life Injury	❑ Against Medical Advice*
❑ Ambiguous	❑ Sensory Dermatome	❑ Lymphatic	❑ Other *(List in 'Comments')*	
❑ Unknown	❑ Muscle Weakness	❑ Hypotension		
❑ Other *(Comments)*				

Discharge Destination
❑ Home   ❑ Other *(where?)* _____

Print Name of Chamber Representative for IDAN follow-up

_____

Date _____

Please send this form to:

Divers Alert Network
The Peter B. Bennet Center
6 West Colony Place
Durham, NC 27705

How did you feel before your last dive?	❏ Good	❏ Fair	❏ Tired	❏ Exhausted	❏ Hungover

Did you have symptoms before your last dive? ❏ Yes ❏ No *If yes, explain in 'Comments.'*

Did you have symptoms underwater or at altitude? ❏ Yes ❏ No *If yes, explain in 'Comments.'*

Were you given emergency oxygen? ❏ Yes ❏ No *If yes, list date, time, method, flowrate & duration in 'Comments.*

Were you treated in a chamber for this dive series? ❏ Yes ❏ No *If yes, list where and when in 'Comments.'*

In order of onset, what were your symptoms and their severities on a scale of 1 *(minor)* **to 10** *(worst possible)* **?**	**Where were the symptoms in your body?**	**What dates and times did the symptoms occur?**
1st:		
2nd:		
3rd:		
4th:		
5th:		
6th:		

COMMENTS *(other symptoms, changes in symptoms, of dive profile, emergency O2, recompression, etc.)*

RELEASE FOR RESEARCH STATEMENT I understand that this form is for research only and not for insurance purposes. All information will be kept strictly CONFIDENTIAL. I understand that International Divers Alert Network (IDAN) may contact me for clarification. This release authorizes any hospital, medical clinic, physician, nurse and/or the keeper of medical records to divulge, give, and/or permit to copy any information pertaining to the medical condition or history of the undersigned to IDAN only. I agree that a copy of this statement shall have the same validity as the original.

*Diver Signature*_____ *Date* _____

Signature of Witness to Release _____ *Date* _____

Appendix D
Knots and Splicing

The rope work described and illustrated in this appendix will meet most ordinary needs in lifesaving. Lifeguards must learn these knots and practice them until they can be tied with speed and certainty. Supervisors should regularly test these skills. It is better to know these few knots expertly than to have superficial knowledge of many.

A knot or splice is never as strong as the rope itself. The average efficiency of knots varies from 50-60% of the rope's strength. However, a well-made splice has about 85-95% of this strength. Splices are therefore preferred for heavy loads.

The strength of a rope is derived largely from the friction that exists between the individual fibers, yarn, and strands of which the rope is made. The twisting of these fibers into yarn, then into strands, and finally into cables is done in such a manner as to increase the amount and effectiveness of the friction between the rope elements.

Knots

Knots use friction to keep two or more pieces of line together. Properly tied knots create a level of friction adequate to keep the end of a line secure (fastened) when a load is placed on the line. Knots that can be tied and untied swiftly can make the difference between life and death, or the saving and destruction of property.

The square or reef knot (Figure D-1) is perhaps the most useful knot known. It should not be used to tie together lines of different sizes, as it will slip. The square knot is used for tying light lines together, not for tying heavy hawsers. Although simple and effective, the square knot has one serious flaw — it jams and is difficult to untie after being heavily stressed.

The sheet or becket bend (Figure D-2) is used for tying two lines of different sizes together. It will not slip, even if there are great differences in the size of the lines.

The bowline (Figure D-3) will not slip, does not pinch or kink the rope as much as some other knots, and does not jam and become difficult to untie. This knot is the most desirable knot for carrying heavy loads and is the most useful and important knot for lifeguarding purposes.

The clove hitch (Figure D-4) is actually composed of two half hitches, tied in such a way that they work together. This knot is used for making line fast temporarily to a piling or bollard.

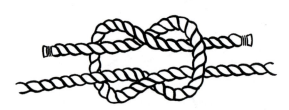
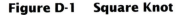

Figure D-1   Square Knot

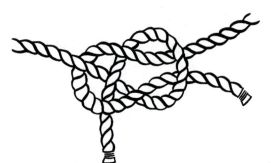
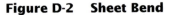

Figure D-2   Sheet Bend

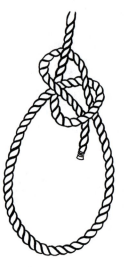

Figure D-3   Bowline

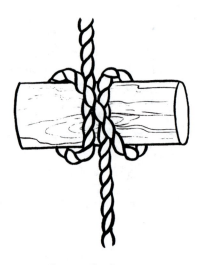

Figure D-4   Clove Hitch

The fisherman's bend (Figure D-5), also called the anchor bend, is handy for making fast to a buoy or the ring of an anchor.

Cleats (Figure D-6) are found on most boat docks, on flagpoles, and in other places. They allow the free end of a line to be quickly and securely fastened, and detached with equal ease. Tying a line to a cleat involves running the line around the base of the cleat, and then tying a half hitch around one of the horns. Usually, an additional half hitch is tied to the other horn in such a way that the line falls together on the cleat.

Splicing

Splicing essentially involves weaving a rope back into itself. It is stronger than a knot and cleaner, without a large bulge that might catch on something as the line plays out. Splicing is usually done to

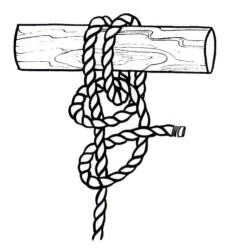

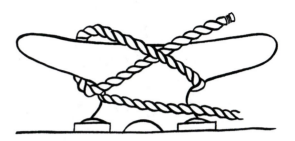

Figure D-5   Fisherman's Bend

Figure D-6   Tying to a Cleat

create a loop in the line (eye splice), or to join the ends of two lines. The following explanations cover the splicing of twisted, not braided, line. For purposes of explaining splicing and knots rope is said to have a *standing portion* and a *free end*. The free end is the end of the rope in which the knot is tied or the splice is made. The standing part is the remainder of the rope, away from the free end.

End-Splice

An end splice (Figure D-7) is used to permanently join the ends of two lines to create a single line. The splice will be much stronger than any knot and much cleaner. This enlarges the rope's diameter at the splice, but much less so than would a knot.

Step 1 — To start the end splice, the splicer first unlays the strands of both rope ends for a short distance as described for the eye splice. The six strand ends are taped to prevent unraveling. In this type of splice, it may also be helpful to wind a small piece of tape or string around the standing end of each line at the junction where unlaying of the strands was started. Next, the ends are married together so that the strands of each rope lie alternately between strands of the other.

Step 2 — Working with any one of the three free strands on one line, it is tucked under a strand on the other line just above where the unlaying was done and past the tape or string. Then the next strand is tucked under the next adjacent strand in the standing line, and finally the third. It may be easiest to fully splice one line into the other in one direction, until the ends are fully tucked, before beginning the splice in the other direction.

Step 3 — Once the splice has continued in both directions until all six strands are fully tucked, the splice is complete. For adequate strength, there should be at least five tucks per strand. After the splice is finished, it can be rolled under foot to smooth it up, then a strain put on it, and finally the excess ends cut off.

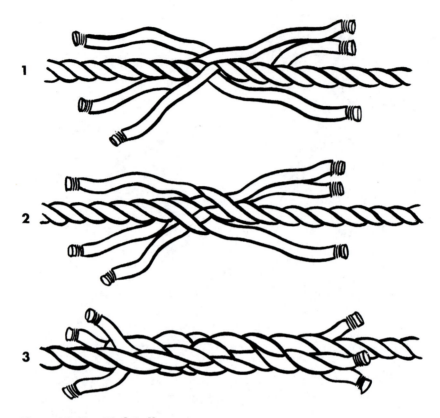

Figure D-7   End Splice

Eye Splice

The eye splice (Figure D-8) creates a permanent loop in the end of a line. The loop can be spliced around a fixed object, such as the end of a rescue buoy, to create a permanent attachment or simply left in the end of a line for other purposes. One end of a boat tow, for example, is a spliced loop.

The eye splice is started by separating (unlaying) the twisted strands about six inches to a foot or more back from the end of the line, depending on the size of rope being spliced. The ends should be taped using masking tape or similar to prevent unraveling of the strands during splicing.

Next a loop is formed in the rope by laying the free end back along the standing portion of line so that the center strand lies over and directly along the standing part. The size of the loop is determined by the point where the opened strands are first tucked back into the line.

Step 1 — The splicer starts by selecting the topmost strand of the standing part of the line and tucking B under it. It should be pulled up snugly, but not so tight as to distort the natural lay of the strands in the standing part of the line. Note that the tuck is made from right to left, against the lay of the standing part. Next, the left strand (A) is tucked under a different strand of the standing line, which lies to the left of strand under which B was pulled. The splicer tucks from right to left in every case.

Step 2 — The loop should be turned over as has been done in Step 2 of Figure D-8. Strand C is now pulled under the third strand of the standing part of the line. The greatest risk of starting a splice incorrectly is in the first tuck of strand C. It should go under from right to left. If the first tuck of each of the strands A, B, and C, is correctly made, the splice at this point will look as shown in Step 2.

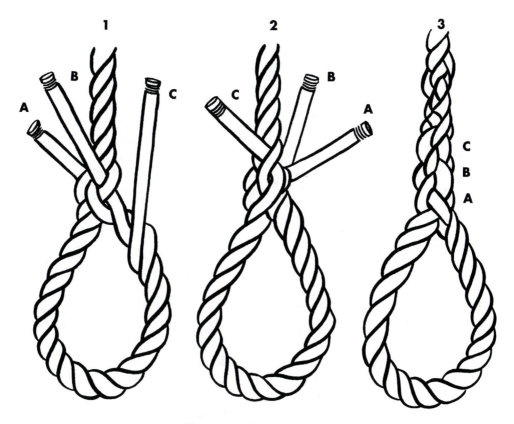

Figure D-8   Eye Splice

Step 3 —The splicer then returns to strand A, lays it over the next strand up the standing part of the line, and then tucks it under the one after that. The same is then done with B and C in order. This process is repeated, one tuck at a time, until the ends have been woven (spliced) fully into the standing part of the line with no significant end left. When complete, the splice should appear as in Step 3 of Figure D-8.

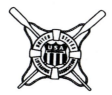

Glossary

abaft—aft of, to the rear of

abeam—on the side of the vessel, amidships, or at right angles

about—to go on the opposite tack, change directions

abyss—an extraordinarily deep part of the ocean

accretion—gradual build-up of sand or shoreline due to current or tidal action

adrift—floating at the mercy of wind or current

aft—toward the stern of a vessel

aground—a vessel which has struck bottom; also known as grounded, beached

air embolism—in scuba diving, a serious disorder caused by rapid expansion of air in the lungs during a fast ascent

all terrain vehicle (ATV)—a small three or four wheel vehicle with oversized tires or treads designed for use on rough terrain

alveoli—small sacs in the lungs where exchange of carbon dioxide and oxygen takes place

amidships—middle point of a vessel between bow and stern

anoxia (also anoxemia)—absence of oxygen

antifouling paint—a substance applied to a the hull of a vessel which is intended to chemically resist attachment of marine organisms

antimicrobial—a substance which is capable of destroying or inhibiting growth of microorganisms

Aqualung (TM)—see scuba

artificial respiration—inflating the lungs of a person by mechanical means or by blowing into the airway of the victim

ash breeze—absence of wind; calm

aspirate—to inhale a substance into the lungs; a typical finding in a near drowning incident is *water aspiration*

aspirator—tool used to clear fluid or food regurgitation from the air passages of an asphyxiated or non-breathing patient

astern—behind a vessel

atmosphere—(physics) a unit of pressure equal to the air pressure at sea level; pressure at sea level (one atmosphere) is 14.7 pounds per square inch (psi), but it doubles at 33 feet in water depth (two atmospheres), triples at 66 feet in depth (three atmospheres), and so on

awash—covered by water; usually the state of a vessel overcome by waves or tide

backboard—see spineboard

backrush—seaward return of water following the uprush of a wave on the beach backup—safety personnel who respond to assist the primary rescuer(s) to assist or stand-by a rescue operation

backwash—see backrush

backwater—(1) water turned back by an obstruction, opposing current, or the like; (2) to propel a rowboat or dory in a stern first direction using a reverse rowing or boating stroke

bag-valve-mask resuscitator (BVM)—a hand-held ventilation device used for artificial respiration consisting of a self inflating bag, a one-way valve, and a face mask; used with or without oxygen

bailout bottle—a small scuba tank with limited air supply that can be strapped to the waist and used for a rapid underwater search (also known as a pony tank)

ballast—broken stone, gravel, or other heavy material used in a vessel to improve stability or control the draft

bar—a submerged or emerged embankment of sand, gravel, or mud built on the sea floor in shallow water by waves and currents

barometer—an instrument for measuring atmospheric pressure and generally used for predicting changes in the weather

bar port—a harbor that can be entered only when the tide rises sufficiently to permit passage of vessels over a bar

bather—(dated term) a swimmer or wader

bathymetric chart—a map delineating the form of the bottom of a body of water, usually by means of depth contours

BC, BCD—see buoyancy compensator

beach break—waves breaking hard on a sharply sloping sand beach

beach erosion—the carrying away of beach material by wave action, tidal currents, littoral currents, or wind

beam—(1) a vessel's maximum width (2) the side of a vessel

beam sea—wind at right angles to a vessel's keel

bearings—the position of one location with respect to another; for example, lifeguards may get their bearings by noting their location in the water as compared to several fixed points on shore

becalm—a sailing vessel is becalmed when there is no wind adequate to propel the vessel forward; also known as being "in irons"

bellyboard—a small surfboard or similar inflexible object ridden in the surf in a prone position, also known as paipo board, Boogie Board,® or bodyboard

bends—see decompression sickness

berm—a narrow shelf, path, or ledge created by wave action on the sand

bilge—lower internal part of vessel's hull

billow—usually a great wave or surge of water; any wave

bitt—a vertical post (usually one of a pair) fitted into a vessel's deck for securing lines for towing, mooring, or other purposes

blind rollers—long, high swells that have increased in height almost to the breaking point as they pass over shoals or run in shoaling water

bloodborne pathogen—an agent carried in the blood, particularly a living microorganism, capable of causing disease

blown out—the state of waves which have been knocked down by wind

board surfing—any activity that involves riding waves with the use of a surfboard; also known as surfing, riding

boating—the standing, forward facing rowing position used by the stern rower of a dory

boat tow—a short length of line with a fastener at each end that enables a swimming lifeguard to tow a boat in distress

bodyboard—see belly board

body skimming—sliding along the beach on thin water in a prone position after gaining momentum from running and leaping forward; also known as body whomping

bodysurfing—riding a wave without the aid of a floating device

boil—upwelling of water caused by a swell riding or striking shallow water or rock formations, causing a visual disturbance on the water surface; also known as up-swelling, swirls

Boogie Board®—see bellyboard

bosun's chair—a seat in which a person hangs while being moved from one vessel to another or to shore

bow—the forward part of a vessel

breaking wave—a wave breaking on the shore, over shoal water or reef; a wave which makes an audible noise as it spills over; also known as a breaker or crasher

breakwater—a structure protecting a shore area, harbor, anchorage, or basin from waves or current; also known as seawall, jetty

broach—to veer sideways to the wind or swell; a vessel which broaches in the surf is in great danger

buddy system—two persons, usually divers, swimming together for mutual support and safety

bulkhead—(1) any upright partition separating compartments on a vessel; (2) a wall or embankment for holding back earth and protecting a shoreline from erosion due to wave action

buoy line—(1) a line supported by buoys, used to delineate a boundary in the water; (2) separated buoys placed in a line to delineate a water boundary

buoyancy compensator (BC)—an inflatable vest-like device used by divers to compensate for changing buoyancy when descending and ascending; also known as a buoyancy compensator device (BCD)

Burnside, Bob—inventor of the modern plastic rescue buoy, still known to some as the *Burnside buoy*

calm—the state or condition of the water surface when there is no wind, waves or surface disturbance

can rack—storage rack for rescue buoys

cataracts—a clouding of the lens of the eye, associated with long term exposure to sunlight

cat's paw—a puff of wind; a light breeze affecting a small area, as one that causes patches of ripples on the surface of a water area

certification officer—(USLA) person appointed by the USLA to evaluate whether an applying agency adheres to the recommended USLA open water lifeguard guidelines

chafe—to rub or damage by rubbing

chafing gear—anything used to prevent chafing

channel—(1) a natural or artificial waterway that periodically or continuously contains moving water, or that forms a connecting link between two bodies of water; (2) the part of a body of water deep enough to be used for navigation through an area otherwise too shallow for navigation; (3) the deepest portion of a stream, bay, or rip current through which the main volume or current of water flows

chock—a heavy casting of metal or wood with two short horn-shaped arms curving inward between which ropes or hawser may pass for towing, mooring, etc.

chop—disturbed surface of water usually caused by strong wind or after-effects of waves; white caps

cleat—a metal fitting with two horns pointing in opposite directions and used for temporarily fastening a line; usually attached to a dock, pier, or vessel

close hauled—setting a sail such that the boom roughly parallels the length of a vessel, when sailing in the direction of the wind; also known as reefing

coast—the general region of indefinite width that extends from the sea inland to the first major change in terrain features

coastal current—a relatively uniform drift usually flowing parallel to the shore in the deep water adjacent to the surf line; may be related to tides, winds, or distribution of mass; also known as offshore current

Code III—the code in many states for an expedited emergency response; requires emergency lights and siren for an emergency vehicle

Code X—(1) the USLA approved code word which signifies a missing (submerged) swimmer, causes implementation of an emergency plan for locating and retrieving a missing swimmer; (2) the USLA approved signal for a missing (submerged) swimmer formed by crossing the arms overhead in the form of an X

comber—a deep water wave whose crest is pushed forward by strong wind

coral—(1) a rocklike structure or reef formed of the hard calcareous skeleton of various anthozoans; (2) a polyp of the family Anthozoa

coral head—a mushroom or pillar-shaped coral growth

countercurrent—a current flowing adjacent to the main current but in an opposing direction

crasher—a wave breaking hard from top to bottom; also known as pounder, coming over, heavy, sand buster, cruncher

crest—the highest part of a wave

crest width—the length of a wave along its crest

critical incident stress debriefing—a meeting of those involved in a life-threatening incident to help workers cope with related stress, usually led by a mental health professional,

curl—curved portion of a wave which tumbles forward

current—a stream of flowing water

daily information board—sign displayed by lifeguards advising the public of ambient weather and surf conditions, as well as other topical information

davit—a small crane-like device on a vessel used for launching a small boat over the side or hoisting cargo; usually used in tandem with one holding the bow and the other the stern of the small boat

dead reckoning—a method of navigation utilizing only the speed and heading of the craft, without reference to astronomical observations or mechanical positioning devices

decompression illness—a scuba diving affliction which occurs when compressed gases in the body produce bubbles which form in the cells or circulatory system

defibrillator—a device that sends an electric shock through the chest to the heart to attempt to change the rhythm of an ineffectively beating heart to a productive rhythm

degree—(1) a unit of temperature; (2) a unit of angular distance; 1/360 of a circle

demand valve—a valve attached to a face mask that delivers 100% oxygen to a breathing person on demand

diver's flag—a flag generally flown on a floating device, intended to warm boaters of submerged scuba divers; standard appearance of the diver's flag is either square red with a white diagonal bar running across from one corner to other or alpha flag (burgee) with inner half blue, outer half white

dive tables—chart of rules for scuba divers to use in avoiding decompression sickness; also known as decompression tables

documented vessel—vessel registered with the U. S. Bureau of Customs or the U. S. Coast Guard

dorsal fin—the main fin located along the back of many fish and marine mammals

dory—(lifeguard) boat with narrow flat bottom and high flaring sides propelled by rowing and designed for use in surf

draft—the depth of a vessel below the water line

drowning—asphyxiation by submersion in water or other liquid

dry suit—diver's suit designed to protect and retain body heat without allowing water to permeate

ebb current—outgoing tidal current associated with a decrease in the height of a tide

ebb tide—outgoing tide

eddy—a circular movement of water usually formed where currents pass obstructions, between two adjacent currents flowing counter to each other, or along the edge of a permanent current

Eight Plate®—descent device shaped like the number 8 which, when properly used, exerts friction on line passing through it and allows control of line with a load placed on it; used in cliff rescue; also known as: figure eight electrolysis—(nautical) chemical decomposition of metals or alloys by the action of an electric current caused by contact with salt water

embayment—an indentation in a shore line forming an open bay

Emergency Medical System (EMS)—network of community resources and medical personnel to provide emergency care to victims of sudden illness or injury

emergency operation plan—a plan for efficient response to an anticipated emergency situation

equalize—to bring air pressure in the sinuses to a point equal to ambient air pressure; necessary primarily in scuba diving and flying; also known as clearing

equatorial tides—tides occurring approximately every two weeks when the moon is over the equator

erosion—a natural processes by which sand, soil, or rock is broken up and transported, usually by wind and water

estuary—the area where a river meets a tidal bay; also known as drowned river mouth, branching bay, firth, forth

exostosis—an abnormal bony growth on the surface of a bone or tooth (sometimes a complication in the ear canal of swimmers due to long term exposure to cold water)

fake—(n) one coil of a rope; (v) to lay out line in such a way that it will easily play out when one end is thrown or otherwise pulled

fathom—six-foot measure of water depth

fathometer—device used to measure the depth of the water; also known as depth gauge, depth finder, depth sounder

feathering—(1) a wave just beginning to break, blowing white water on the peak of a wave caused by wind or momentum; also known as knifer, hanging up; (2) rowing technique involving dropping the wrists to cause the oar blades to be parallel to the water on the return stroke

feeder channels—channels parallel to shore along which feeder currents flow before converging to form the neck of a rip-current

feeder—current of water moving along the shore providing water to a rip current; usually created by wave action and gravity

feeling bottom—the action of a deep water wave on running into shallow water and beginning to be influenced by the bottom

fender—cushion to protect a boat from bumping against a dock or another boat; also, bumper

ferry angle—an upstream angle against a current taken in an effort to reach a specific point ashore

fetch—(1) an area of the sea surface over which seas are generated by a wind having constant direction and speed; (2) the length of the fetch area, measured in the direction of the wind in which the seas are generated

first responder—(1) a medical aid provider first to the scene of a medical emergency; (2) an emergency medical aid course produced by the National Highway Traffic Safety Administration

flag system—consistently colored flags used to designate certain water activity or surf conditions

flotation device—any device that a person uses for support on the water surface

flood—the incoming tide

flotsam—floating debris, driftwood, etc.

flow—the combination of tidal and nontidal current that represents the actual water movement

free ascent—an emergency skill used by scuba divers in reaching the surface when air supply is unexpectedly available; a free ascent is likely to result in decompression illness

free diver—a diver operating without the benefit of scuba equipment; skin diver

freeboard—the vertical distance from the water to the gunwale of a vessel

full time lifeguard—lifeguard appointed to a full time, year round position as a lifeguard at an open water beach

fully developed sea—the maximum height to which ocean waves can be generated by a given wind force

gang grapnel—A series of hooks set in a parallel pattern and used in the same fashion as a grappling hook

glassy—smooth, unrippled sea surface caused by absence of wind

grappling hook—a device with four, five, or more flukes or claws used to drag on the bottom to snag corpses or other objects

groin—a small jetty, extending at roughly right angles to the shore, usually designed to trap lateral drift and/or retard erosion of the shoreline

ground swell—a long, high ocean swell

guarded area—water recreational area with lifeguards on duty; a guarded beach

guide lines—lines secured to an object to prevent it from being damaged; lines attached to aid in control of a floating or suspended object

guidelines—(USLA) The Guidelines for Open Water Lifeguard Training & Standards promulgated by the USLA for use in the national Lifeguard Agency Certification Program or Aquatic Rescue Response Team program

gully—a relatively narrow ravine in the ocean bed

gunwale (gun-el)—the upper edge of the side of a vessel; also known as the rail

gutter rip—a short, powerful, fast-moving rip current found on a scalloped, steep, sloping beachfront; gutter rips can sweep people off their feet by surprise and into the next wave; the sweeping underwater current action is often confused with the misnomer "undertow"

harbor—an area of water affording natural or manufactured protection for vessels

hawser—a heavy line used to moor or tow a vessel

head of a rip—area where the neck of a rip widens and disperses and the power of the rip ends

heavy sea—severe water disturbance caused by winds or swell; also known as rough sea

heavy surf—large breaking waves; also known as heavies, surf's up, crashers, blue birds on the horizon

helm—wheel or tiller by which a vessel is steered

helmsman—one who steers a vessel; also known as driver, operator, pilot

high siding—leaning body weight toward that side of a boat that is broadside and being pushed by a wave in an effort to avoid capsizing

high water mark—the highest point that water reaches during a tidal phase

hurricane wave—a sudden rise in the level of the sea associated with a hurricane; also known as hurricane surge, hurricane tide

hydrofoil—a vessel equipped with planes that provide lift when the vessel is propelled forward

hypertonic—having a higher osmotic pressure than the surrounding medium; when seawater is aspirated, its salt content is higher than that of fluids in the tissues of the lungs (hypertonic) and can draw that fluid into the lungs

hyperventilation—excessive breathing in and out; skin divers hyperventilate when preparing to hold their breath; hyperventilation purges the breathing stimulant, carbon dioxide, out of the respiratory system and to a minor degree increases the percentage of oxygen in the lungs; hyperventilation can cause unconsciousness and drowning

hypoxia—lack of oxygen in the tissues of the body

incident command system (ICS)—a system used to control and direct resources at the scene of an emergency; commonly used by emergency providers

incident commander (IC)—the person in charge of an emergency incident; most often used when the incident command system has been formally implemented

inflatable rescue boat (IRB)—an inflatable soft hulled boat powered by an outboard engine capable of carrying several lifeguards and rescue equipment; also known as an inshore rescue boat

inhalator—machine used to administer a fresh flow of oxygen or air on demand to a breathing patient in irons—a condition that prevents a sailing vessel to move forward; the operator of a sailing vessel that is in irons is unable to change the position of the vessel to allow the sails to fill

inlet—a short, narrow waterway connecting a bay or lagoon with the sea

inside—area between the breaking waves and the shoreline; usage: "he was caught inside by large surf"

intersecting waves—one of the component waves that, when superimposed on others, produces cross-swells; also known as sugarloaf sea, pyramidal sea

intertidal zone—that portion of the shoreline lying between the high and low tide marks

intramuscular—within a muscle (ex: an intramuscular injection involves first inserting a needle into the muscle)

intravenous—within a vein or administered into a vein (ex: intravenous fluids are administered by first inserting a needle into a blood vein)

inversion layer—a layer of water in which temperature increases with depth

invertebrate—an organism that lacks a spine, such as a sea urchin or mollusk

isthmus—a narrow strip of land, bordered on both sides by water, that connects two larger bodies of land

jettison—to throw objects overboard, especially to lighten a craft in distress; to remove articles from a person to allow more buoyancy, such as the weight belt from a scuba diver

jetty—a structure, usually of rock, extending into a body of water to protect a harbor or shoreline from erosion and storm activity; also known as groin

junior lifeguard—adolescent or younger person involved in a program taught by professional lifeguards to learn lifeguarding techniques; also known as nipper, J.G., junior guard

keel—a longitudinal structure extending along the center of the bottom of a vessel that gives main support to the vessel's hull bottom; the keel often projects below the bottom; also known as center line, skeg

kelp—the general name for large species of seaweeds; kelp forests are common along the West Coast with single plants extending 60 or more feet from the bottom; also known as seaweed

Kimball, Sumner Increase—first and only leader of the U.S. Lifesaving Service during its existence from 1878 to 1915; formerly chief of the Revenue Marine Division which (included lifesaving services) from 1871 to 1878

knee board—a type of belly board designed and used to surf in a kneeling position

knot—one nautical mile per hour (a nautical mile is 1.15 times a statute mile)

lagoon—a shallow sound, pond, or lake generally separated from the open ocean

landline—line swum out to a victim or victims in distress and used to pull them back to shore; also known as reel, line, lifeline

landmarks—a conspicuous object on land or sea that marks a locality; a visual line-up of two or more fixed objects on the beach to obtain a precise location on the water surface; also known as marks

last seen point—the last place a victim was observed before submerging

lead line—(1) a line, wire, or cord used in sounding; (2) a light line which is thrown, shot, or swim to make a connection between two points and to then pull a larger line, such as a hawser, between them (usually for towing purposes)

leash—a short line used to secure a surfboard, belly board, bodyboard, or similar flotation device to the user's wrist or ankle; also known as a tether, surf leash

leeward—the side (usually of a vessel) away from the wind

lifeguard boat—vessel used by lifeguards to save lives and property or to patrol an assigned area; also known as rescue boat, patrol boat, surf boat

life car—a device used by the first lifesavers in conjunction with the breeches buoy apparatus to evacuate several victims at a time from a distressed ship

lifeguard stand—a primitive elevated observation post used by lifeguards, lacking first aid or storage facilities; usually staffed only in the busy season; also known as seasonal tower, bird cage, supplementary tower, perch, bench lifeguard vehicle—vehicle used to transport backup lifeguards and lifesaving equipment to needed areas and to patrol an assigned area; also known as a jeep, rescue vehicle, four-wheel drive vehicle, mobile unit, area unit, lifeguard truck

life ring—a floating ring which can be thrown to a person in distress, often including rope around the edges

littoral drift—the material moved in the littoral zone under the influence by waves and currents

littoral transport—the movements of material along the shore in the littoral zone by waves and currents

littoral zone—the nearshore zone

log book—book kept at main stations, on rescue boats, and in emergency vehicles listing pertinent daily activities and times; used as a record of lifeguard activity

low water—the lowest limit of the surface water level reached by the lowering or outgoing tide

lull—period of lower waves between sets of unusually large waves

lunar tide—that part of the tide caused solely by the tide-producing forces of the moon as distinguished from that part caused by the forces of the sun

Lyle, David—originator of the Lyle gun used by early lifesavers to deploy the breeches buoy apparatus

macular degeneration—loss of central vision, associated with long term exposure to sunlight

main tower—a lifeguard station, usually staffed all year, that supplies assistance to other lifeguard facilities in a given area; also known as tower zero, mother station, central vantage tower, control tower

make fast—to secure the end of a line by tying it to a fixed point

mass rescue—a rescue involving multiple victims, usually more than two or three; also known as multiple victim rescue

mat surf—surfing waves with the aid of an air-filled, semi-flexible object; also known as air mattress, rubber raft, float

mean high water (MHW)—the average height of all high

mechanical resuscitation—resuscitation done with the aid of a mechanical device, as opposed to mouth-to-mouth

mooring—an anchored buoy to which a boat is secured when not in use

mouth-to-mouth—resuscitation of a non-breathing victim by blowing air from the mouth of the rescuer into a nonbreathing victim's airway; also known as rescue breathing

mouthpiece—the breathing end of a snorkel

mud flat—a muddy or sandy coastal strip usually submerged by high tide

narcosis (nitrogen narcosis)—an sense of stupor or drunkenness felt by deep sea divers due to increased levels of dissolved nitrogen in the blood; also known as rapture of the deep

neck—portion of a rip where most drownings and rescues take place

nematocyst—stingers, found in jellyfish and Portuguese man-of-war, which are intended to paralyze prey and ward off attackers

nontidal current—any current that is caused by other than tidal forces

notice to mariners—a periodic notice containing information affecting the safety of navigation

observer—a person in a vessel delegated to watch a person or object being towed by the vessel

offshore wind—a wind blowing seaward from the land in a coastal area; also known as land breeze, opposing wind

off-gassing—in scuba diving, the release of nitrogen from body tissues upon ascending, which is necessary to avoid decompression sickness (DCS)

one-feeder rip—rip current fed by a current coming from only one direction

onshore wind—a wind blowing landward from the sea in a coastal area; also known as a sea breeze

open water—any sizable natural body of water such as a lake, river, ocean, lake, or bay

OSHA—acronym for the Occupational Safety and Health Administration of the U.S. Department of Labor, charged with ensuring that workplaces are safe

outflow—the flow of water from a river or its estuary to the sea

outside—anything on the offshore side of the surfline; also known as back side, out back

over the falls—object or person falling without control from wave peak to the wave bottom; also known as a wipeout

painter—a short line attached to bow of a small boat primarily for purposes of fastening to a dock or towing

parenteral—brought into the body other than through the digestive tract, such as by intravenous or intramuscular injection

passage—a narrow navigable pass or channel between two land masses or shoals

pathogens—an agent, particularly a living microorganism, which causes disease

patrol—walking or driving in an emergency vehicle or rescue boat, with ready rescue gear, to observe and inspect a beach and water area; also known as a beach check, beach run, down to the line

peak—the top of a wave at the maximum point before breaking

pendulum technique—a rescue technique in swiftwater that involves throwing a line to a victim who is then pulled to shore in an arc by the natural flow of the current

permanent lifeguard—(see full time lifeguard)

personal flotation device (PFD)—a buoyant device designed to be held or worn to keep a person afloat; a life jacket

Peterson, Pete—the Santa Monica lifeguard who designed the first rescue tube, still known to some as the *Peterson tube*

photokeratitis—damage to the cornea of the eye from exposure to intense light

plunging wave—wave that tends to curl over and break with a crash; also known as crasher, heavy, breaker

pod—a school of marine mammals, such as seals or whales

porpoise—(lifeguarding) an action taken by a lifeguard to move through water, particularly incoming surf, during the transition from high stepping through shallow water to swimming; the arcing motion of repeatedly diving forward in a surface dive, grabbing the sand, crouching, and then diving forward again

port—side of a vessel to left when facing the bow

posted area—area that has signs, flags, or signals regulating water and beach activities; also known as designated area, signed area

pothole—a hole in the ocean floor in the surf line a few feet or yards in diameter; also known as hole, inshore hole

prevailing current—the flow most frequently observed during a given period, usually a month, season, or year; also known as prevailing drag

preventive action—providing verbal commands or advice to people to help them avoid or extricate themselves from a dangerous area; note: a preventive action is not a rescue; see rescue

primary zone—a lifeguard's assigned water zone of responsibility

protocol—standardized method

psi—acronym for pounds per square inch

pterygium—a callous-like growth that can spread over the white of the eye, caused by exposure to sunlight, wind, and dust or blowing sand; requires surgery to remove

race—a very fast current flowing through a relatively narrow channel

radio code—numbers used in place of often used words or phrases for purposes of abbreviating radio conversations and masking their meaning; also known as code list, codes, code

rail—the edge of a rescue board or surfboard running lengthwise

ready about—warning by the operator of a sailing vessel to the crew to prepare for a change of tack and swing of the boom

recompression—the treatment of decompression sickness or air embolism in a recompression chamber, which simulates returning the injured diver to an underwater depth

recurring training—training conducted cyclically to maintain proficiency in rescue, physical, and EMS skills

red tide—rust-coloring in the ocean caused by a natural dinoflagellate plankton bloom, usually in the spring and summer

reef—any hard geographical structure that is underwater at high tide

reef break—isolated waves breaking over shallow waters of a reef; also known as peak break

reflected wave—a wave that is returned seaward when it impinges upon a very steep beach, barrier, or other reflecting surface; also known as back wash

refraction of water waves—a phenomenon by which wave trains approaching a beach from an acute angle tend to wrap to a direct, perpendicular angle prior to striking the shoreline

regulator—a mechanical device for adjusting the high pressure flow of air from a compressed air cylinder to the current atmospheric pressure so that it can be comfortably breathed

repetitive dive—more than one saturation dive over thirty-three feet using scuba gear; also known as repeat

rescue—any case in which a lifeguard physically assists a victim in extrication from the water when the victim lacks apparent ability to do so alone; also known as a run, save, pull out, jump, job (see preventive action)

rescue board—a large, wide surfboard over ten feet long, usually with handles, used to make rescues; also known as a paddle board

rescue boat—a boat used in the observation and rescue of swimmers, surfers, or boats; may be motorized or manually powered; some rescue boats are used in firefighting and related functions; also known as a patrol boat or lifeguard boat

rescue breathing—resuscitation of a non-breathing victim by blowing air from the mouth of the rescuer into a nonbreathing victim's airway; also known as mouth-to-mouth

rescue buoy—cylindrical flotation device with handles, secured by a line to a shoulder sling, harness, or belt to a lifeguard and used to effect a swimming rescue or an assist; modern rescue buoys have handles for victims to grab and are made of hard plastic; also known as: torpedo buoy, torp, can, or can buoy

rescue flotation device (RFD)—elongated flotation device secured by a line to a shoulder sling, harness, or belt to a lifeguard and used to effect a swimming rescue; the two major types of RFDs are the rescue buoy and rescue tube

rescue tube—a flexible foam rubber RFD which can be wrapped around a victim's chest, fastened, and used by a lifeguard to tow the victim to safety

resting stroke—swimming stroke used to rest the body without losing buoyancy or forward motion; may indicate fatigue; common resting strokes are: sidestroke, breaststroke

resurgence—the continued rising and falling of a bay or semi-enclosed water body many hours after the passage of a severe storm

resuscitation—process of rhythmically inflation the lungs of an asphyxiated victim with oxygen or air

resuscitator—machine used to rhythmically inflate the lungs of an asphyxiated victim with oxygen from a tank

retardation—the amount of time by which corresponding tidal phases grow later day by day

RFD—acronym for "rescue flotation device"

rhumb line—the path of a vessel or swimmer that maintains a straight and true course without variation

rip current—current of water traveling away from shore generated by wave action; also known as: rip, hole, seaward current, run, runout; note: the rip current is commonly misnamed a "rip tide", though tides have only a peripheral impact on rip currents

roller—(1) one of a series of waves, usually a long-crested wave that rolls up a beach; (2) an air-filled fabric cylinder used to facilitate moving small boats on the land

rowboat—a small boat designed to be propelled with oars

rudder—the device used for steering and maneuvering a boat, particularly a sailboat or a large motorized boat

run—lifeguard or equipment en route to a rescue or assist; assist or rescue in progress; also known as: rescue assist, emergency, code III

runback—a colloquial term for backwash

sandbar—a ridge of sand in the sea bottom, normally submerged depending upon tides and other factors; also known as bar, shoal

scuba—self-contained underwater breathing apparatus which involves the use of a tank of compressed air and a regulator which reduces the pressure of the air to a breathable pressure

scull—(1) an oar used at the stern of a boat to propel it forward with a back and forth motion; (2) either of two oars at the side of a light boat used by a single rower; (3) a light racing boat propelled by rowing; (4) to propel a boat using a scull or sculls

sea anchor—device attached to a vessel by a line which traps water, thus creating a drag; used to retard the drift of a vessel, usually in the open ocean where depths do not allow anchoring

seaboard—a general term for an extensive expanse of coastal region bordering the sea; ex: the Eastern Seaboard refers to the East Coast of the United States

sea level—the height of the surface of the sea at a given point in time; also known as: water level

sea wall—a manufactured structure of rock, concrete, or wood built along a portion of coast to prevent wave erosion of the beach

search pattern—present pattern used by personnel in locating person or objects on the surface or submerged; also known as search line

seasonal current—a current that changes with seasonal winds or swell direction

seasonal lifeguard—lifeguard employed during the summer months, vacations, weekends, and holidays, usually an hourly employee; also known as recurrent guard, weekend guard, part-time guard, guard as needed, temporary guard, summer guard

seaward—the direction away from shore and toward the sea

seaweed—any macroscopic marine algae, such as seagrass or kelp

sediment—any natural material carried in suspension by water which causes underwater visibility obstruction

seiche—an occasional and sudden oscillation of the water of a lake, bay, or estuary resulting in dramatic changes in the water level caused by wind or change in barometric pressure; may result in sudden shoreline flooding

senior guard—a lifeguard who by virtue of experience, knowledge, and/or maturity has been assigned to a key station, tower, area, or special departmental function that carries with it added responsibility and/or supervisory duties

set—series of waves larger than the norm

shallow water blackout—loss of consciousness of a free diver while under water due to lack of oxygen or an imbalance of carbon dioxide; normally occurs when a free diver attempt to stay submerged too long on a single breath of air

shallow water wave—a wave moving from sea toward shore, influenced by the decreasing water depth of the shoreline; wavelength decreases, wave height increases, and velocity is reduced, but the period remains unchanged

shelf—a rock ledge, reef, or sandbank in the sea

shoal—a submerged ridge, bank, or bar consisting of or covered by mud, sand, or gravel that is at or near enough to the water surface and constitutes a danger to navigation; if composed of rock or coral, it is called a reef

shoaling effect—the alteration of a wave as it passes over a shoal

shorebreak—waves which quickly peak and break onshore to a sharply sloping beach; also known as: inside break, insiders

side current—body of water traveling parallel to shore, generated by wave action, wind, or tide; also known as drag, parallel drag, feeder, trough, lateral drift, long shore current

skeg—the fin on the bottom of a surfboard or bodyboard which helps provide stability in the water; a timber that connects the keel and sternpost of a ship; also known as a keel

skim board—a flat, thin board, usually round, ridden after being thrown into very shallow water over a flat sand beach

skindiver—see free diver

slack water—the interval when the speed of the tidal current is very weak or zero; usually refers to the period of reversal between ebb and flood currents; also known as: slack tide

slider—wave breaking with its white water sliding in an even motion down its face; also known as a feathering wave

slough—a marshy or reedy pool, pond, inlet, backwater, etc.

small craft warning—storm signal warning pleasure craft vessels of dangerous water surface conditions caused by strong wind

snorkel—a J-shaped tube held in the mouth and used in conjunction with a mask that permits breathing when a person's face is just at water level or just under the surface

snub—to quickly secure a rope by wrapping it around a cleat, post, etc.; also known as make fast, secure

solar tide—the tide caused solely by the tide-producing forces of the sun

sounding—the measurement of the depth of water beneath a ship

spilling wave—wave breaking gradually over a considerable distance; also known as a slider

spineboard—a rigid board used to immobilize and transport victims suspected of having suffered spinal injury; also known as a backboard

stand-by—a state of readiness during which a lifeguard prepares for an imminent a fixed location in preparation for emergency response; a stand-by may proceed to an emergency response or be canceled if the emergency is resolved

starboard—side of vessel to right when standing on the vessel and facing the bow

stern—the rear end of a vessel; also known as transom, aft

Stokes Basket®—a contour stretcher constructed of tubular frame woven with wire mesh; also known as: litter, litter basket, Stokes stretcher

storm surge—increased water level due to storm activity and resultant surf

storm tide—a regular tide exaggerated by storm surge

stretcher—portable platform or body contour platform used to transport any injured or deceased person in a lying position; also known as gurney, litter

surf (noun)—breaking waves; (verb) to be propelled or gain momentum using the forward motion of a swell or wave with or without the aid of a floating device; to board surf; to body surf

surface dive—the act of submerging underwater in a forward motion, usually a forward rolling motion

surface wave—a wave on the surface of the water; most often formed by wind, but may be formed by seismic activity or the gravitational pull of the moon and sun

surfboard—any rigid, inflexible device upon which or with the use of aid which a person can ride waves or be carried along or propelled by the action of waves; also known as: board, stick surfline—the offshore point along a beach where waves are breaking at a given time, bordered on the outside by the most offshore break and on the inside by the most shoreward break; the distance of the surfline from shore varies with the size of the waves since larger waves break further offshore than smaller waves

surf zone—area between the furthest outside waves that are just beginning to break and the edge of the water on the beach

surf's down—waves breaking smaller than normal; no surf at all

surf's up—waves breaking larger than normal

surfing area—area open to surfboarding only, no swimming unless incidental to surfboarding

surfing—riding or being propelled by the action of a wave with the aid of a surfboard; also known as: board surf, surfboarding

surge—a swelling or sweeping rush of water, a violent rising and falling of water

swell—a surface wave in open water before it strikes a beach

swim fins—flat, webbed rubber footwear worn by swimmers to gain power and speed out of their kick by artificially elongating the feet; also known as fins, flippers

swimming area—water area open to swimming only

tertiary zone—area of responsibility checked by a lifeguard in less frequent pattern than primary and secondary zones

tether—a short line used to secure a surfboard, belly board or similar flotation device to the user; also known as a leash, surf leash

thermocline—a layer of water in a lake or similar body of water that is of distinctly different temperature than the layer above or below; most often used to refer to a sudden and dramatic lowering in temperature when descending in a lake; most likely in still water, since current tends to adversely effect formation

three points of a rescue—the three components of every water rescue as identified by USLA: 1) recognize and respond; 2) contact and control; and 3) signal and save

thwart—a seat that runs across the beam of a boat or vessel

tide—alternating horizontal movement of water associated with the rise and fall of the tide caused by the astronomical tide producing forces; tidal current

tidal delta—sand bars or shoals formed in the entrance of inlets by reversing tidal currents

tidal flat—a marsh or sandy or muddy coastal flatland covered and uncovered by the rise and fall of the tide; a mud flat

tidal wave—a disfavored term for a tsunami

tide mark—(1) a high water mark left by tidal water; (2) the highest point reached by a high tide; (3) a visual mark indicating any specified state of tide

tide pool—a pool of water remaining in the intertidal area after recession of the tide

tide race—a very rapid tidal current in a narrow channel or passage

tide tables—tables that give daily predictions, of the times and heights of the tide

tideway—a channel through which a tidal current flows

tiller—bar or handle for turning a vessel's rudder

topside—upon the upper deck of a vessel; also known as above deck

trainee—a lifeguard in training; (USLA: A lifeguard trainee may work only under the direct and immediate supervision of an Open Water Lifeguard with 1,000 hours experience or a Full time Open Water Lifeguard with a ratio of one trainee to one experienced lifeguard)

transverse bars—slightly submerged sand ridges that extend at right angels to the shoreline

treading water—maintaining a stationary position on the surface of the water by using the legs and arms

trough—parallel inshore channel in the ocean floor running a few to many yards in length which may help foster development of a rip current; also known as hole, feeder, trench, drop-off, channel

tsunami—very large wave created by an event that causes a sudden shift in the sea, such as earthquakes, volcanoes, landslides, or the crash of a meteorite; tsunamis generally have extraordinarily long periods which make them almost invisible in the open ocean, but deadly when they arrive onshore and break; also known as a tidal wave or seismic wave

two-feeder rip—rip current generated by two currents which merge, feeding the neck of the rip current

undertow—a misnomer which suggests a current pattern (not known to exist) that drags a person under the water; this word is not used by knowledgeable lifeguards except to correct others; usage note: this term may have been coined to refer to a combination of phenomena involving a person being knocked down by a wave, pulled offshore by a backrush or rip current, and submerged due to lack of swimming ability

underway—vessel in motion

universal precaution—an approach to infection control which assumes that all blood and human bodily fluids are infectious

uplifted reef—a coral reef exposed above the water

uprush—the rush of water up onto the beach following the breaking of a wave

up-welling—bottom water reaching the surface because of disturbance caused by swells, waves, or current

victim—any person who is imperiled or injured and (usually) requires the assistance of a lifeguard; a person caught in a rip current is considered to be a victim; depending on circumstances; a victim may also be known as a casualty, accident victim, or patient

wake—path of disturbed water left behind a moving vessel or moving object in water

warning—verbal contact by voice or electronic equipment explaining an existing danger

water ability—personal performance and endurance in all types of water conditions, such as surfing, diving, swimming, paddling, etc.

waterspout—a tornado occurring over water

wave—a ridge or swell, representing a force of energy, moving through water, surface waves are most often caused by wind on the water

wave crest—The highest part of a wave

wave generation—the creation of waves by natural or mechanical means

wave train—a continual series of water waves moving in the same direction and generated by the same source

wave trough—the lowest part of a wave; the area between two ocean swells

weight belt—belt containing varying weights worn by a diver to compensate for surface buoyancy

wetsuit—foam neoprene rubber suit that fits snugly to the body and helps insulate a swimmer, surfer, or diver from cold water

white cap—wind-blown surface chop that has white froth or foam appearance

whitewater—in the surf zone, water that is mixed with air causing it to turn white; also known as: soup, surge, slop, fizz, foam

wind-driven current—a current fed by the force of a wind

wind-mixing—mechanical stirring of water due to motion induced by the surface wind

windward—the direction from which the wind is blowing

wind wave—a wave formed by wind

Index